# Pancreatic Pathology

*Editors*

LAURA D. WOOD
LODEWIJK A.A. BROSENS

# SURGICAL PATHOLOGY CLINICS

www.surgpath.theclinics.com

*Consulting Editor*
JASON L. HORNICK

December 2016 • Volume 9 • Number 4

**ELSEVIER**

1600 John F. Kennedy Boulevard • Suite 1800 • Philadelphia, Pennsylvania, 19103-2899

http://www.theclinics.com

**SURGICAL PATHOLOGY CLINICS Volume 9, Number 4**
**December 2016 ISSN 1875-9181, ISBN-13: 978-0-323-47753-6**

Editor: Lauren Boyle
Developmental Editor: Donald Mumford

*Surgical Pathology Clinics* (ISSN 1875-9181) is published quarterly by Elsevier Inc., 360 Park Avenue South, New York, NY 10010. Months of issue are March, June, September, and December. Business and Editorial Office: Elsevier Inc., 1600 John F. Kennedy Blvd., Ste. 1800, Philadelphia, PA 19103-2899. Accounting and Circulation Offices: Elsevier Inc., 3251 Riverport Lane, Maryland Heights, MO 63043. Periodicals postage paid at New York, NY and at additional mailing offices. Subscription prices are $200.00 per year (US individuals), $263.00 per year (US institutions), $100.00 per year (US students/residents), $250.00 per year (Canadian individuals), $300.00 per year (Canadian Institutions), $250.00 per year (foreign individuals), $300.00 per year (foreign institutions), and $120.00 per year (international & Canadian students/residents). Foreign air speed delivery is included in all *Clinics'* subscription prices. All prices are subject to change without notice. **POSTMASTER:** Send address changes to *Surgical Pathology Clinics*, Elsevier, 3251 Riverport Lane, Maryland Heights, MO 63043. **Customer Service: 1-800-654-2452 (US). From outside the United States, call 1-314-447-8871. Fax: 1-314-447-8029. E-mail: JournalsCustomerServiceusa@elsevier.com (for print support) and JournalsOnlineSupport-usa@elsevier.com (for online support).**

*Reprints.* For copies of 100 or more, of articles in this publication, please contact the Commercial Reprints Department, Elsevier Inc., 360 Park Avenue South, New York, NY 10010-1710. Tel. 212-633-3874; Fax: 212-633-3820; E-mail: reprints@elsevier.com.

*Surgical Pathology Clinics of North America* is covered in *MEDLINE/PubMed (Index Medicus).*

# Contributors

## CONSULTING EDITOR

**JASON L. HORNICK, MD, PhD**
Director of Surgical Pathology, Director,
Immunohistochemistry Laboratory, Brigham
and Women's Hospital, Associate Professor of
Pathology, Harvard Medical School, Boston,
Massachusetts

## EDITORS

**LAURA D. WOOD, MD, PhD**
Assistant Professor of Pathology and
Oncology, Department of Pathology, The Sol
Goldman Pancreatic Cancer Research Center,
Johns Hopkins University School of Medicine,
Baltimore, Maryland

**LODEWIJK A.A. BROSENS, MD, PhD**
Assistant Professor, Department of Pathology,
University Medical Center Utrecht, Utrecht,
The Netherlands

## AUTHORS

**SYED Z. ALI, MD, FRCPath, FIAC**
Professor, Department of Pathology, The
Johns Hopkins Hospital, The Johns Hopkins
University School of Medicine, Baltimore,
Maryland

**GOKCE ASKAN, MD**
Memorial Sloan Kettering Cancer Center,
New York, New York

**OLCA BASTURK, MD**
Memorial Sloan Kettering Cancer Center,
New York, New York

**MARC G.H. BESSELINK, MD, MSc, PhD**
Department of Surgery, Academic Medical
Center, Amsterdam, The Netherlands

**LODEWIJK A.A. BROSENS, MD, PhD**
Assistant Professor, Department of Pathology,
University Medical Center Utrecht, Utrecht,
The Netherlands

**OLIVIER R.C. BUSCH, MD, PhD**
Department of Surgery, Academic Medical
Center, Amsterdam, The Netherlands

**PAOLA CAPELLI, MD**
Department of Diagnostics and Public Health,
University and Hospital Trust of Verona,
Verona, Italy

**JENNIFER A. COLLINS, DO, MPH**
Clinical Fellow, Department of Pathology, The
Johns Hopkins Hospital, The Johns Hopkins
University School of Medicine, Baltimore,
Maryland

**IVAR PRYDZ GLADHAUG, MD, PhD**
Department of Hepato-Pancreato-Biliary
Surgery, Oslo University Hospital; Institute of
Clinical Medicine, University of Oslo, Oslo,
Norway

**SEUNG-MO HONG, MD, PhD**
Associate Professor, Department of Pathology,
Asan Medical Center, University of Ulsan
College of Medicine, Songpa-gu, Seoul,
Republic of Korea

**WAKI HOSODA, MD, PhD**
Department of Pathology, Johns Hopkins
University, Baltimore, Maryland

**SUN-YOUNG JUN, MD, PhD**
Associate Professor, Department of Pathology, Incheon St. Mary's Hospital, The Catholic University of Korea, Bupyeong-gu, Incheon, Republic of Korea

**ANNE MARIE LENNON, MD, PhD**
Benjamin Baker Scholar, Associate Professor of Medicine and Surgery, Division of Gastroenterology and Hepatology, The Johns Hopkins Medical Institutions, Baltimore, Maryland

**SHU LIU, PhD**
Department of Pathology, University of Pittsburgh Medical Center, Pittsburgh, Pennsylvania

**CLAUDIO LUCHINI, MD**
Department of Diagnostics and Public Health; ARC-Net Research Center, University and Hospital Trust of Verona, Verona, Italy; Surgical Pathology Unit, Santa Chiara Hospital, Trento, Italy

**ISAAC Q. MOLENAAR, MD, PhD**
Department of Surgery, University Medical Center Utrecht, Utrecht, The Netherlands

**SAOWANEE NGAMRUENGPHONG, MD**
Assistant Professor of Medicine, Division of Gastroenterology and Hepatology, The Johns Hopkins Medical Institutions, Baltimore, Maryland

**MICHAËL NOË, MD**
Department of Pathology, University Medical Center Utrecht, Utrecht, The Netherlands

**MEREDITH E. PITTMAN, MD**
Assistant Professor, Department of Pathology and Laboratory Medicine, Weill Cornell Medical College, New York, New York

**STEFFI J.E. ROMBOUTS, MD**
Department of Surgery, University Medical Center, Utrecht, The Netherlands

**SAFIA N. SALARIA, MD**
Department of Pathology, Microbiology, and Immunology, Vanderbilt University Medical Center, Nashville, Tennessee

**ALDO SCARPA, MD, PhD**
Department of Diagnostics and Public Health; ARC-Net Research Center, University and Hospital Trust of Verona, Verona, Italy

**CHANJUAN SHI, MD, PhD**
Department of Pathology, Microbiology, and Immunology, Vanderbilt University Medical Center, Nashville, Tennessee

**AATUR D. SINGHI, MD, PhD**
Department of Pathology, University of Pittsburgh Medical Center, Pittsburgh, Pennsylvania

**MICHELLE STRAM, MD**
Department of Pathology, University of Pittsburgh Medical Center, Pittsburgh, Pennsylvania

**JOHANNA A. TOL, MD, PhD**
Department of Surgery, Academic Medical Center, Amsterdam, The Netherlands

**MARC J. VAN DE VIJVER, MD, PhD**
Department of Pathology, Academic Medical Center, Amsterdam, The Netherlands

**CASPER H.J. VAN EIJCK, MD, PhD**
Department of Surgery, Erasmus Medical Center, Rotterdam, The Netherlands

**LENNART B. VAN RIJSSEN, MD**
Department of Surgery, Academic Medical Center, Amsterdam, The Netherlands

**CHRISTOPHER J. VANDENBUSSCHE, MD, PhD**
Assistant Professor, Department of Pathology, The Johns Hopkins Hospital, The Johns Hopkins University School of Medicine, Baltimore, Maryland

**CAROLINE SOPHIE VERBEKE, MD, PhD**
Institute of Clinical Medicine, University of Oslo, Oslo, Norway; Department of Pathology, Oslo University Hospital, Oslo, Norway; Department of Pathology, Karolinska University Hospital, Stockholm, Sweden

**JOANNE VERHEIJ, MD, PhD**
Department of Pathology, Academic Medical Center, Amsterdam, The Netherlands

**JANTIEN A. VOGEL, MD**
Department of Surgery, Academic Medical Center, Amsterdam, The Netherlands

**MARIEKE S. WALMA, MD**
Department of Surgery, University Medical Center, Utrecht, The Netherlands

**LAURA D. WOOD, MD, PhD**
Assistant Professor of Pathology and Oncology, Department of Pathology, The Sol Goldman Pancreatic Cancer Research Center, Johns Hopkins University School of Medicine, Baltimore, Maryland

Contributors

JANTIEN A. VOGEL, MD
Department of Surgery, Academic Medical Center, Amsterdam, The Netherlands

MARIJKE B. WALMA, MD
Department of Surgery, University Medical Center, Utrecht, The Netherlands

LAURA D. WOOD, MD, PhD
Assistant Professor of Pathology and Oncology, Department of Pathology, The Sol Goldman Pancreatic Cancer Research Center, Johns Hopkins University School of Medicine, Baltimore, Maryland

# Contents

Specimen grossing is a key step in the pathology examination of pancreatic resection specimens. Optimal display of pathologic changes and extensive tissue sampling are important determinants of the quality of pathology reporting. Divergence in macroscopic examination practice has led to considerable variation in the reporting of factors that are of clinical and prognostic significance. This article provides a detailed account of the macroscopic examination procedure with reference to current (inter-)national guidelines and recommendations.

Recent advances in pancreatic surgery have the potential to improve outcomes for patients with pancreatic cancer. We address 3 new, trending topics in pancreatic surgery that are of relevance to the pathologist. First, increasing awareness of the prognostic impact of intraoperatively detected extraregional and regional lymph node metastases and the international consensus definition on lymph node sampling and reporting. Second, neoadjuvant chemotherapy, which is capable of changing 10% to 20% of initially unresectable, to resectable disease. Third, in patients who remain unresectable following neoadjuvant chemotherapy, local ablative therapies may change indications for treatment and improve outcomes.

Pancreatic cancer represents the seventh leading cause of cancer death in the world, responsible for more than 300,000 deaths per year. The most common tumor type among pancreatic cancers is pancreatic ductal adenocarcinoma, an infiltrating neoplasm with glandular differentiation that is derived from the pancreatic ductal tree. Here we present and discuss the most important macroscopic, microscopic, and immunohistochemical characteristics of this tumor, highlighting its key diagnostic features. Furthermore, we present the classic features of the most common variants of pancreatic ductal adenocarcinoma. Last, we summarize the prognostic landscape of this highly malignant tumor and its variants.

To better understand pancreatic ductal adenocarcinoma (PDAC) and improve its prognosis, it is essential to understand its origins. This article describes the pathology of the 3 well-established pancreatic cancer precursor lesions: pancreatic intraepithelial neoplasia, intraductal papillary mucinous neoplasm, and mucinous cystic neoplasm. Each of these precursor lesions has unique clinical findings, gross and microscopic features, and molecular aberrations. This article focuses on histopathologic diagnostic criteria and reporting guidelines. The genetics of these lesions are briefly discussed. Early detection and adequate treatment of pancreatic cancer precursor lesions has the potential to prevent pancreatic cancer and improve the prognosis of PDAC.

## Nonductal Pancreatic Cancers

Sun-Young Jun and Seung-Mo Hong

Nonductal pancreatic neoplasms, including solid pseudopapillary neoplasms, acinar cell carcinomas, and pancreatoblastomas, are uncommon. These entities share overlapping gross, microscopic, and immunohistochemical features, such as well-demarcated solid neoplasms, monotonous cellular tumor cells with little intervening stroma, and abnormal beta-catenin expression. Each tumor also has unique clinicopathologic characteristics with diverse clinical behavior. To differentiate nonductal pancreatic neoplasms, identification of histologic findings, such as pseudopapillae, acinar cell features, and squamoid corpuscles, is important. Immunostainings for acinar cell or neuroendocrine markers are helpful for differential diagnosis. This article describes the clinicopathologic and immunohistochemical features of nonductal pancreatic cancers.

## Pancreatic Neuroendocrine Tumors

Safia N. Salaria and Chanjuan Shi

Pancreatic neuroendocrine neoplasms include well-differentiated pancreatic neuroendocrine tumors (PanNETs) and neuroendocrine carcinomas (NECs) with well-differentiated PanNETs accounting for most cases. Other pancreatic primaries and metastatic carcinomas from other sites can mimic pancreatic neuroendocrine neoplasms. Immunohistochemical studies can be used to aid in the differential diagnosis. However, no specific markers are available to differentiate PanNETs from NETs of other sites. Although NECs are uniformly deadly, PanNETs have variable prognosis. Morphology alone cannot predict the tumor behavior. Although some pathologic features are associated with an aggressive course, Ki67 is the only prognostic molecular marker routinely used in clinical practice.

## Benign Tumors and Tumorlike Lesions of the Pancreas

Olca Basturk and Gokce Askan

The pancreas is a complex organ that may give rise to large number of neoplasms and non-neoplastic lesions. This article focuses on benign neoplasms, such as serous neoplasms, and tumorlike (pseudotumoral) lesions that may be mistaken for neoplasm not only by clinicians and radiologists, but also by pathologists. The family of pancreatic pseudotumors, by a loosely defined conception of that term, includes a variety of lesions including heterotopia, hamartoma, and lipomatous pseudohypertrophy. Autoimmune pancreatitis and paraduodenal ("groove") pancreatitis may also lead to pseudotumor formation. Knowledge of these entities will help in making an accurate diagnosis.

Chronic pancreatitis is a debilitating condition often associated with severe abdominal pain and exocrine and endocrine dysfunction. The underlying cause is multifactorial and involves complex interaction of environmental, genetic, and/or other risk factors. The pathology is dependent on the underlying pathogenesis of the disease. This review describes the clinical, gross, and microscopic findings of the main subtypes of chronic pancreatitis: alcoholic chronic pancreatitis, obstructive chronic pancreatitis, paraduodenal ("groove") pancreatitis, pancreatic divisum, autoimmune pancreatitis, and genetic factors associated with chronic pancreatitis. As pancreatic ductal adenocarcinoma may be confused with chronic pancreatitis, the main distinguishing features between these 2 diseases are discussed.

Pancreatic cytopathology, particularly through the use of endoscopic ultrasound-guided fine-needle aspiration (FNA), has excellent specificity and sensitivity for the diagnosis of pancreatic lesions. Such diagnoses can help guide preoperative management of patients, provide prognostic information, and confirm diagnoses in patients who are not surgical candidates. Furthermore, FNA can be used to obtain cyst fluid for ancillary tests that can improve the diagnosis of cystic lesions. In this article, we describe the cytomorphological features and differential diagnoses of the most commonly encountered pancreatic lesions on FNA.

Pancreatic cysts are extremely common, and are identified in between 2% to 13% on abdominal imaging studies. Most pancreatic cysts are pseudocysts, serous cystic neoplasms, mucinous cystic neoplasms, or intraductal papillary mucinous neoplasms. The management of pancreatic cysts depends on whether a cyst is benign, has malignant potential, or harbors high-grade dysplasia or invasive carcinoma. The diagnosis of pancreatic cysts, and assessment of risk of malignant transformation, incorporates clinical history, computed tomography (CT), magnetic resonance imaging (MRI), endoscopic ultrasound, and fine-needle aspiration of cyst fluid. This article reviews the cyst fluid markers that are currently used, as well as promising markers under development.

Pancreatic neoplasms have a wide range of histologic types with distinct clinical outcomes. Recent advances in high-throughput sequencing technologies have greatly deepened our understanding of pancreatic neoplasms. Now, the exomes of major histologic types of pancreatic neoplasms have been sequenced, and their genetic landscapes have been revealed. This article reviews the molecular changes underlying pancreatic neoplasms, with a special focus on the genetic changes that characterize the histologic types of pancreatic neoplasms. Emphasis is also made on the molecular features of key genes that have the potential for therapeutic targets.

Meredith E. Pittman, Lodewijk A.A. Brosens, and Laura D. Wood

Although the pancreas is affected by only a small fraction of known inherited disorders, several of these syndromes predispose patients to pancreatic adenocarcinoma, a cancer that has a consistently dismal prognosis. Still other syndromes are associated with neuroendocrine tumors, benign cysts, or recurrent pancreatitis. Because of the variability of pancreatic manifestations and outcomes, it is important for clinicians to be familiar with several well-described genetic disorders to ensure that patients are followed appropriately. The purpose of this review is to briefly describe the hereditary syndromes that are associated with pancreatic disorders and neoplasia.

# SURGICAL PATHOLOGY CLINICS

RELATED INTEREST

*Clinics in Laboratory Medicine* June 2015 (Volume 35, Issue 2)
**Diagnostic Testing for Enteric Pathogens**
Alexander J. McAdam, *Editor*

**THE CLINICS ARE AVAILABLE ONLINE!**
Access your subscription at:
www.theclinics.com

# Preface
# The Changing Landscape of Pancreatic Pathology

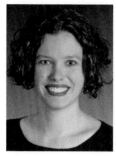
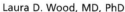
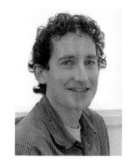

Laura D. Wood, MD, PhD    Lodewijk A.A. Brosens, MD, PhD

*Editors*

The practice of pancreatic pathology has evolved significantly in recent years. In this issue, we provide an update into the major diagnostic entities in the pancreas, including both neoplastic and nonneoplastic diseases. In addition, we provide correlations with other specialties of relevance to the practicing pathologist. We first focus on gross dissection of pancreatic resection specimens, as this process lays the groundwork for accurate diagnosis. We then discuss the process that resulted in the gross specimen by highlighting advances in surgery that are relevant to the practicing pathologist. Then, we turn to the tumors of the pancreas, which represent the entities encountered most commonly in practice—these include pancreatic adenocarcinoma (and variants), precursor lesions, nonductal cancers, and neuroendocrine tumors. Next, we cover benign pancreatic lesions, including pancreatitis and benign masses. We then focus on other pathologic analyses that are commonly used on the pancreas, including cytopathology and cyst fluid analysis. Finally, we highlight the molecular genetics of pancreatic neoplasms, a field that has advanced greatly in recent years, and discuss genetic syndromes with pancreatic manifestations. This broad update is intended for practicing pathologists in order to capture the critical advances in recent years.

Laura D. Wood, MD, PhD
Sol Goldman Pancreatic Cancer Research Center
Johns Hopkins University School of Medicine
CRB2 Room 345
1550 Orleans Street
Baltimore, MD 21231, USA

Lodewijk A.A. Brosens, MD, PhD
Department of Pathology (H04-312)
University Medical Center Utrecht
Heidelberglaan 100
3584 CX Utrecht, The Netherlands

E-mail addresses:
ldwood@jhmi.edu (L.D. Wood)
l.a.a.brosens@umcutrecht.nl (L.A.A. Brosens)

Surgical Pathology 9 (2016) xiii
http://dx.doi.org/10.1016/j.path.2016.10.001
1875-9181/16/© 2016 Published by Elsevier Inc.

# Dissection of Pancreatic Resection Specimens

Caroline Sophie Verbeke, MD, PhD[a,b,c,*], Ivar Prydz Gladhaug, MD, PhD[a,d]

## KEYWORDS

- Pathology • Dissection • Pancreatoduodenectomy • Pancreatic cancer

## ABSTRACT

Specimen grossing is a key step in the pathology examination of pancreatic resection specimens. Optimal display of pathologic changes and extensive tissue sampling are important determinants of the quality of pathology reporting. Divergence in macroscopic examination practice has led to considerable variation in the reporting of factors that are of clinical and prognostic significance. This article provides a detailed account of the macroscopic examination procedure with reference to current (inter-)national guidelines and recommendations.

## OVERVIEW

Dissection of pancreatic resection specimens is the initial step of the pathology examination procedure. Its purpose is to bring to light all tissue changes and to facilitate sampling. As such, it is an important determinant of the overall quality of the pathology examination. Optimal visualization of findings is also important for case discussion with surgical colleagues and correlation with preoperative imaging.

Despite the crucial role of specimen dissection, recommendations related to specimen grossing are usually not included in (inter-)national pathology guidelines.[1–5] Although there is broad consensus on which data items should be included in the macroscopic part of a pathology report, guidelines do not usually recommend how this information should be obtained. The current lack of guidance and consensus has resulted in nonuniform reporting of data items as crucial as cancer origin, tumor size and extent, and margin status.[6–9]

In this article, the procedures for specimen handling and dissection, macroscopic examination, and tissue sampling will be discussed. Where relevant, reference will be made to local anatomic detail or surgical technique for the pathology report to provide an accurate and clinically meaningful record of macroscopically visible changes. Specimen handling is described for cancer specimens, but can be equally well applied to pancreatic resection specimens for any other neoplastic or non-neoplastic pathology occurring in the pancreas, ampulla, common bile duct, or periampullary duodenum. A summary of the grossing procedure is provided in **Box 1**.

## SPECIMEN ORIENTATION AND EXTERNAL INSPECTION

For orientation of pancreatoduodenectomy specimens (PDES), it is easiest to start with the identification of the pancreatic transection margin, which has typically an ovoid shape and shows lobulated pancreatic parenchyma with a more or less centrally placed main pancreatic duct. The next structure to identify is the groove of the superior mesenteric vein (SMV), which lies immediately posterior to the transection margin, has a slightly curved shape, and a smooth, sometimes slightly shiny surface. The extrapancreatic stump of the common bile duct, which may be of varying length and closed with a surgical suture, can be found at the cranial end of the SMV groove. Medial to the

Disclosure Statement: The authors have no conflicting interests to declare.
[a] Institute of Clinical Medicine, University of Oslo, Postboks 1171, Blindern, Oslo 0318, Norway; [b] Department of Pathology, Oslo University Hospital, Sognsvannsveien 20, Oslo 0372, Norway; [c] Department of Pathology, Karolinska University Hospital, F42, Stockholm 14186, Sweden; [d] Department of Hepato-Pancreato-Biliary Surgery, Oslo University Hospital, Sognsvannsveien 20, Oslo 0372, Norway
* Corresponding author. Department of Pathology, Oslo University Hospital, Sognsvannsveien 20, Oslo 0372, Norway.
E-mail address: c.s.verbeke@medisin.uio.no

Surgical Pathology 9 (2016) 523–538
http://dx.doi.org/10.1016/j.path.2016.05.001

**Box 1**
**Handling of pancreatoduodenectomy specimens**

- Before fixation
  - Open stomach, duodenum, and gallbladder longitudinally and rinse.
  - For biobanking of fresh tumor tissue, identify the tumor site and incise in the axial plane.
- Fixation (in formalin for up to 48 hours)
- Following fixation
  - Orientate the specimen and inspect externally.
  - Record measurements: pancreas, stomach, duodenum, gallbladder, extrapancreatic common bile duct, possibly other resected structures (eg, vein).
  - Record externally visible abnormalities.
  - Carefully remove surgical sutures, clips, staples.
  - Sample transection margins of the pancreatic neck, extrapancreatic common bile duct, stomach/duodenum.
  - Inspect and sample the gallbladder and cystic duct.
  - Ink according to an agreed color code
    - The pancreatic surfaces: SMV, SMA, anterior, posterior
    - Important other structures, for example, venous resection.
  - Slice in the axial plane (thickness: 3 mm).
  - Lay slices out in sequential order, caudal surface facing up.
  - Take photographs: overview, close-ups.
  - Describe the tumor and any other pathology.
  - Take tissue samples following the sequential order of the specimen slices.
  - Block key: record the specimen slice number from which the samples are taken.
  - Use at least one whole-mount block, best where the tumor is at its largest extension.
  - For standard tissue cassettes, sample the tumor en bloc with anatomic structures (including a venous resection) and margins.
  - Sample lymph nodes en bloc with the specimen surface or anatomic landmarks.

smoothly surfaced SMV groove lies the roughly textured specimen surface that has been sharply dissected from the superior mesenteric artery (SMA), hereafter called the SMA margin (see also section "Inking of the specimen surface").

Because of the complex anatomy of PDES, specimen orientation and identification of the various resection margins and specimen surfaces may be difficult for the less experienced pathologist. Therefore, some guidelines recommend that the surgeon inks or places a suture on one of the specimen surfaces, usually the SMV groove or SMA margin.[3–5] Although this may be helpful, it has not yet become established practice.[8] If inking is the preferred method, this should be limited to one surface, such that it does not interfere with external specimen inspection, which is important, for example,

for biobanking (see section "Biobanking of fresh tissue").

Following the identification of the previously mentioned key structures, the PDES can be inspected externally. Attention should be paid to the possible presence of a resected segment or sleeve of the SMV or portal vein (PV), which obviously will be adherent to the SMV groove. Changes that can guide biobanking of fresh tumor tissue are described in the section "Biobanking of fresh tissue".

Distal pancreatectomy specimens (DPES) usually include the spleen, which facilitates specimen orientation. Further helpful is the localization of the splenic vessels, which run along the superior-posterior aspect of the pancreatic body and tail.

## SPECIMEN FIXATION

On receiving a fresh PDES, the stomach and/or duodenum and gallbladder should be opened longitudinally and rinsed. To avoid potential transection of a tumor involving the periampullary duodenum, the duodenum should be carefully probed with a finger before opening it along the antimesenteric side. Formalin fixation should not be longer than 48 hours. Pinning of the specimen to a cork plate is not necessary and will delay fixation.

## INKING OF THE SPECIMEN SURFACE

Multicolored inking of the surfaces of the pancreatic head has a dual purpose. It facilitates specimen orientation during grossing and allows unequivocal identification of the tissue surface during microscopic examination.

In PDES, the following surfaces can be discerned[3,5,10] (**Fig. 1**):

- SMV surface: the shallow and slightly curved, groovelike impression of the SMV and PV on the medial aspect of the pancreatic head. The groove has a smooth surface and is most concave in its cranial part, that is behind the pancreatic neck and along the extrapancreatic common bile duct. Further caudally, the groove usually flattens out, and the border to the anterior surface may not be that distinct.
- SMA surface: the roughly textured surface medial and posterior to the SMV surface, which the surgeon sharply dissects from the SMA. It usually has a broader (caudal) base and tapers toward a narrower cranial end.
- Posterior surface: the fibrous but relatively smooth, flat surface between the posterior duodenal wall and the SMA/SMV surface.
- Anterior surface: the smooth, peritoneum-lined surface between the anterior duodenal wall and the SMV groove. This is not a surgical margin, but the anatomic surface facing the lesser sac. Tumor involvement of this surface portends an increased risk for local recurrence and poorer survival.[11]

PDES resulting from an extended surgical procedure include additional structures (eg, blood vessels, colon, small bowel) and associated resection margins that require inking. Especially if a

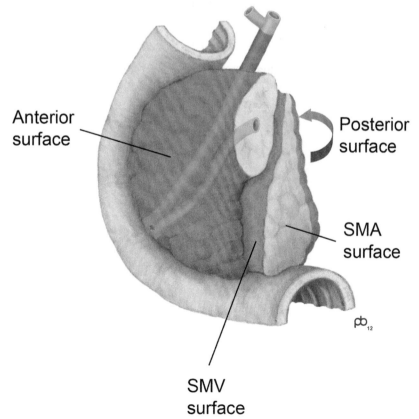

*Fig. 1.* Circumferential margins in a PDES, inked in different colors: red, anterior; green, facing the SMV; yellow, facing the SMA; blue, posterior. (*From* Campbell F, Verbeke CS. Pathology of the pancreas – a practical approach. London: Springer; 2013; with permission of Springer.)

Anterior surface

Posterior surface

SMA surface

SMV surface

venous (sleeve) resection is very small, it may be helpful to ink it with a different color.

For DPES, the anterior and posterior surface of the pancreatic body and tail are inked.

Inking is best performed after specimen fixation, as the ink usually sticks better to fixed tissues. Depending on the ink that is used, spraying 10% acetic acid onto the freshly applied ink may reduce bleeding of colors. When inking an unfixed specimen, application of dry ground pigment dissolved in acetone ensures that the inks dry quickly and reduces the risk of bleeding of colors.

Before inking, surgical sutures, clips, or staples should be removed without tissue disruption. If a metal stent is inserted in the common bile duct and cannot be removed by gentle traction, the metal mesh should be cut with small pliers and wires pulled out individually to prevent tissue disruption.

## SPECIMEN DISSECTION

Worldwide, *4* different approaches to the dissection of PDES are being used: the multivalving, bread-loafing, and axial slicing techniques, as well as a technique based on slicing perpendicular to the axis that follows the curvature of the pancreatic head.[12–15] The axial slicing technique is described in this section and compared with the other techniques in the section "Advantages of the Axial Slicing Technique."

### SAMPLING OF TRANSECTION MARGINS

Before proceeding with the actual specimen dissection, the transection margins of PDES

should be sampled as full-face sections: the proximal gastric/duodenal margin, the distal duodenal margin, the margin at the pancreatic neck and the margin of the extrapancreatic bile duct (see also section "Sampling Technique"). In DPES resulting from a laparoscopic procedure, the staple line on the transection margin must be carefully removed, and the immediately adjacent tissue is to be sampled.

## DISSECTION OF OTHER STRUCTURES INCLUDED IN STANDARD RESECTION SPECIMENS

It is usually easier to examine and sample the gallbladder and cystic duct before dissecting the pancreatic head, unless these structures are involved by a tumor that extends from the pancreatic head or common bile duct. In most DPES, the spleen can be dissected from the tip of the pancreatic tail, once external specimen examination and inking of the surfaces are completed. If the tumor or another lesion is located close to the spleen, the latter should be dissected en bloc with the pancreatic tail.

## AXIAL SLICING OF PANCREATODUODENECTOMY SPECIMENS

The pancreatic head is sliced in the axial plane, that is perpendicular to the descending part of the duodenum (Fig. 2). The dissection plane is therefore the same as that of computerized tomography (CT) scanning. Dissection should

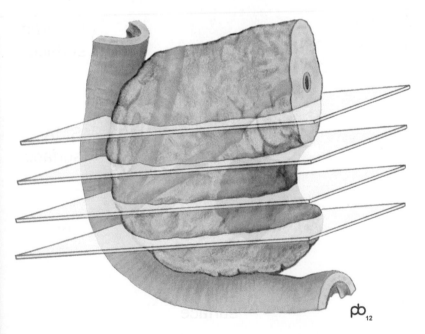

Fig. 2. Axial specimen dissection. The PDES is sliced in a plane perpendicular to the longitudinal axis of the descending duodenum. (*From* Campbell F, Verbeke CS. Pathology of the pancreas – a practical approach. London: Springer; 2013; with permission of Springer.)

include the entire head of pancreas, the extrapancreatic common bile duct, and any adherent structures, such as a venous resection. Specimen slices should be approximately 3-mm thick to allow good views on the small anatomic structures of the pancreatic head and periampullary region. A PDES will usually result in 10 to 14 or more axial slices (Fig. 3). As illustrated in Fig. 4, axial specimen slices have characteristic outlines that correspond to the various specimen surfaces. The anterior surface has typically a convex curved shape and may overlie a copious amount of adipose tissue. The latter is especially present in the cranial part of the pancreatic head and may blend with the transverse mesocolon and infrapyloric fat. The SMV groove has a shallow concave shape and usually overlies directly the pancreatic parenchyma without an intervening layer of peripancreatic fat. The posterior surface is flat.

## ADVANTAGES OF THE AXIAL SLICING TECHNIQUE

Two other main dissection techniques for PDES are being used, the so-called bivalving or multivalving and bread-loafing techniques. According to the first technique, the pancreatic and common bile ducts are probed, and the specimen is sliced along the plane defined by both probes. This approach may be technically challenging, especially if one or both ducts are narrowed by tumor. Furthermore, as the dissection plane is determined by the configuration of both ducts, and this varies between cases, specimen slices do not always display the anatomy in the same fashion. With the bread-loafing technique, the pancreatic head is serially sliced parallel to the pancreatic transection margin. With this technique, dissection of the ampulla and periampullary region may be difficult and suboptimal, because the descending part of the duodenum is sliced longitudinally. In contrast, the axial specimen slices provide good views on the ampullary region (Figs. 5 and 6).

An important advantage of the axial slicing technique is the technical ease with which it can be performed and the fact that it can be used for any PDES, irrespective of the pathology that is encountered. Furthermore, as it results in a fully standardized rendition of the local anatomy

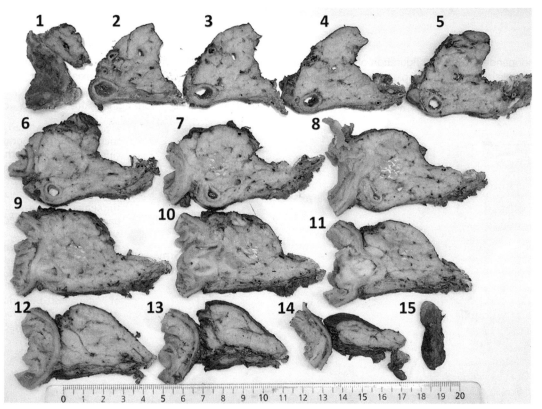

*Fig. 3.* Axial specimen slices lined up in sequential order (*1*, most cranial; *15*, most caudal slice). Slices are laid out with the inferior cut surface facing upward, such that the anatomy is seen as on a CT scan. Details of slices 7 to 11 are shown in Fig. 6.

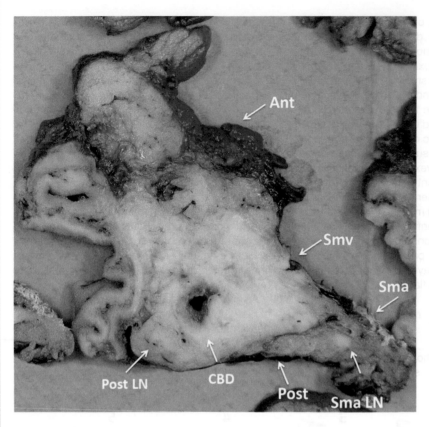

*Fig. 4.* Typical configuration of an axial specimen slice. Specimen surfaces are inked as described in **Fig. 2.** A small lymph node can be seen within the peripancreatic fat under the posterior and SMA-facing surface, respectively. The axial slice stems from a specimen with a large pancreatic ductal adenocarcinoma involving the common bile duct and SMV groove. Ant, anterior; CBD, common bile duct; Post LN, posterior lymph node; Post, posterior surface; Sma, surface facing SMA; Sma LN, lymph node in peripancreatic fat facing SMA; Smv, surface facing SMV.

independent of the configuration of the pancreatic and bile ducts, macroscopic images of axial specimen slices are "readable" by all pathologists, in a similar way as CT images can be interpreted worldwide. Moreover, margin assessment seems to be more accurate with the axial slicing technique.[16–19] Further advantages are summarized in **Box 2.** The International Study Group for

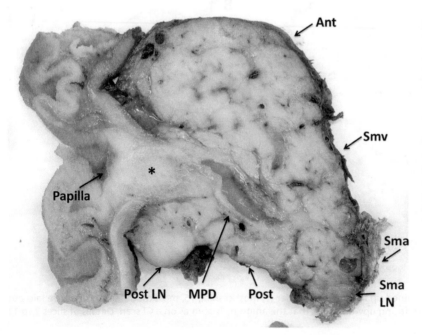

*Fig. 5.* Axial slice from a specimen with adenocarcinoma infiltrating the papilla and ampulla of Vater. Note prestenotic dilatation and mild wall thickening of the main pancreatic duct (*MPD*) and metastatic involvement of a posterior peripancreatic lymph node (*Post LN*). Ant, anterior surface; asterisk, ampulla of Vater; Post, posterior surface; Sma, surface facing SMA; Smv, surface facing SMV.

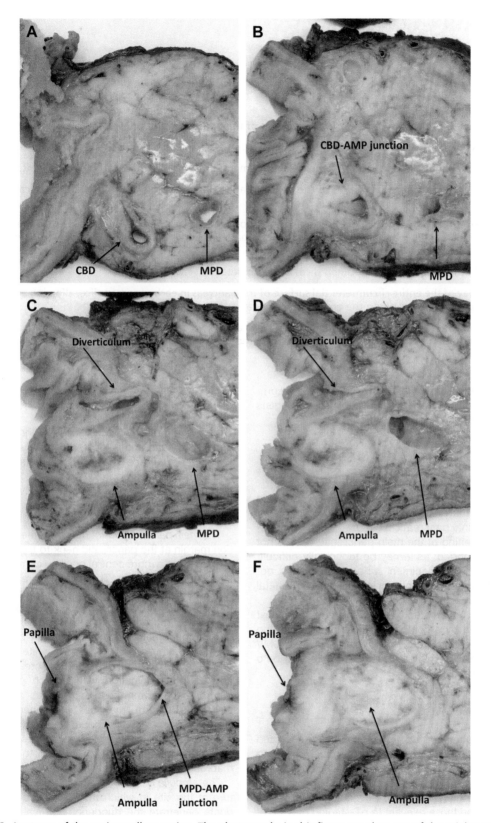

*Fig. 6.* Anatomy of the periampullary region. The photographs in this figure are close-ups of the axial specimen slices 7 to 11 shown in **Fig. 3** (*E* shows the back side of slice 10). (*A*) The common bile duct (*CBD*) and main pancreatic duct (*MPD*) are dilated. (*B*) The junction of the CBD with the ampulla (*CBD-AMP junction*) is infiltrated by tumor, causing irregular wall thickening. (*C*) The ampulla is infiltrated by tumor. A duodenal diverticulum lies anterior to the ampulla. (*D*) Note the polypous tumor protrusion into the dilated distal MPD. (*E*, *F*) Tumor occludes the ampulla and junction with the MPD (*MPD-AMP junction*). Note the plaquelike tumor infiltration of the papilla.

---

**Box 2**
Advantages of axial slicing of pancreatoduodenectomy specimens

- Technically easy to perform.

- No need for probing or longitudinal opening of the pancreatic and/or common bile duct.

- Pancreatic surface remains intact, facilitating margin assessment.

- Applicable to all pancreatoduodenectomy specimens, irrespective of the pathology encountered.

- Fully standardized visualization of the pancreas and related structures, facilitating identification of anatomic variation and pathologic change.

- Straightforward cross-sectional slicing of the duodenal wall providing detailed views on the intact (peri-)ampullary region. No need for additional dissection of the periampullary region with "releasing cuts."[20]

- Yield of numerous thin-specimen slices allowing detailed views.

- Display of the entire circumferential surface of the pancreas in each specimen slice, allowing accurate margin assessment along the entire craniocaudal length of the pancreatic head.

- Visualization of the pancreatic head and related anatomy in the same (axial) plane as on computed tomography imaging, facilitating pathological-radiological correlation.

---

Pancreatic Surgery (ISGPS) endorses the recommendation of the Royal College of Pathologists UK to use the axial slicing technique.[2,19]

## DISSECTION OF DISTAL AND TOTAL PANCREATECTOMY SPECIMENS

The pancreatic body and tail are serially sliced in the sagittal plane; that is, perpendicular to the longitudinal pancreatic axis.[2,3,10,14,21,22] Longitudinal opening of the main pancreatic duct is not recommended, as it may be technically difficult, disrupts the specimen surface, and does not result in a better display of lesions than by sagittal slicing.[5]

Total pancreatectomy specimens are best dissected by a combined approach of axial and sagittal slicing. In case of resection of the SMV and/or SMA, axial slicing may be extended onto the proximal body.

## MACROSCOPIC EXAMINATION

Identification and documentation of a tumor and its relationship to anatomic structures and specimen margins is the main goal of macroscopic examination and key to correct pT-staging and pR-staging. Furthermore, the relation to structures other than those relevant to pT-staging may be of interest to surgical and radiology colleagues regarding resectability and patient selection. The following sections provide guidance for the identification of such anatomic structures (see **Figs. 5** and **6**; **Figs. 7–12**).

## IDENTIFICATION OF ANATOMIC STRUCTURES IN PANCREATODUODENECTOMY SPECIMENS

*The common bile duct* runs obliquely through the pancreatic head and is located relatively close to the posterior surface (see **Fig. 7**). The extrapancreatic part measures approximately 5 to 15 mm in length, lies at the cranial end of the SMV groove, and is commonly surrounded by one or several, often large lymph nodes.

*The main pancreatic duct* runs from the transection margin at the pancreatic neck to the ampulla and takes up a more central position compared to the common bile duct. The main pancreatic duct joins the ampulla just caudal to the junction of the ampulla with the common bile duct. The main pancreatic duct can be distinguished from the intrapancreatic common bile duct based on its membranous (<0.5-mm thick) white wall, its more medial location within the pancreatic head and its communication with branch ducts. In contrast, the common bile duct has a thicker wall (1.0–1.5 mm), may be bile-stained and is located closer to the duodenal wall and posterior surface of the pancreatic head (see **Fig. 7**). Branch ducts are normally too small to be seen macroscopically.

*The ampulla of Vater* is the olive-shaped structure at the site in which the bile and pancreatic ducts penetrate the duodenal wall (see **Figs. 5** and **6**). The ampulla is usually located approximately midway the craniocaudal length of the pancreatic head. The papilla of Vater represents the orifice of the ampullary channel, which is lined with duodenal mucosa.

*Fig. 7.* Axial slice from a PDES showing a dilated common bile duct (*CBD*) with an irregularly thickened wall. The main pancreatic duct (*MPD*) is smaller, has a thin membranous wall and lies medial to the CBD. The minor ampulla forms a small nodular structure that interrupts the duodenal muscularis propria. Part of the Santorini duct is seen in longitudinal section.

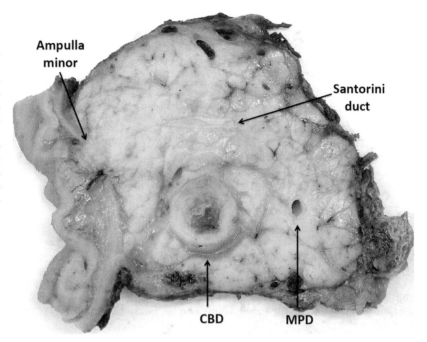

*The Santorini duct* is usually 1.0-mm to 1.5-mm wide and therefore not often exposed by serial slicing (see **Fig. 7**). *The minor ampulla* is identified as a 2-mm to 3-mm nodular structure that interrupts the duodenal muscularis propria. The *minor papilla* lies 10 to 15 mm proximal to the papilla of Vater.

*The gastroduodenal artery* runs through the peripancreatic adipose tissue that covers the anterior-superior part of the pancreatic head. A suture is often seen on the short stump that protrudes from the specimen surface (see **Figs. 8** and **9B**). The smaller *inferior pancreatoduodenal artery* is found in the peripancreatic adipose tissue close

*Fig. 8.* A short stump of the gastroduodenal artery (*GDA*) is seen on the cranial aspect of the pancreatic head. Note the axial incision (*asterisk*) for biobanking.

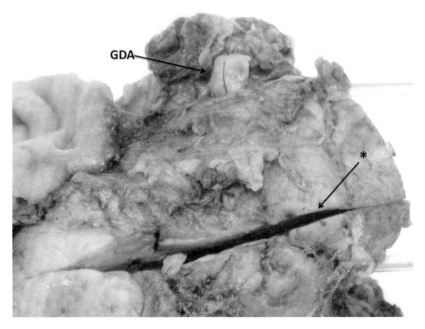

A

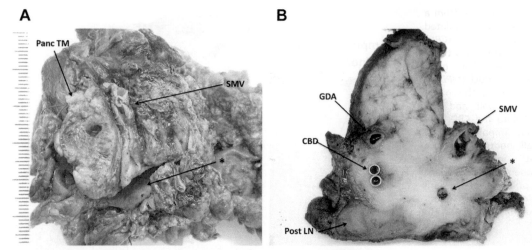

B

*Fig. 9.* Pancreatoduodenectomy specimen with superior mesenteric vein (*SMV*) resection. (*A*) A 50-mm-long vein segment is adherent to the SMV groove, behind the transection margin of the pancreatic neck (*Panc TM*). Note the axial incision (*asterisk*) for biobanking of fresh tumor tissue. (*B*) An axial specimen slice shows a large tumor, which infiltrates the stented common bile duct (*CBD*), superior mesenteric vein (*SMV*) and a posterior peripancreatic lymph node (*Post LN*). The tumor lies close to the gastroduodenal artery (*GDA*). Note the site of biobanking (*asterisk*).

to the SMA margin of caudal specimen slices, where it often forms a small plexus (see **Fig. 10**).

A *resection of the SMV or PV* is located along the SMV groove (see **Fig. 9**). As the confluence of the SMV and splenic vein into the PV is located behind the pancreatic neck, a venous resection located in the top part of the venous groove stems from the PV.

A *resection of the hepatic artery* measures usually only a few millimeters in length and lies in the peripancreatic soft tissue on the superior aspect of the pancreatic head (see **Fig. 11**).

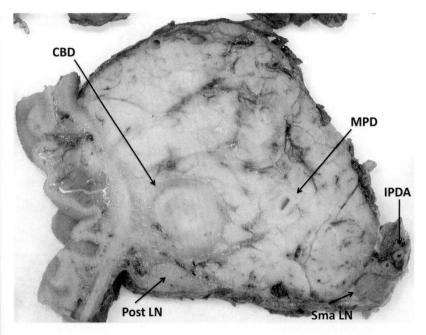

*Fig. 10.* Axial slice from a specimen with an obstructing distal common bile duct (*CBD*) cancer. Note the presence of the inferior pancreato-duodenal artery (*IPDA*; 2 cross sections) in the peripancreatic fat facing the SMA. MPD, main pancreatic duct; Post LN, posterior lymph node; Sma LN, lymph node in the peripancreatic fat facing the SMA.

*Fig. 11.* Axial slice from a PDES with ductal adeno-carcinoma of the pancreas infiltrating the duodenum and hepatic artery.

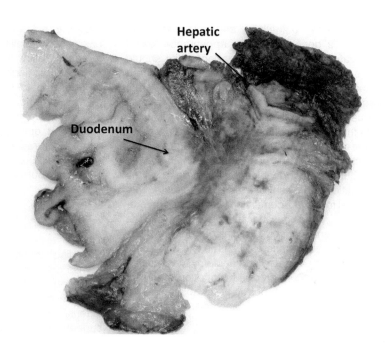

## IDENTIFICATION OF ANATOMIC STRUCTURES IN DISTAL PANCREATECTOMY SPECIMENS

The *splenic artery and vein* run along the superior-dorsal aspect of the pancreatic body and tail (see **Fig. 12**). Proximally, both vessels run midway along the posterior aspect of the pancreatic body before reaching the junction with the celiac trunk and SMV, respectively.

## MACROSCOPIC DESCRIPTION

Recording of findings during macroscopic examination should be in accordance with

*Fig. 12.* Sagittal slices from a distal pancreatec-tomy specimen with a large ductal adenocarci-noma infiltrating the splenic vein (*SPV*). The splenic artery (*SPA*) shows atherosclerotic change but is clear of tumor.

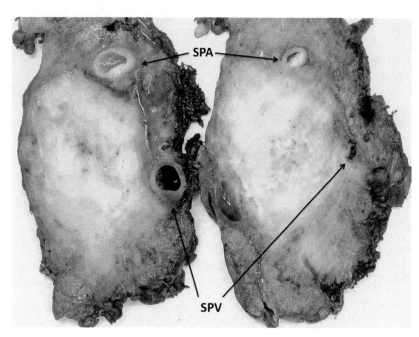

(inter-)national guidelines and minimum data sets. As a general rule, the appearance, exact localization, and size of any abnormality should be recorded. Two dimensions can be measured in the specimen slice in which the lesion is at its largest extent, whereas the third dimension can be calculated by multiplying the slice thickness with the number of slices involved by the lesion.

The anatomic structures described in the previous 2 sections are not only helpful for specimen orientation, but also important landmarks to describe the localization and extent of a lesion. Both factors are essential for careful correlation with findings on preoperative imaging and during surgery. The frequently encountered, but clinical irrelevant statement of "head of pancreas" as the site of a tumor removed by pancreatoduodenectomy, can thus be replaced by a more precise description of the tumor's 3-dimensional position, for example, the cranial-medial part of the pancreatic head, close to, but not infiltrating the common bile duct at its point of entrance into the pancreatic head.

## PHOTODOCUMENTATION

Photodocumentation of the specimen slices is highly recommended, because it provides useful guidance during microscopic examination and

excellent material for demonstration during multidisciplinary meetings.[3,10,13] Moreover, such photographs allow retrospective review of the macroscopic findings, which is particularly important for the identification of the cancer origin (pancreas, ampulla, or distal common bile duct) and complements slide review for the provision of second opinion or systematic quality assurance.[9] Pictures should be taken in close-up (eg, see **Figs. 5–7**). A photograph of all axial specimen slices laid out in sequential order is also helpful (see **Fig. 3**).

## TISSUE SAMPLING

Sampling should be extensive, because carcinomas are often poorly circumscribed, and their size and extent is easily underestimated on naked-eye inspection.[18,20,23] The importance of extensive sampling from the specimen margins is supported by molecular studies.[24]

### SAMPLING TECHNIQUE

The use of at least one whole-mount block is recommended, because this facilitates accurate microscopic measurement of tumor dimensions in the axial plane.[2,10] When using standard tissue

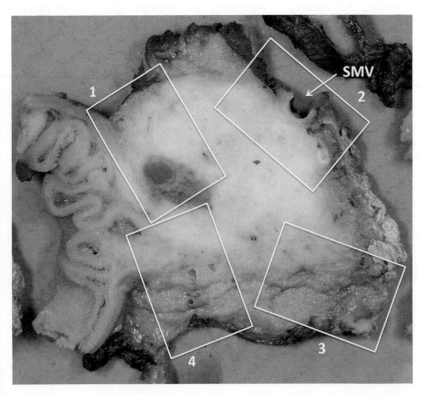

*Fig. 13.* Samples should be taken by rectilinear incisions and include at least 2 anatomic reference points. Sample *1* includes the duodenal wall and anterior surface (*inked red*). Sample *2* includes the anterior surface (*red*), the margin facing the superior mesenteric artery (*SMA; yellow*) and a sleeve resection of the superior mesenteric vein (*SMV*). Sample *3* includes the posterior (*blue*) and SMA-facing surfaces (*yellow*). Sample *4* includes the posterior surface (*blue*) and duodenal wall adjacent to the ampulla of Vater.

cassettes, the following principles should be observed (**Fig. 13**):

- The tumor should be sampled en bloc with adjacent structures or any of the previously described specimen surfaces.[2,3,5,10,22] Tumor should not be dissected out from the surrounding tissues.
- Peripancreatic lymph nodes should be sampled en bloc with the specimen surface. Dissection of individual lymph nodes from the peripancreatic fat, or removal of the peripancreatic fat layer from around the pancreas (so-called orange-peeling method[20]) is not recommended, as this may interfere with assessment of the circumferential margins. Furthermore, because the pancreas is not always well circumscribed, it may be difficult to dissect along the correct tissue plane.
- Lymph nodes should be embedded in their entirety, unless a metastasis is macroscopically visible.[3,13]
- To facilitate tissue orientation during microscopic examination, samples should include at least one anatomic landmark; for instance, an inked margin or parts of the duodenal muscle layer, bile duct, or ampulla. Samples taken from the center of a tumor, without adjacent anatomic structures or margins are of limited value, and do not provide information regarding pT-staging or pR-staging.
- Division of an axial specimen slice into 4 or 5 tissue samples is an easy way to allow optimal orientation and reconstruction of findings.

A number of tissues are routinely sampled:

- For PDES, the transection margins of the pancreatic neck, common bile duct, and stomach and/or duodenum are sampled en face. If the stomach and duodenum are macroscopically unremarkable, the samples from the transection margins may suffice. The gallbladder and cystic duct are sampled as per local protocol.
- For DPES, the pancreatic transection margin is sampled en face. In addition, one sample suffices for a macroscopically unremarkable spleen, whereas one or more samples are required from background pancreatic parenchyma, depending on the pathology that is encountered.

## BLOCK KEY

Tissue samples are best taken from the specimen slices in sequential order, as it facilitates 3-dimensional reconstruction of the tumor and prevents double-counting or triple-counting of large lymph nodes that are present in 2 or 3 consecutive specimen slices. With the help of close-up photographs of the specimen slices, anatomic landmarks and inks on specimen surfaces, identification of the sampled tissues is easy and requires no further information in the block key other than the slice number from which the samples are taken. Identification of the position of lymph nodes can be based on the inked overlying margin or the position to key anatomic structures (see **Figs. 4**, **5** and 9B, **10**, **13**).

## SPECIMENS WITH VENOUS RESECTION

Venous resections, segmental or sleeve resections, are sampled en bloc with the adjacent tissues (see **Figs. 9** and **13**). As it may not always be clear whether the vein is infiltrated by tumor or only tethered by fibrosis, (sub-)total sampling of the vein and the adjacent tissues is recommended.[3,25]

## SPECIMENS FROM EXTENDED PANCREATIC RESECTIONS

An extended PDES may include a segment of small bowel (**Fig. 14**), large bowel, or mesocolon. Extended DPES may include for example, the left adrenal gland, left-sided colon, or stomach (**Fig. 15**). Sampling should aim at demonstrating whether the resected structure is involved by tumor or determining the minimum clearance. Sampling of the transection margins of a segment of colon or stomach is often irrelevant.

## BIOBANKING OF FRESH TISSUE

Banking of fresh tissue samples is often part of routine specimen grossing. For PDES, incisions should be made in the axial plane, such that dissection of the formalin-fixed specimen is not interfered with. To limit the number of incisions required to expose the tumor, it is important to look for tumor-related changes, for example, bulging of the pancreatic surface, irregularity of the SMV groove, adherence of a segment of vein, and irregularity or ulceration of the duodenal mucosa or papilla of Vater. A normal-sized common bile duct and main pancreatic duct may indicate a tumor in the caudal half of the pancreatic head. Information from preoperative imaging may be helpful for targeted biobanking. Sampling of the tumor should avoid areas that are relevant for evaluation of the T-, N-, and R-descriptors.

536

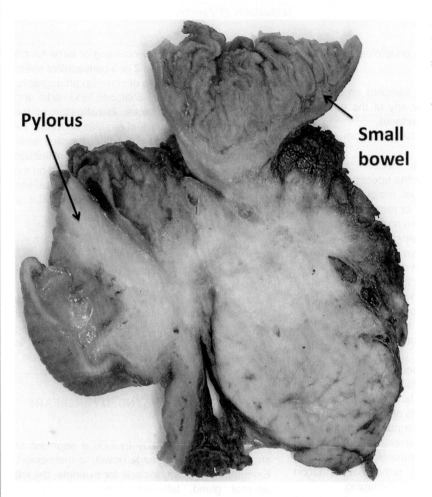

**Pylorus**

**Small bowel**

*Fig. 14.* Axial slice from an extended PDES including a segment of small bowel. Note tumor infiltration of the outer layer of the bowel wall and pylorus.

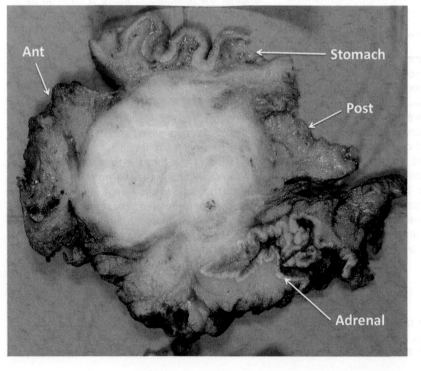

Ant

Stomach

Post

Adrenal

*Fig. 15.* Sagittal slice from an extended distal pancreatectomy specimen including the left adrenal gland and stomach. Note tumor infiltration of the gastric wall and periadrenal fat. Ant, anterior surface; Post, posterior surface.

## SUMMARY

Specimen grossing is an important step in the pathology examination of pancreatic resection specimens, and a major determinant of the quality of the overall process. A fully standardized and detailed approach is required to ensure accurate and reproducible reporting. Dissection of PDES by axial slicing combines technical ease with full standardization, and optimal display of the local anatomy and pathologic changes in a similar fashion as on CT images, which facilitates communication of findings among pathologists, radiologists, and surgeons.

## ACKNOWLEDGMENTS

The authors thank Øystein H. Horgmo, medical illustrator, University of Oslo, for assistance with the illustrations.

## REFERENCES

1. Washington K, Berlin J, Branton P, et al. Protocol for the examination of specimens from patients with carcinoma of the exocrine pancreas. College of American Pathologists; 2013. Available at: www.cap.org.
2. Campbell F, Foulis AK, Verbeke CS. Dataset for the histopathological reporting of carcinomas of the pancreas, ampulla of Vater and common bile duct. The Royal College of Pathologists; 2010. Available at: www.rcpath.org.
3. Cancer of the exocrine pancreas, ampulla of Vater and distal common bile duct. The Royal College of Pathologists of Australasia; 2014. Available at: https://www.rcpa.edu.au/.
4. Seufferlein T, Porzner M, Heinemann V, et al. Ductal pancreatic adenocarcinoma. Dtsch Arztebl Int 2014; 111:396–402.
5. Pancreatic adenocarcinoma. NCCN Clinical Practice Guidelines in Oncology. 2015. Available at: www.nccn.org/patients. Accessed June 14, 2016.
6. Feakins R, Campbell F, Verbeke CS. Survey of UK histopathologists' approach to the reporting of resection specimens for carcinomas of the pancreatic head. J Clin Pathol 2013;66: 715–7.
7. Westgaard A, Laronningen S, Mellem C, et al. Are survival predictions reliable? Hospital volume versus standardisation of histopathologic reporting for accuracy of survival estimates after pancreatoduodenectomy for adenocarcinoma. Eur J Cancer 2009; 45:2850–9.
8. Katz MH, Merchant NB, Brower S, et al. Standardization of surgical and pathologic variables is needed in multicenter trials of adjuvant therapy for pancreatic cancer: results from the ACOSOG Z5031 trial. Ann Surg Oncol 2011;18: 337–44.
9. Verbeke CS, Gladhaug IP. Resection margin involvement and tumour origin in pancreatic head cancer. Br J Surg 2012;99:1036–49.
10. Björnstedt M, Franzén L, Glaumann H, et al. Gastrointestinal pathology pancreas and peri-ampullary region. KVAST Study Group for hepatopancreatobiliary pathology; 2012. Available at: http://svfp.se/node/222. Accessed June 14, 2016.
11. Nagakawa T, Sanada H, Inagaki M, et al. Long-term survivors after resection of carcinoma of the head of the pancreas: significance of histologically curative resection. J Hepatobiliary Pancreat Surg 2004;11: 402–8.
12. Verbeke CS. Resection margins and R1 rates in pancreatic cancer–are we there yet? Histopathology 2008;52:787–96.
13. Hruban RH, Klimstra DS, Pitman MB. Tumors of the pancreas. AFIP atlas of tumor pathology. 6th edition. Washington, DC: American Registry of Pathology in collaboration with the Armed Forces Institute of Pathology; 2007.
14. Campbell F, Verbeke CS. Pathology of the pancreas - a practical approach. London: Springer; 2013.
15. Japan Pancreas Society. Classification of pancreatic cancer. 2nd edition. Tokyo: Kanehara; 2003.
16. Chandrasegaram MD, Goldstein D, Simes J, et al. Meta-analysis of radical resection rates and margin assessment in pancreatic cancer. Br J Surg 2015; 102:1459–72.
17. Esposito I, Kleeff J, Bergmann F, et al. Most pancreatic cancer resections are R1 resections. Ann Surg Oncol 2008;15:1651–60.
18. Jamieson NB, Foulis AK, Oien KA, et al. Positive mobilization margins alone do not influence survival following pancreatico-duodenectomy for pancreatic ductal adenocarcinoma. Ann Surg 2010;251: 1003–10.
19. Verbeke CS, Leitch D, Menon KV, et al. Redefining the R1 resection in pancreatic cancer. Br J Surg 2006;93:1232–7.
20. Verbeke CS, Knapp J, Gladhaug IP. Tumour growth is more dispersed in pancreatic head cancers than in rectal cancer: implications for resection margin assessment. Histopathology 2011;59:1111–21.
21. Verbeke CS. Resection margins in pancreatic cancer. Surg Clin North Am 2013;93:647–62.
22. Nelson H, Hunt KK, Veeramachaneni N, et al. Operative standards for cancer surgery. Volume 1: breast, lung, pancreas, colon. Philadelphia: American College of Surgeons; Alliance for Clinical Trials in Oncology; Wolters Kluwer; 2015. p. 181–272.

23. Kim J, Reber HA, Dry SM, et al. Unfavourable prognosis associated with K-ras gene mutation in pancreatic cancer surgical margins. Gu 2006;55:1598–605.

24. Bockhorn M, Uzunoglu FG, Adham M, et al. Borderline resectable pancreatic cancer: a consensus statement by the International Study Group of Pancreatic Surgery (ISGPS). Surgery 2014;155:977–88.

25. Adsay NV, Basturk O, Saka B, et al. Whipple made simple for surgical pathologists: orientation, dissection, and sampling of pancreaticoduodenectomy specimens for a more practical and accurate evaluation of pancreatic, distal common bile duct, and ampullary tumors. Am J Surg Pathol 2014;38: 480–93.

# Recent Advances in Pancreatic Cancer Surgery of Relevance to the Practicing Pathologist

Lennart B. van Rijssen, MD[a], Steffi J.E. Rombouts, MD[b],
Marieke S. Walma, MD[b], Jantien A. Vogel, MD[a], Johanna A. Tol, MD, PhD[a],
Isaac Q. Molenaar, MD, PhD[b], Casper H.J. van Eijck, MD, PhD[c],
Joanne Verheij, MD, PhD[d], Marc J. van de Vijver, MD, PhD[d],
Olivier R.C. Busch, MD, PhD[a], Marc G.H. Besselink, MD, MSc, PhD[a],*,
For the Dutch Pancreatic Cancer Group

## KEYWORDS

- Whipple • Pancreatoduodenectomy • Pancreas • Surgery • Pathology • Lymph node
- Neoadjuvant • Radiofrequency ablation

## Key points

- Pancreatic cancer remains one of the most deadly cancers, and only 20% of patients are eligible for surgery.
- Both the total number and the ratio of lymph node metastases are strong prognostic factors in pancreatic cancer, but extended lymphadenectomy does not improve survival.
- Initially borderline resectable and nonresectable disease may be downstaged to resectable disease in approximately 30% to 40% of patients following neoadjuvant chemotherapy.
- Local ablative therapies for locally advanced disease, such as radiofrequency ablation and irreversible electroporation, may offer a survival benefit compared with current standard palliative chemotherapy but trials will have to be awaited.

## ABSTRACT

Recent advances in pancreatic surgery have the potential to improve outcomes for patients with pancreatic cancer. We address 3 new, trending topics in pancreatic surgery that are of relevance to the pathologist. First, increasing awareness of the prognostic impact of intraoperatively detected extraregional and regional lymph node metastases and the international consensus definition on lymph node sampling and reporting. Second, neoadjuvant chemotherapy, which is capable of changing 10% to 20% of initially unresectable, to resectable disease. Third, in patients who remain unresectable following neoadjuvant chemotherapy, local ablative therapies may change indications for treatment and improve outcomes.

## OVERVIEW

Pancreatic cancer remains one of the deadliest forms of cancer, with an overall 5-year survival

Financial Declarations/Conflicts of Interest: None to declare.
[a] Department of Surgery, Academic Medical Center, Meibergdreef 9, Amsterdam 1105 AZ, The Netherlands;
[b] Department of Surgery, University Medical Center, Heidelberglaan 100, Utrecht 3584 CX, The Netherlands;
[c] Department of Surgery, Erasmus Medical Center, Gravendijkwal 230, Rotterdam 3015 CE, The Netherlands;
[d] Department of Pathology, Academic Medical Center, Meibergdreef 9, Amsterdam 1105 AZ, The Netherlands
* Corresponding author. Department of Surgery, Academic Medical Center, G4-196, Meibergdreef 9, Amsterdam 1105 AZ, The Netherlands.
E-mail address: m.g.besselink@amc.uva.nl

rate of 3% to 6%.[1–3] By 2030, pancreatic cancer is projected to become the number 2 cause of cancer-related deaths in Western countries.[4] Although patients with resectable disease relatively have the best prognosis, they represent only 20% of the population with pancreatic cancer, and overall survival following surgery in these patients is still only 20 months.[5–8] Patients with nonresectable disease may be divided into patients with locally advanced or metastatic disease, each representing approximately 40% of the total population. Locally advanced pancreatic cancer (LAPC) precludes a resection due to extensive involvement of important vascular structures, such as the celiac trunk, superior mesenteric artery, superior mesenteric vein, and portal vein.[9] Survival of patients with LAPC is approximately 10 months following standard chemotherapy treatment with gemcitabine.[10–12] In patients with metastatic disease, survival is approximately 7 months following palliative treatment with gemcitabine.[13]

There have been several recent advances in treatment for patients with pancreatic cancer. For example, FOLFIRINOX (a combination of 5-fluorouracil [5-FU], oxaliplatin, irinotecan, and leucovorin) is a relatively new chemotherapy regimen and has demonstrated a significant survival benefit up to approximately 11 months in the metastatic setting, although it is generally reserved for fitter patients (World Health Organization performance status 0–1) due to the increased toxicity profile.[13] In surgical patients, postoperative mortality has dropped to approximately 1% to 2% in very high volume centers, although the complication rate remains high at approximately 50%.[6] As research is progressing rapidly, we describe 3 new and trending topics in pancreatic surgery, which are of relevance to the practicing pathologist. These include the intraoperative assessment of lymph nodes, neoadjuvant treatment to induce tumor resectability in patients with initially nonresectable or borderline resectable disease, and 2 emerging local ablative therapies for LAPC: irreversible electroporation (IRE) and radiofrequency ablation (RFA).

## EXAMINATION OF LYMPH NODES

Nodal metastases are a strong prognostic factor for survival after surgery in patients with pancreatic cancer.[14] Recent studies have however demonstrated that the lymph node ratio, the number of lymph nodes with metastases divided by the total number of excised lymph nodes, and the total amount of resected positive nodes have significant prognostic value.[15,16] This stresses the importance of identifying all lymph nodes in surgical specimens with pancreatic cancer. There is, however, no therapeutic impact of extensive lymphadenectomy. Five randomized controlled trails found no survival benefit when comparing extended to standard lymphadenectomy during pancreatoduodenectomy for pancreatic cancer.[17–21]

Until recently, the interpretation of these data was difficult due to different definitions of "standard" and "extended" lymphadenectomy in pancreatoduodenectomy. Hence, in 2014, the International Study Group of Pancreatic Surgery (ISGPS) published a definition of a standard lymphadenectomy based on the available literature and consensus statements formulated during several expert meetings.[22] The consensus statement included the following lymph nodes (classified according to the Japanese Pancreas Society, **Fig. 1**) as part of a standard lymphadenectomy: 5, 6, 8a, 12b1-2, 12c, 13a-b, 14a-b and 17a-b.[23]

The ISGPS definition was designed for pancreatic ductal adenocarcinoma, but is advised for all pancreatoduodenectomies. According to the current seventh edition of the TNM classification, however, not all lymph nodes included in the ISGPS standard lymphadenectomy are always considered as regional nodes.[24] For example, lymph node 8a (hepatic artery) is regarded as a regional node in case of pancreatic carcinoma, but as an extraregional node in case of an ampullary tumor. This would imply that the impact of frozen section analysis of this lymph node during pancreatoduodenectomy could depend on the type of cancer, which, however, may be difficult to determine at that stage.

Furthermore, the ISGPS did not include para-aortic lymph nodes in the standard resection, as para-aortic lymph node metastases are strongly related to decreased survival.[25–28] Available evidence on survival following pancreatic resection in the presence of various intraoperatively detected lymph node metastases consists of small, retrospective studies with selection bias. It has become clear that especially para-aortic lymph node metastases predict poor survival after pancreatoduodenectomy. Large prospective studies are needed to create clinical risk models to determine whether exploration should be aborted once these lymph node metastases are detected.

Standardized pathologic examination of lymph nodes, and of lymph node classification is crucial to allow valid comparison of study results. To optimize this process, lymph nodes could be sent for pathologic analysis separately, by the surgeon. A clear description of the total amount of identified nodes, both positive and negative, and which

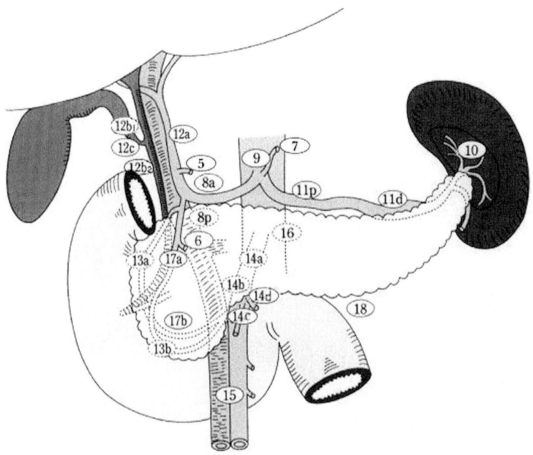

**Fig. 1.** Japan Pancreas Society nomenclature of peripancreatic lymph nodes. (*From* Tol JA, Gouma DJ, Bassi C, et al. Definition of a standard lymphadenectomy in surgery for pancreatic ductal adenocarcinoma: a consensus statement by the International Study Group on Pancreatic Surgery (ISGPS). Surgery 2014;156:591–600; *adapted from* Japan Pancreas Society. Classification of pancreatic carcinoma. 2nd English edition. Tokyo: Kanehara & Co. Ltd; 2003.)

lymph node stations were involved are of great prognostic value to the practicing clinicians and patients alike.

## SHIFTING NONRESECTABLE TO RESECTABLE DISEASE

Microscopically radical (R0) surgery offers the best survival rates for patients with pancreatic cancer. With the introduction of the axial slicing technique, the R1 resection rate has increased markedly from 53% to 85%.[29] This finding, in combination with the ineffectiveness of extended lymphadenectomy demonstrates the need for strategies to reduce tumor extension, perineural, and other microscopic invasion.[17–21] Therefore, various studies are ongoing that investigate neoadjuvant therapy (mainly chemo-radiotherapy) in this setting.[30]

Especially in patients with LAPC and borderline resectable disease, neoadjuvant treatment is of importance, because it may downstage the tumor to such an extent that it becomes eligible for resection. A recent systematic review found a 33% resection rate (of which 79% R0) in patients with borderline resectable disease or LAPC, following treatment with varying, mostly 5-FU or gemcitabine-based neoadjuvant treatment regimens. FOLFIRINOX already demonstrated a significant survival benefit compared with standard gemcitabine in patients with metastatic disease.[13] Resection rate increased to 43% (of which 92% R0) in patients with borderline resectable or LAPC after neoadjuvant treatment with FOLFIRINOX.[31] Evidence on the survival times after neoadjuvant FOLFIRINOX in patients with initially nonresectable disease is scarce, but after resection, survival rates comparable to primarily resectable patients have been described.[32] It has, however, to be considered that most studies report on highly selected groups of patients with LAPC. Usually, only patients who have completed FOLFIRINOX chemotherapy are included. A recent systematic review

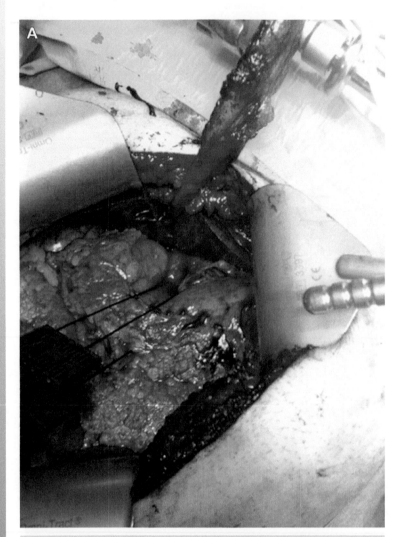

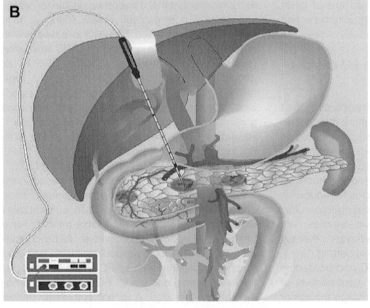

*Fig. 2.* Local ablative therapies. (*A*) IRE: intraoperative detail. (*B*) RFA: schematic.

addressed the specific pathologic challenges when assessing a pancreatic resection specimen after neoadjuvant chemotherapy.[33]

Future prospective multicenter studies will elucidate the benefits of these and other neoadjuvant treatments in the setting of initially resectable, borderline resectable disease or LAPC.[34,35]

## LOCAL ABLATIVE THERAPIES FOR NONRESECTABLE DISEASE

For patients with LAPC, local ablative therapies are currently being studied as a treatment option. Local ablation is mostly applied in LAPC that has remained stable, but still unresectable, after 2 to 3 months of chemotherapy. RFA and IRE have herein been the most extensively studied ablative therapies.[36] In both procedures, needles are inserted in the tumor, either directly in the center (RFA) or at the edges (IRE) of the tumor. Both techniques may be performed either during exploratory laparotomy, or percutaneously (Fig. 2).

RFA is an ablative method in which heat is produced through the application of a high-frequency alternating current, which leads to thermal coagulation and protein denaturation and thus tumor destruction.[37,38] Complications seen after RFA are pancreatitis, fistulas, portal vein thrombosis, duodenal ulcers, and bleeding. In a series of 100 pancreatic RFAs, a morbidity rate of 24% and a mortality rate of 3% were reported, with a median overall survival from diagnosis of 20 months.[39]

IRE is a nonthermal technique, in which the ablative effect is based on creating so called "nanopores" in the lipid bilayer of the cell membrane due to an electric field. These pores are suggested to disrupt intracellular homeostasis, thereby inducing apoptosis.[40,41] As a result of the lack of thermal effect, in contrast to RFA, the connective tissue matrix supposedly remains unaffected, which may lead to preservation of vascular and ductal structures within the treatment field of IRE.[42,43] In a recently published case series of 200 patients treated with IRE, IRE was either used solely (n = 150) or as "margin accentuation" in combination with resection (n = 50) to improve tumor clearance at the resection margins. Morbidity consisted of 100 complications in 54 patients, of which 32 grade ≥3 in the IRE-only group and 49 complications in 20 patients, of which 15 grade ≥3 in the IRE + resection group within 90 days after the procedure.[44] Postoperative mortality rate was 1.5%. Overall survival was 23 months for patients treated with IRE only and 28 months for the combination treatment. Some studies have also reported the use of percutaneous IRE.[45]

As such, the addition of local ablative therapies to the standard treatment of patients with LAPC seems safe and feasible, and could increase life expectancy by several months. Furthermore, local ablative therapies as a primary treatment strategy in LAPC also have been described to increase survival in patients not eligible for chemotherapy.[46] Randomized studies are currently lacking but clearly required, especially because selection bias makes it virtually impossible to value current outcomes. It may well be that only the least aggressive pancreatic cancers are currently selected for these ablation strategies, making comparison with overall survival in patients with LAPC impossible. In the Netherlands, the PELICAN trial is currently ongoing in which patients with LAPC first undergo 2 months of chemotherapy, preferably FOLFIRINOX.[34] If the disease remains stable but unresectable (which may require exploratory laparotomy to confirm), patients are randomized to undergo either RFA followed by chemotherapy or continue with chemotherapy alone.

## SUMMARY

Three new, trending topics in pancreatic surgery that are of relevance to the practicing pathologist include the examination of lymph nodes, neoadjuvant treatment with FOLFIRINOX to induce tumor resectability, and local ablative therapies, such as RFA and IRE, for LAPC.

## REFERENCES

1. Coupland VH, Kocher HM, Berry DP, et al. Incidence and survival for hepatic, pancreatic and biliary cancers in England between 1998 and 2007. Cancer Epidemiol 2012;36:e207–14.
2. Klint A, Engholm G, Storm HH, et al. Trends in survival of patients diagnosed with cancer of the digestive organs in the Nordic countries 1964-2003 followed up to the end of 2006. Acta Oncol 2010; 49:578–607.
3. Karim-Kos HE, de Vries E, Soerjomataram I, et al. Recent trends of cancer in Europe: a combined approach of incidence, survival and mortality for 17 cancer sites since the 1990s. Eur J Cancer 2008;44:1345–89.
4. Rahib L, Smith BD, Aizenberg R, et al. Projecting cancer incidence and deaths to 2030: the unexpected burden of thyroid, liver, and pancreas cancers in the United States. Cancer Res 2014;74: 2913–21.
5. Garcea G, Dennison AR, Pattenden CJ, et al. Survival following curative resection for pancreatic

ductal adenocarcinoma. A systematic review of the literature. JOP 2008;9:99–132.

6. Cameron JL, He J. Two thousand consecutive pancreaticoduodenectomies. J Am Coll Surg 2015; 220:530–6.

7. Oettle H, Post S, Neuhaus P, et al. Adjuvant chemotherapy with gemcitabine vs observation in patients undergoing curative-intent resection of pancreatic cancer: a randomized controlled trial. JAMA 2007; 297:267–77.

8. Ueno H, Kosuge T, Matsuyama Y, et al. A randomised phase III trial comparing gemcitabine with surgery-only in patients with resected pancreatic cancer: Japanese Study Group of Adjuvant Therapy for Pancreatic Cancer. Br J Cancer 2009; 101:908–15.

9. Edge SB, Byrd DR, Compton CC, et al. AJCC cancer staging manual. 7th edition. New York: American Joint Committee on Cancer: Springer-Verlag; 2010.

10. Louvet C, Labianca R, Hammel P, et al. Gemcitabine in combination with oxaliplatin compared with gemcitabine alone in locally advanced or metastatic pancreatic cancer: results of a GERCOR and GISCAD phase III trial. J Clin Oncol 2005;23:3509–16.

11. Poplin E, Feng Y, Berlin J, et al. Phase III, randomized study of gemcitabine and oxaliplatin versus gemcitabine (fixed-dose rate infusion) compared with gemcitabine (30-minute infusion) in patients with pancreatic carcinoma E6201: a trial of the Eastern Cooperative Oncology Group. J Clin Oncol 2009;27:3778–85.

12. Rocha Lima CM, Green MR, Rotche R, et al. Irinotecan plus gemcitabine results in no survival advantage compared with gemcitabine monotherapy in patients with locally advanced or metastatic pancreatic cancer despite increased tumor response rate. J Clin Oncol 2004;22:3776–83.

13. Conroy T, Desseigne F, Ychou M, et al. FOLFIRINOX versus gemcitabine for metastatic pancreatic cancer. N Engl J Med 2011;364:1817–25.

14. Hatzaras I, George N, Muscarella P, et al. Predictors of survival in periampullary cancers following pancreaticoduodenectomy. Ann Surg Oncol 2010;17: 991–7.

15. Tol JA, Brosens LA, van Dieren S, et al. Impact of lymph node ratio on survival in patients with pancreatic and periampullary cancer. Br J Surg 2015;102: 237–45.

16. Malleo G, Maggino L, Capelli P, et al. Reappraisal of nodal staging and study of lymph node station involvement in pancreaticoduodenectomy with the Standard International Study Group of Pancreatic Surgery definition of lymphadenectomy for cancer. J Am Coll Surg 2015;221:367–79.e4.

17. Pedrazzoli S, DiCarlo V, Dionigi R, et al. Standard versus extended lymphadenectomy associated with pancreatoduodenectomy in the surgical treatment of adenocarcinoma of the head of the pancreas: a multicenter, prospective, randomized study. Lymphadenectomy Study Group. Ann Surg 1998;228:508–17.

18. Farnell MB, Pearson RK, Sarr MG, et al. A prospective randomized trial comparing standard pancreatoduodenectomy with pancreatoduodenectomy with extended lymphadenectomy in resectable pancreatic head adenocarcinoma. Surgery 2005; 138:618–28, [discussion: 28–30].

19. Nimura Y, Nagino M, Takao S, et al. Standard versus extended lymphadenectomy in radical pancreatoduodenectomy for ductal adenocarcinoma of the head of the pancreas: long-term results of a Japanese multicenter randomized controlled trial. J Hepatobiliary Pancreat Sci 2012;19:230–41.

20. Jang JY, Kang MJ, Heo JS, et al. A prospective randomized controlled study comparing outcomes of standard resection and extended resection, including dissection of the nerve plexus and various lymph nodes, in patients with pancreatic head cancer. Ann Surg 2014;259:656–64.

21. Yeo CJ, Cameron JL, Sohn TA, et al. Pancreaticoduodenectomy with or without extended retroperitoneal lymphadenectomy for periampullary adenocarcinoma: comparison of morbidity and mortality and short-term outcome. Ann Surg 1999;229:613–22, [discussion: 22–4].

22. Tol JA, Gouma DJ, Bassi C, et al. Definition of a standard lymphadenectomy in surgery for pancreatic ductal adenocarcinoma: a consensus statement by the International Study Group on Pancreatic Surgery (ISGPS). Surgery 2014;156:591–600.

23. Japanese Pancreas Society. Classification of pancreatic carcinoma. 2nd edition. Tokyo: Kanehara & Co; 2003.

24. Sobin LH, Gospodarowicz MK, Wittekind C, International Union Against Cancer (UICC), editors. TNM classification of malignant tumours. 7th edition. Hoboken (NJ): Wiley-Blackwell; 2010.

25. Yamada S, Nakao A, Fujii T, et al. Pancreatic cancer with paraaortic lymph node metastasis: a contraindication for radical surgery? Pancreas 2009;38:e13–7.

26. Schwarz L, Lupinacci RM, Svrcek M, et al. Paraaortic lymph node sampling in pancreatic head adenocarcinoma. Br J Surg 2014;101:530–8.

27. Nappo G, Borzomati D, Perrone G, et al. Incidence and prognostic impact of para-aortic lymph nodes metastases during pancreaticoduodenectomy for peri-ampullary cancer. HPB (Oxford) 2015;17: 1001–8.

28. Paiella S, Malleo G, Maggino L, et al. Pancreatectomy with para-aortic lymph node dissection for pancreatic head adenocarcinoma: pattern of nodal metastasis spread and analysis of prognostic factors. J Gastrointest Surg 2015;19:1610–20.

29. Verbeke CS, Leitch D, Menon KV, et al. Redefining the R1 resection in pancreatic cancer. Br J Surg 2006;93:1232–7.

30. Gillen S, Schuster T, Meyer Zum Buschenfelde C, et al. Preoperative/neoadjuvant therapy in pancreatic cancer: a systematic review and meta-analysis of response and resection percentages. PLoS Med 2010;7:e1000267.

31. Petrelli F, Coinu A, Borgonovo K, et al. FOLFIRINOX-based neoadjuvant therapy in borderline resectable or unresectable pancreatic cancer: a meta-analytical review of published studies. Pancreas 2015;44:515–21.

32. Bickenbach KA, Gonen M, Tang LH, et al. Downstaging in pancreatic cancer: a matched analysis of patients resected following systemic treatment of initially locally unresectable disease. Ann Surg Oncol 2012;19:1663–9.

33. Verbeke C, Lohr M, Karlsson JS, et al. Pathology reporting of pancreatic cancer following neoadjuvant therapy: challenges and uncertainties. Cancer Treat Rev 2015;41:17–26.

34. Pancreatic Locally advanced Irresectable Cancer Ablation in the Netherlands (PELICAN trial; www.pelicantrial.nl). Central Committee on Research Involving Human Subjects (CCMO) registration number NL50467.018.14. Available at: https://www.toetsingonline.nl. Accessed January 3, 2016.

35. Preoperative radiochemotherapy versus immediate surgery for resectable and borderline resectable pancreatic cancer: a multicentre randomized phase III clinical trial (PREOPANC). Central Committee on Research Involving Human Subjects (CCMO) registration number NL40472.078.12. Available at: https://www.toetsingonline.nl. Accessed January 3, 2016.

36. Rombouts SJ, Vogel JA, van Santvoort HC, et al. Systematic review of innovative ablative therapies for the treatment of locally advanced pancreatic cancer. Br J Surg 2015;102:182–93.

37. Coster HG. A quantitative analysis of the voltage-current relationships of fixed charge membranes and the associated property of "punch-through". Biophys J 1965;5:669–86.

38. Weaver JC, Vaughan TE, Chizmadzhev Y. Theory of electrical creation of aqueous pathways across skin transport barriers. Adv Drug Deliv Rev 1999;35:21–39.

39. Girelli R, Frigerio I, Giardino A, et al. Results of 100 pancreatic radiofrequency ablations in the context of a multimodal strategy for stage III ductal adenocarcinoma. Langenbecks Arch Surg 2013;398:63–9.

40. Tarek M. Membrane electroporation: a molecular dynamics simulation. Biophys J 2005;88:4045–53.

41. Delemotte L, Tarek M. Molecular dynamics simulations of lipid membrane electroporation. J Membr Biol 2012;245:531–43.

42. Davalos RV, Mir IL, Rubinsky B. Tissue ablation with irreversible electroporation. Ann Biomed Eng 2005;33:223–31.

43. Maor E, Ivorra A, Leor J, et al. The effect of irreversible electroporation on blood vessels. Technol Cancer Res Treat 2007;6:307–12.

44. Martin RC 2nd, Kwon D, Chalikonda S, et al. Treatment of 200 locally advanced (stage III) pancreatic adenocarcinoma patients with irreversible electroporation: safety and efficacy. Ann Surg 2015;262:486–94, [discussion: 92–4].

45. Narayanan G, Hosein PJ, Arora G, et al. Percutaneous irreversible electroporation for downstaging and control of unresectable pancreatic adenocarcinoma. J Vasc Interv Radiol 2012;23:1613–21.

46. Giardino A, Girelli R, Frigerio I, et al. Triple approach strategy for patients with locally advanced pancreatic carcinoma. HPB (Oxford) 2013;15:623–7.

# Pancreatic Ductal Adenocarcinoma and Its Variants

Claudio Luchini, MD[a,b,c,*], Paola Capelli, MD[a],
Aldo Scarpa, MD, PhD[a,b]

## KEYWORDS

- Pancreatic ductal adenocarcinoma • Pancreatic cancer • PDAC • Ductal • Adenosquamous
- Colloid • Osteoclast

## Key points

- Pancreatic cancer was the seventh leading cause of cancer death in the world in the past 3 years.
- There are classic morphologic features to be used for the diagnosis of pancreatic ductal adenocarcinoma.
- There is not an unequivocal immunohistochemical panel for the diagnosis of this tumor.
- Chronic/autoimmune pancreatitis is an important differential diagnosis

## ABSTRACT

Pancreatic cancer represents the seventh leading cause of cancer death in the world, responsible for more than 300,000 deaths per year. The most common tumor type among pancreatic cancers is pancreatic ductal adenocarcinoma, an infiltrating neoplasm with glandular differentiation that is derived from pancreatic ductal tree. Here we present and discuss the most important macroscopic, microscopic, and immunohistochemical characteristics of this tumor, highlighting its key diagnostic features. Furthermore, we present the classic features of the most common variants of pancreatic ductal adenocarcinoma. Last, we summarize the prognostic landscape of this highly malignant tumor and its variants.

## OVERVIEW

Pancreatic cancer is a lethal malignancy; it was the seventh leading cause of cancer death in the world in the past 3 years, responsible for more than 300,000 deaths per year.[1,2] The 5-year survival of pancreatic cancer is approximately 5%, a figure that has remained constant in recent decades. The most common type among malignant tumors is pancreatic ductal adenocarcinoma (PDAC), an infiltrating neoplasm with glandular differentiation, which is derived from the pancreatic ductal tree. The highest incidence of PDAC is recorded among African Americans and indigenous population in Oceania (approximately 1 per 10,000).[3] Moreover, high-resource countries and urban populations have a higher incidence than low-income countries and rural populations.[3] Studies of migrant populations suggest that environmental and dietary factors play an important role in the etiology.[4] PDAC is associated with nutritional and dietary factors like high intake of fats and obesity, low physical activity, and heavy alcohol drinking.[3,5] However, the best-known risk factor for PDAC is tobacco smoking, which is associated with a 2 to 3 times greater risk than

Disclosure Statement: Prof. Scarpa is supported by Ministry of University (FIRB RBAP10AHJB) and AIRC (grant n. 12182). The other authors have nothing to disclose.
[a] Department of Diagnostics and Public Health, University and Hospital Trust of Verona, Piazzale Scuro, 10, Verona 37134, Italy; [b] ARC-Net Research Center, University and Hospital Trust of Verona, Piazzale Scuro, 10, Verona 37134, Italy; [c] Surgical Pathology Unit, Santa Chiara Hospital, Largo Medaglie D'oro, Trento 38122, Italy
* Corresponding author. Department of Diagnostics and Public Health, University and Hospital Trust of Verona, Piazzale Scuro, 10, Verona 37134, Italy.
E-mail addresses: claudio.luchini@katamail.com; claudio.luchini@univr.it

Surgical Pathology 9 (2016) 547–560
http://dx.doi.org/10.1016/j.path.2016.05.003

surgpath.theclinics.com

in nonsmokers.[6] Other significant conditions associated with a higher risk of PDAC are diabetes mellitus, with a risk of approximately twofold, and a history of chronic pancreatitis, above all if this condition is hereditary, as it is associated with an increased risk of PDAC of more than 10-fold.[7] Clinical features include back pain, jaundice for pancreatic head tumor, unexplained weight loss, pruritus, diabetes mellitus, and occasionally migratory thrombophlebitis, acute pancreatitis, hypoglycemia, and hypercalcemia.[3,8–10] For the radiological study of pancreas, one of the best imaging modalities is represented by computed tomography (CT), in which PDAC appears as a hypodense mass in up to 92% of cases; on endoscopic ultrasonography (EUS), most PDACs are echo-poor and nonhomogeneous.[3,11,12] Variants of conventional PDAC are the following: (1) adenosquamous carcinoma, (2) colloid carcinoma, (3) undifferentiated or anaplastic carcinoma, (4) undifferentiated carcinoma with osteoclastlike giant cells (UCOCGC), (5) signet-ring carcinoma, (6) medullary carcinoma and (7) hepatoid carcinoma.[3,13] Another important entity is represented by carcinomas with mixed differentiation. This heterogeneous group is composed of mixed acinarductal carcinoma, mixed acinar-neuroendocrine carcinoma, mixed acinar-neuroendocrine-ductal carcinoma and mixed adeno-neuroendocrine carcinoma (MANEC).[3]

## GROSS FEATURES

## CONVENTIONAL PANCREATIC DUCTAL ADENOCARCINOMA

Most (60%–70%) PDACs are located in the head of the gland, and the remainder, with a similar rate (approximately 15% each), in the body and/or tail.[11] Generally, PDAC is a solitary lesion, but it may also occasionally present as a multifocal disease.[3,13] PDACs are firm, hard, sclerotic and poorly defined masses, which replace the normal lobular architecture of the gland. The cut surface is usually whitish (Fig. 1). Sometimes, a microcystic area can be present, particularly in large tumors; hemorrhage and necrosis are very rare. Most PDACs of the head range from 1.5 to 5.0 cm, whereas PDACs of body/tail are usually larger. PDACs of the head usually invade the common bile duct and/or the Wirsung duct, producing stenosis that results in proximal dilatation of both duct systems. More advanced PDACs in the head can involve the papilla of Vater and the duodenal wall. In the body/tail, PDAC usually causes obstruction of the Wirsung duct, with secondary changes in the upstream pancreatic

parenchyma, including retention-cyst formation, duct dilatation, and fibrous atrophy of the parenchyma. At the time of the diagnosis, most PDACs have already spread beyond the pancreatic parenchyma, and are not operable; conversely, the typical TNM status at diagnosis of the operable PDACs is T3N1 (T3 indicates that the tumor has grown outside the pancreas into nearby surrounding tissues, but not yet into major blood vessels or nerves, and N1 indicates the presence of metastasis in regional lymph nodes) highlighting also the rapidity of tumor growth and of metastasis. Common extensions of PDAC of the head are the following: intrapancreatic portion of the common bile duct, peripancreatic or retroperitoneal (posterior lamina) adipose tissue, papilla of Vater, and duodenum. Perineural invasion is a very common mechanism by which PDAC reaches these structures. PDACs of body and tail can first invade spleen, stomach, left adrenal gland, peritoneum, and colon. The lymph nodes most commonly involved by PDAC are the peripancreatic lymph nodes. Furthermore, for PDACs of the head, an important site of metastasis is represented by the chains of lymph nodes along the superior mesenteric and common hepatic arteries, and the hepatoduodenal ligament. For PDACs of body and tail, frequent sites of involvement are the superior and inferior body and tail lymph node groups, and the lymph nodes of the splenic hilus.[3] Metastasis of the para-aortic area is associated with a worse prognosis.[14]

## PANCREATIC DUCTAL ADENOCARCINOMA VARIANTS

The variants of conventional PDAC have some peculiar macroscopic aspects, but there are no definitive criteria to distinguish such variants grossly. *Adenosquamous carcinoma* is usually represented by a white-gray firm and multinodular mass (see Fig. 1). *Colloid carcinoma* is characterized by large pools of mucin, usually arising in association with an intraductal mucinous papillary neoplasm (IMPN) of intestinal-type (see Fig. 1). *Undifferentiated or anaplastic carcinoma* is larger than conventional PDAC but has very similar macroscopic features; *the variant with osteoclastlike giant cells* has very often several foci of hemorrhage and necrosis (see Fig. 1). *Signet-ring* and *medullary carcinoma* are grossly very similar to conventional PDAC and *hepatoid carcinoma* is characterized by white-yellowish, multi-lobed masses. Last, mixed carcinomas usually consist in large masses with necrotic foci.

## Pathologic Key Features

*Conventional PDAC*

1. Glandular and ductlike structures with haphazard pattern of growth (well and moderately differentiated tumors).

2. Small and poorly formed glands, individual infiltrating cells, solid pattern (poorly differentiated tumors).

3. Marked desmoplastic stromal reaction.

4. Production of sialo-type and sulfated acid mucins (well and moderately differentiated tumors).

5. Scanty or null production of mucins (poorly differentiated tumors).

6. Cytologically: atypical cells with pleomorphic, enlarged nuclei, with prominent, huge irregular nucleoli.

7. Mitoses, particularly atypical mitoses.

8. Glandular necrotic debris.

9. Lympho-vascular invasion, perineural infiltration, lymph node metastasis are very common.

10. Extranodal extension of tumor metastasis is common (approximately 60% of node-positive cases).

*Variants*

1. Adenosquamous carcinoma: ductal plus squamous differentiation in at least 30% of the tumor.

2. Colloid carcinoma: presence of large extracellular stromal mucin pools with suspended neoplastic cells in at least 80% of the neoplasm.

3. Undifferentiated carcinoma: does not show a definitive pattern of differentiation.

4. UCOCGC: is composed of 2 cellular types: spindle and pleomorphic cells are the real neoplastic cells, and osteoclastlike giant cells, that have not a malignant behavior.

5. Signet-ring carcinoma: almost exclusively constituted of signet-ring cells.

6. Medullary carcinoma: poor differentiation, prominent syncytial growth pattern.

7. Hepatoid carcinoma: a significant cellular population with hepatocellular differentiation.

## MICROSCOPIC FEATURES

Most PDACs are composed of well/moderately differentiated glandular and ductlike structures, infiltrating the pancreatic parenchyma (**Fig. 2**). They are characterized by a haphazard pattern of growth and are associated with a desmoplastic stromal reaction (see **Fig. 2**). These tumors produce sialo-type and sulfated acid mucins, which stain with Alcian blue and periodic acid-Schiff. Poorly differentiated PDACs usually form small and poorly formed glands; cytologically, these structures are composed of cells with pleomorphic, atypical nuclei, individual infiltrating cells, and solid patterns. They produce much less sialo-type and sulfated acid mucin than the more differentiated PDACs.

## WELL-DIFFERENTIATED PANCREATIC DUCTAL ADENOCARCINOMA

Well-differentiated PDACs are composed of haphazardly arranged infiltrating and medium-size glandular and ductlike structures; the contours of ductlike structures may be irregular or angular, and especially pronounced in the "large-duct" variant.[15] The neoplastic cells are cuboidal or columnar, forming a single cell layer; rarely, papillary projections can be seen. The cytoplasm is usually eosinophilic, and the nuclei are round or oval and may be even 4 times larger than non-neoplastic nuclei. This comparison is often possible and easy because many PDACs have entrapped normal ducts; otherwise normal endothelium or lymphocyte nuclei can be used to this

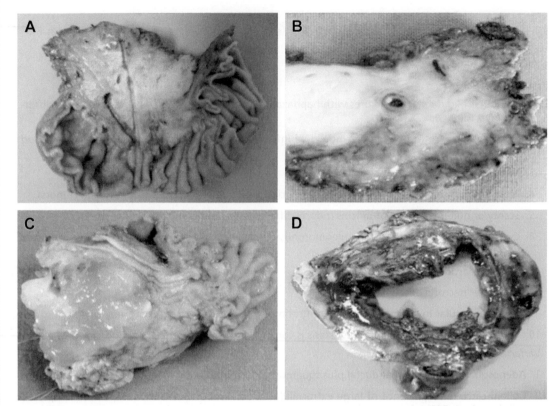

**Fig. 1.** Gross features of PDAC and its variants. Conventional PDAC is usually represented by firm, hard, sclerotic, and poorly defined masses, that replace the normal lobular architecture of the gland. The surface of cut is usually white. In this case, a PDAC of the head of the pancreas invades the common bile duct and the Wirsung duct with stenosis (*A*). Adenosquamous variant is generally a white-gray firm and multinodular mass, often larger than conventional PDAC at the time of diagnosis. In this case the multinodular architecture is clearly evident (*B*). Colloid carcinoma is distinguished by large pools of mucin, usually arising in association with an IMPN, intestinal-type. In this case it is clearly present an abundant deposit of thick mucin (*C*). Undifferentiated or anaplastic carcinoma is larger than conventional PDAC but has very similar macroscopic features; the variant with osteoclastlike giant cells has very often several foci of hemorrhage and necrosis, and can show, like in this case, a cystic appearance (*D*).

aim. Colonization of normal ducts by neoplastic cells is also common (**Fig. 3**). However, it has to be clarified that the size, shape, and location of the nuclei can vary widely among cells, even within the individual neoplastic glands. The nuclear membranes are sharp and the distinct nucleoli, generally 2 or more, are often large; mitoses are not so common. Lympho-vascular invasion, perineural infiltration (**Fig. 4**) as well as lymph node metastasis are very common features. The neoplastic epithelium can even entirely replace the endothelium, re-lining the vessel by well-differentiated epithelial cells. Furthermore, a particular morphologic feature of lymph node metastasis, that is the extra-nodal extension of neoplastic cells in the peri-nodal adipose tissue, has recently been associated with worse prognosis in many cancer types, also including PDAC.[16–19] The grading of PDAC is based on the combined assessment of histologic and cytologic features, and mitotic activity

(**Table 1**), and also plays an important role in the prognostic stratification of patients[3,20]; the grading systems is based on a 3-tiered scale: well-differentiated (G1), moderately differentiated (G2), and poorly differentiated (G3) PDAC. Summarizing the most important features, grade 1 is characterized by well-differentiated glands, intensive production of mucin, and 0 to 5 mitoses per 10 high-power fields (HPF); nuclei have a little polymorphism and a marked polar arrangement (**Fig. 5**).

## MODERATELY DIFFERENTIATED PANCREATIC DUCTAL ADENOCARCINOMA

Moderately differentiated PDACs are very similar to the well-differentiated PDACs, but they produce a mixture of medium-sized ductlike structures and small tubular glands of variable shape and size. There is a greater variation in cellular and nuclear size, chromatin structure, and prominence of

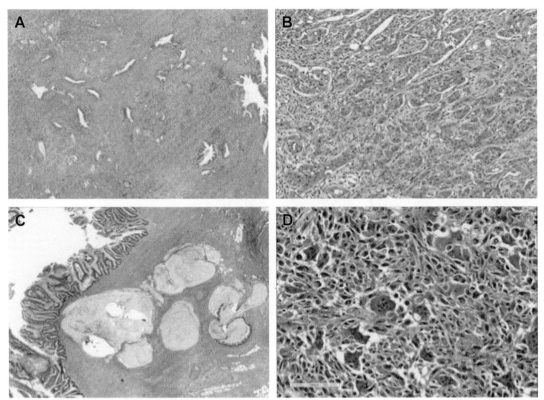

*Fig. 2.* Microscopic features of PDAC and its variants. Most PDACs are composed of well-developed or moderately developed glandular and ductlike structures, which infiltrate the adjacent pancreatic parenchyma. In this picture is present the typical haphazard pattern of growth as well as the classic desmoplastic stromal reaction (*A*). Adenosquamous carcinoma has both significant ductal and significant squamous differentiation, at least of 30%. This photograph shows the overt squamous differentiation (*B*). Colloid carcinoma is characterized by the presence of large extracellular stromal mucin pools with suspended neoplastic cells in at least 80% of the neoplasm. In this picture, the typical association with intestinal-type IPMN has been shown (*C*). Undifferentiated carcinoma does not show a definitive direction of differentiation; the UCOCGC variant is composed of 2 cellular types: spindle and pleomorphic cells, the real neoplastic cells, and osteoclastlike giant cells, that can have more than 20 nuclei each, but without a malignant behavior. Furthermore, as shown in this picture, the osteoclastlike giant cells can show a clear phagocytosis (*D*). Original magnification, A = ×4, B = ×10, C = ×2, D = ×20.

nucleoli; usually, there are more mitotic figures. Mucin production appears to be lower than in well-differentiated PDAC. Foci of poor and irregular glandular formation are often found at the advancing front of the tumor, particularly where the carcinoma invades the normal pancreatic parenchyma. Summarizing the most important microscopic aspects, grade 2 is characterized by moderately differentiated ductlike structures and tubular glands, irregular mucin production (lower than grade 1), and 6 to 10 mitoses per 10 HPF; nuclei have moderate polymorphism (see **Fig. 5**).

## POORLY DIFFERENTIATED PANCREATIC DUCTAL ADENOCARCINOMA

Poorly differentiated PDACs are composed of densely packed, small irregular glands, solid sheets, and nests, as well as many individual cells. The desmoplastic response to the neoplasm can be minimal, and foci of hemorrhage and necrosis may occur. The cells forming glands and solid cellular sheets show marked nuclear pleomorphism, scanty or no mucin production, and high mitotic activity. Summarizing this concept, to reach a standardization about the grading issue (it lacks a high interobserver agreement among pathologists about grading, thus highlighting standard parameters is very important), grade 3 is characterized by poorly differentiated glands, solid areas and single cells patterns, abortive mucoepidermoid and pleomorphic structures, scanty or absent mucin production, and more than 10 mitoses per 10 HPF; nuclei have marked pleomorphism and increased size (see **Fig. 5**).

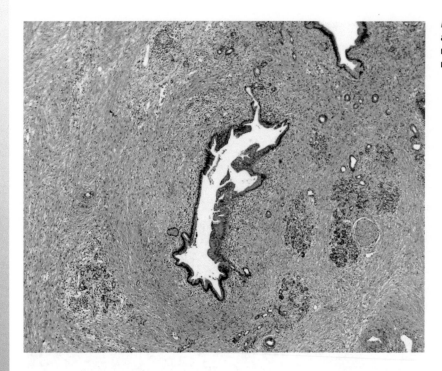

*Fig. 3.* A normal pancreatic duct colonized by neoplastic cells (original magnification ×10).

## PANCREATIC DUCTAL ADENOCARCINOMA VARIANTS

Peculiar microscopic features define the diverse PDAC variants. *Adenosquamous carcinoma* has both significant ductal and squamous (at least 30%) differentiation (see **Fig. 2**). *Colloid carcinoma* is characterized by the presence of large extracellular stromal mucin pools with suspended neoplastic cells in at least 80% of the neoplasm (see **Fig. 2**). *Undifferentiated or anaplastic carcinoma* shows a significant part of the neoplasm

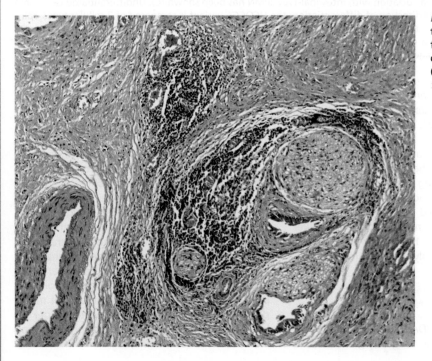

*Fig. 4.* Perineural infiltration is a classic microscopic feature of pancreatic ductal adenocarcinomas (original magnification ×20).

**Table 1**
Histopathologic grading of pancreatic ductal adenocarcinoma

| Tumor Grade | Glandular/Ductal Differentiation | Mucin Production | Mitoses (× 10 HPF) | Nuclear Atypia |
|---|---|---|---|---|
| 1 | Well-differentiated ductlike glands | Intensive and diffuse | ≤5 | Mild atypia, polar arrangement |
| 2 | Moderately differentiated ductlike glands and tubular glands | Irregular and focal | 6–10 | Moderate pleomorphism |
| 3 | Poorly differentiated glands, solid nests, single cells infiltration, pleomorphic structures | Abortive | >10 | Marked pleomorphism and increased nuclear size, prominent huge nucleoli |

Abbreviation: HPF, high-power field.

that does not show a definitive direction of differentiation. The *UCOCGC* variant is composed of 2 cellular types: spindle and pleomorphic cells (the real neoplastic cells) and osteoclastlike giant cells that can have more than 20 nuclei each (nonneoplastic reactive cells) (see **Fig. 2**); pure *undifferentiated carcinoma* is a very rare entity and can show highly anaplastic cells (**Fig. 6**). *Signet-ring carcinoma* is composed almost exclusively of poorly cohesive neoplastic cells with intracytoplasmic mucin that displaces the nuclei toward the periphery (see **Fig. 6**); notably, a breast or gastric primary should be excluded. *Medullary carcinoma* is characterized by poor differentiation and prominent syncytial growth pattern immersed in an intense inflammatory infiltrate composed of leukocytes; an increased number of tumor-infiltrating CD3-positive lymphocytes can be present. Last, *hepatoid carcinoma* is composed of a significant cellular population with hepatocellular differentiation. Hepatoid carcinomas are composed of large polygonal cells with abundant eosinophilic cytoplasm, resembling normal and/or neoplastic hepatocytes. These tumors often present a trabecular pattern, very similar to well-differentiated hepatocellular carcinomas. For mixed neoplasms, by definition each component should comprise at least one-third of the neoplastic tissue. The best characterized is MANEC (**Fig. 7**): it can show 2 possible morphologic patterns: (i) neoplastic ductal cells more or less intermingled with neoplastic neuroendocrine cells; (ii) pure neoplastic ductal structures embedded in a solid neuroendocrine cell compartment.[3]

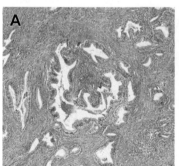 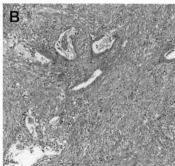 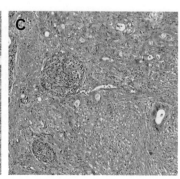

*Fig. 5.* Grading of pancreatic ductal adenocarcinoma. It is based on combined assessment of histologic and cytologic features, and mitotic activity. Grade 1, like in this case (*A*), is characterized by well-glandular-differentiation, intensive production of mucin, and 0 to 5 mitoses per 10 HPF; nuclei have a little polymorphism and a marked polar arrangement. Grade 2 is characterized by moderately differentiated ductlike structures and tubular glands, lower mucin production, and 6 to 10 mitoses per 10 HPF. In this case (*B*), there are few and ruptured glands, without the clear polar arrangement of grade 1. Grade 3 is characterized by poorly differentiated glands, solid areas, and single-cell patterns, abortive muco-epidermoid and pleomorphic structures, scanty or absent mucin production, and more than 10 mitoses per 10 HPF. Nuclei have marked polymorphism and increased size. In this picture (*C*), there is only one gland, very atypical, and it is present the classic single-cell pattern of infiltration of grade 3. Original magnification, A = ×4, B = ×10, C = ×10.

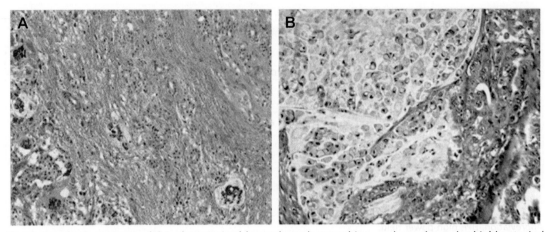

*Fig. 6.* Anaplastic carcinoma (*A*) is characterized by nuclear pleomorphism, and can show also highly atypical cells. Signet-ring carcinoma (*B*) is composed almost exclusively of poorly cohesive neoplastic cells with intracytoplasmic mucin that displaces the nuclei toward the periphery; in this figure, the signet-ring cells are intermingled with neoplastic glands of a conventional pancreatic ductal adenocarcinoma.

## DIFFERENTIAL DIAGNOSIS

### PANCREATITIS

The most important differential diagnosis for conventional PDAC is represented by chronic pancreatitis.[11,21] Grossly, chronic pancreatitis of alcoholic or obstructive etiology usually involves the pancreas more widely than a neoplastic process. The ductal tree may be dilated and a clear lithiasis, with whitish calculi in the ducts, can occur; the pancreatic parenchyma is more rubbery and with a more gritty consistency than PDAC.[3] Groove pancreatitis is a rare form of chronic

pancreatitis affecting the so-called pancreatic groove, that is the space between the pancreatic head, duodenum, and common bile duct. It is strongly associated with long-term alcohol abuse, functional obstruction of Santorini duct and Brunner gland hyperplasia.[22] Characteristic radiologic features of groove pancreatitis are thickening of the medial duodenal wall and cystic spaces between the duodenum and pancreas. Unfortunately, differentiating groove pancreatitis from malignancy on the basis of imaging features, clinical presentation, or laboratory markers can be very difficult, and most of these patients undergo a pancreaticoduodenectomy, because of an

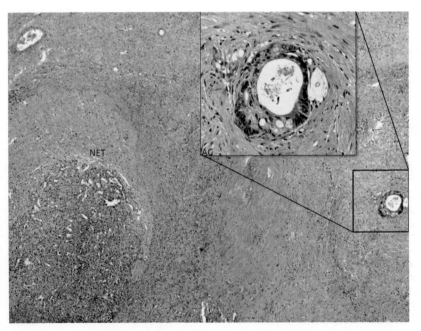

*Fig. 7.* Mixed adeno-neuroendocrine carcinoma is composed of a mixture of neoplastic neuroendocrine cells and neoplastic ductal structures. The neoplastic glands can be more or less intermingled with neuroendocrine elements. AC, adenocarcinoma gland; NET, pancreatic neuroendocrine tumor. original magnification ×4, detail ×20.

inability to completely exclude malignancy. Cytologically, groove pancreatitis can also exhibit numerous multinucleated non-neoplastic cells on smears,[23] extending the issue of the differential diagnosis to the UCOCGC. Autoimmune pancreatitis often mimics PDAC both clinically and grossly, by presenting as a discrete, tumorlike lesion.[24–26] The classic histology of autoimmune pancreatitis includes a cellular fibro-inflammatory stroma with a storiform appearance, a diffuse obliterative venulitis, but pathognomonic is a dense inflammation with abundant plasma cells concentrated around pancreatic ducts. Furthermore, to complete the differential diagnosis, an increased numbers of plasma cells expressing IgG4 (>10–50 cells per HPF) is typical, as well as the presence of antiplasminogen binding protein peptide antibodies.[24]

## REACTIVE GLANDS AND PRECURSOR LESIONS

Microscopically, the most helpful findings in distinguishing PDAC from reactive glands remain the location and the architecture of the glands in addition to the cytologic features.[3] Also the presence of "naked glands in fat" is very suggestive for PDAC, but attention must be paid to the fact that the observed adipose tissue may be derived from adipose involution of normal pancreatic parenchyma; this feature is clearly distinguishable for the presence of remnant of pancreatic islets. Other features that point to a malignant diagnosis are mitotic figures, necrotic luminal debris, stromal desmoplasia, and aberrant DPC4 and/or p53 expression. These latter aspects are very useful also in identifying neoplastic infiltration in surgical specimens with the classic precursor lesions of PDAC: pancreatic intraepithelial neoplasia (PanIN), mucinous cystic neoplasm (MCN), and intraductal papillary mucinous neoplasm (IPMN).

## DIAGNOSIS

### MICROSCOPIC CRITERIA

There are some morphologic features that are fundamental to support a diagnosis of PDAC with a reasonable level of certainty (Fig. 8). They include the haphazard architectural tumor pattern, a marked desmoplastic stromal reaction and "ruptured" or "incomplete" ducts; moreover, perineural or vascular invasions are both highly diagnostic of an infiltrating tumor. A very important microscopic feature, also with a very high diagnostic weight for PDAC, is that the infiltrating malignant glands are often found in abnormal locations, such as immediately adjacent to muscular blood vessels. This criterion is very useful for the diagnosis of PDAC above all in surgical specimens after neoadjuvant therapies, in which the degree of cellular atypia may be very low and usually there are only very few glands in a massive fibrous stroma, and in the differential diagnosis with chronic pancreatitis.[3] Last, it has to be highlighted that knowing the cytologic features of PDAC is fundamental also during histopathologic analysis, especially when PDACs are poorly differentiated and the pathologists have to evaluate single tumor cells. Cytologic features are also important during frozen section examination in which it may be difficult to evaluate the general architecture of the cancer. In these cases, some cytologic features become very useful: the nuclei are enlarged, hyperchromatic, and display irregular nuclear membranes, and the cytoplasm ranges from scant and nonmucinous to abundant and mucinous.[11,27,28] For the PDAC variants, 2 variants have a fixed threshold of peculiar cellular component: adenosquamous carcinoma has to show a squamous differentiation in at least 30% of the neoplasm (the diagnosis is mainly

| △△ | *Differential Diagnosis* |
|---|---|
| **PDAC vs:** | **Useful Features vs PDAC** |
| Chronic pancreatitis | Clear lithiasis, marked inflammatory infiltration, no clear signs of infiltrating tumor (eg, perineural infiltration). |
| Autoimmune pancreatitis | A dense inflammation with abundant plasma cells concentrated around pancreatic ducts, a cellular fibro-inflammatory stroma with a storiform appearance and a diffuse obliterative venulitis. An increased numbers of plasma cells expressing IgG4 (>10–50 cells per HPF) is typical. |
| Reactive glands | Location of the glands (the presence of "naked glands in fat" is very suggestive for PDAC), absence of mitotic figures, of necrotic luminal debris and of stromal desmoplasia. |
| IPMN, MCN | Looking for possible infiltrating component, that lacks in IPMN and MCN. |

morphologic), and *colloid carcinoma* has to present large mucin pools with neoplastic cells in at least 80% of the neoplasm. Last, for mixed carcinomas, each component should represent at least the 30% of all tumor cells.[3]

## IMMUNOHISTOCHEMISTRY OF CONVENTIONAL PANCREATIC DUCTAL ADENOCARCINOMA

There is no unequivocal immunohistochemical panel that can be used to distinguish PDAC from reactive glands or from other extrapancreatic mucin-producing adenocarcinomas (eg, bile duct carcinomas), although some markers may be useful. First of all, PDACs express the same keratins of the normal pancreatic duct epithelium, like keratins 7, 8, 18, and 19.[3] The best of these markers to be used routinely is the classic mixture of keratin 8 and 18. Keratin 20, a typical intestinal-epithelial marker, is often not expressed, or less widely than keratin 7.[29] Among mucins, PDACs usually express MUC1, MUC3, MUC4, and MUC5AC, but not MUC2.[30,31] Furthermore, they express glycoprotein tumor antigens like CA19 to 9, more specific for pancreas disease, CEA and CA125.[3,32] PDACs are usually negative for pancreatic exocrine enzymes, such as trypsin, chymotrypsin, and lipase, for mesenchymal markers like vimentin, and for

neuroendocrine markers, like chromogranin A, CD56, and synaptophysin.[3] However, very rarely, well-differentiated PDACs may contain scattered non-neoplastic neuroendocrine cells in close association with neoplastic glands, without representing a mixed adeno-neuroendocrine carcinoma (so-called MANEC).[33,34] About "immune-molecular" staining, the SMAD4 protein is lost in 55% of PDACs, and aberrant (either overexpression or complete absence of expression) p53 protein expression is seen in most cases.[13] Other markers for PDAC, more recently discovered, are mesothelin, claudin 4, claudin 18, and S100P.[3,13,35,36]

## IMMUNOHISTOCHEMISTRY OF PANCREATIC DUCTAL ADENOCARCINOMA VARIANTS

PDAC variants have classic markers due to their differentiation, which can be very useful for the diagnosis and differential diagnosis. *Adenosquamous*: Cytokeratin 5 and P63 positivity in the squamous component; *colloid*: CDX2 and MUC2 positivity (colloid component: intestinal differentiation); *undifferentiated or anaplastic carcinoma*: positivity for keratin and vimentin but not for E-Cadherin; *UCOCGC*: neoplastic cells are positive for vimentin, keratins and p53, osteoclastlike giant cells are positive for CD68, vimentin, CD45, but are negative for keratins and p53; *hepatoid carcinoma*

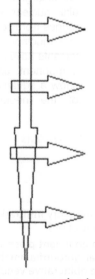

Radiologic - clinic - anamnestic criteria

Microscopic criteria

Immunohistochemistry

Grossly palpable mass

PDAC diagnosis

In case of discordance, exclude pancreatic metastasis from other sites and other possible disease (e.g. chronic pancreatitis, see differential diagnosis box)

*Fig. 8.* Diagnostic algorithm. PDAC, pancreatic ductal adenocarcinoma.

displays positivity for hepatocyte-specific antigen and shows a canalicular pattern of staining with CD10-antibody.[3,13,37–39] *Signet-ring* carcinomas have not a clear-cut immunohistochemistry; at the same time, it has to be noticed that most cases of medullary carcinomas are microsatellite instable and show loss of mismatch repair protein expression. In mixed tumors, classic markers are expressed in each component, and can support the diagnosis, above all in case of poorly differentiated neoplasms. Endocrine component shows typical expression of synaptophysin, chromogranin, and CD56, as well as acinar component of trypsin, chymotrypsin, and Bcl-10.

## MOLECULAR DIAGNOSTIC KEY POINTS

Typical molecular (somatic) alterations in PDAC, also important to support the diagnosis of such tumor, regard 4 key genes: *KRAS*, *CDKN2A*, *TP53,* and *SMAD4*.[2] The most common gene alteration is in *KRAS*, where typical mutations occur in codons 12, 13, and 61.[40,41] Notably, more than 90% of PDAC contains *KRAS* mutations.[3] In addition to these 4 frequently altered genes, various other genes, like *ARID1A*, are mutated at relatively low frequencies in pancreatic cancer, but can play a prognostic role.[42] Molecular genetics of pancreatic cancer and it precursor lesions are discussed in more detail in the article by XXXXX, elsewhere in this issue (see Wood L, Hosoda W: Molecular Genetics of Pancreatic Neoplasms, in this issue).

## PATHOLOGY REPORT

The final pathology report for PDAC should include some important features, to support the diagnosis and to permit an adequate oncologic staging.

For tumors of the head of the pancreas the pathologists should report:

- The grading of the tumor
- The contemporary presence of dysplastic modifications of non-neoplastic ducts (eg, PanIN, that supports the pancreatic origin of the tumor)
- The presence of perineural and/or vascular invasions
- The presence of biliary margin and pancreatic neck margin infiltration
- The presence of choledocic, duodenal (and gastric in Whipple resection specimen), peripancreatic adipose tissue (up to peritoneum), and retroperitoneal (posterior lamina) infiltration
- The nodal status, ideally identifying intestinal (duodenal) nodes, perigastric nodes,

pancreatic-duodenal (dividing them in anterior and posterior is not required by the current TNM staging system) nodes, pericholedocic nodes, and the lymph nodes of the superior mesenteric artery (in the posterior lamina).

For tumors of the body-tail, it should be reported:

- The grading of the tumor
- The contemporary presence of dysplastic modifications of non-neoplastic ducts (eg, PanIN, that supports the pancreatic origin of the tumor)
- The presence of perineural or vascular invasion
- The status of pancreatic neck margin
- The presence of peripancreatic adipose tissue (up to peritoneum) infiltration
- The nodal status, ideally identifying peripancreatic nodes (classically located very closely to splenic vessels on the posterosuperior margin), and the lymph nodes of splenic hilus

Last, following the model of the so called "next-generation histopathologic diagnosis," the most important molecular alterations of cancer will likely be included in the future in the final pathology report.[43]

## PROGNOSIS

Because of the absence of effective methods for early diagnosis and the aggressive nature of this disease, most patients present with locally advanced or metastatic cancer, mostly not eligible for surgical approaches. The 5-year survival rate of PDAC is approximately 5%, a percentage that has remained constant in recent decades. Chemotherapeutic options for advanced PDACs are still limited; gemcitabine has been the standard chemotherapeutic drug for patients with advanced disease for many years, but it provides only a modest survival advantage. The most prevalent oncogenic alteration is mutation in *KRAS*, which seems an obvious target for cancer therapy. However, although great efforts have been made to develop small-molecular inhibitors of mutant *KRAS*, no clinically effective antagonist has been identified yet. In addition to *KRAS*, *SMAD4, TP53,* and *CDKN2A* are also commonly altered in PDAC. However, therapeutic strategies targeting these proteins are considered to be difficult for different reasons, including cellular location and multifunctionality.[2] Overall, pancreatic cancer is characterized by substantial genomic heterogeneity with also numerous infrequently mutated genes.[2] Although the common

## Pitfalls

! Especially on frozen section examination, chronic pancreatitis can mimic very well PDAC; in case of clinical information supporting chronic pancreatitis, the diagnosis of PDAC on frozen sections (eg, pancreatic neck margin) should be avoided in most cases.

! Exclude possible distant metastasis in the pancreas in case of rare variants (eg, signet-ring carcinoma is very rare: exclude a metastasis from breast or stomach) or in case of particular cellular features, even if focal (eg, clear cell: exclude a metastasis from kidney).

! The presence of "naked glands in fat" is very suggestive for PDAC, but attention must be paid to the fact that the adipose tissue may be derived from adipose involution of normal pancreatic parenchyma, so it can represent pancreatic parenchyma in adipose involution rather than peripancreatic adipose tissue. The contemporary presence of Langerhans islets in the fatty tissue indicates an adipose involution.

! In case of mild cellular atypia (eg, surgical specimens after neoadjuvant therapies), it is very important to look for abnormal locations of glands (eg, immediately adjacent to muscular blood vessels, duodenal infiltration, perineural infiltration) to support a diagnosis of PDAC.

! Do not use only immunohistochemistry to support a diagnosis of PDAC, as there is not an unequivocal immunohistochemical profile of such tumor. However, remember that cytokeratins 8 to 18 are the classic keratins expressed by PDAC, and that the aberrant DPC4 and/or p53 immunohistochemical expression is useful to support a diagnosis of cancer.

! Mucin pools without cells represent a pseudo-infiltrative pattern: infiltrating colloid carcinoma also has to present suspended neoplastic cells in mucin pools.

mutations in pancreatic cancer, *KRAS*, *SMAD4*, *TP53*, and *CDKN2A*, are currently not druggable, stratified therapeutic strategies based on genomic alterations that occur at low frequency, as well as multipathway inhibition strategies, might be beneficial for treatment of PDAC. Novel approaches based on genomic information seem likely to revolutionize PDAC therapy over the next few years, following the direction of next-generation histopathologic diagnosis and therapy and of personalized medicine.[43]

The prognosis of PDAC variants is peculiar for some of them. Patients with resected *adenosquamous carcinoma* have a poorer prognosis (median survival of 7–11 months) than do those with conventional PDAC.[3,13,44] *Colloid carcinomas* and *medullary carcinomas* seem to have a better prognosis than classic PDACs, with higher survival indexes.[3,13,45] *Anaplastic carcinomas*, *signet-ring carcinomas*, and *UCOCGC* are characterized by a very poor prognosis.[3,13,46,47]

## REFERENCES

1. Ferlay J, Soerjomataram I, Dikshit R, et al. Cancer incidence and mortality worldwide: sources, methods and major patterns in GLOBOCAN 2012. Int J Cancer 2015;136:E359–86.

2. Takai E, Yachida S. Genomic alterations in pancreatic cancer and their relevance to therapy. World J Gastrointest Oncol 2015;7(10):250–8.

3. Bosman FT, Carneiro F, Hruban RH, et al. WHO classification of tumours of the digestive system. Lyon (France): IARC Press; 2010.

4. Anderson KE, Mack TM, Silverman DT. Cancer of the pancreas. In: Schottenfeld D, Fraumeni JF, editors. Cancer epidemiology and prevention. Oxford (United Kingdom): Oxford University Press; 2006. p. 721–62.

5. World Cancer Research Fund, American Institute for Cancer Research, editors. Food, nutrition, physical activity and the prevention of cancer. A global perspective. Second expert report. Washington, DC: AICR; 2007.

6. Iodice S, Gandini S, Maisonneuve P, et al. Tobacco and the risk of pancreatic cancer: a review and meta-analysis. Langenbecks Arch Surg 2008;393: 535–45.

7. Lowenfelds AB, Maisonneuve P, Dimagno EP, et al. Hereditary pancreatitis and the risk of pancreatic cancer. International Hereditary Pancreatitis Study Group. J Natl Cancer Inst 1997;89:442–6.

8. Holly EA, Chaliha I, Bracci PM, et al. Signs and symptoms of pancreatic cancer: a population-based case-control study in the San Francisco Bay area. Clin Gastroenterol Hepatol 2004;2:510–7.

9. Chari ST, Leibson CL, Rabe KG, et al. Probability of pancreatic cancer following diabetes: a population-based study. Gastroenterology 2005; 129:504–11.

10. Khorana AA, Fine RL. Pancreatic cancer and thromboembolic disease. Lancet Oncol 2004;5:655–63.

11. D'Onofrio M, Capelli P, De Robertis R, et al. Ductal adenocarcinoma. In: D'Onofrio M, Capelli P, Pederzoli P, editors. Imaging and pathology of pancreatic neoplasms: a pictorial atlas. Springer; 2015.

12. Morana G, D'Onofrio M, Tinazzi Martini P, et al. Intraductal papillary mucinous neoplasm (IPMN). In: D'Onofrio M, Capelli P, Pederzoli P, editors. Imaging and pathology of pancreatic neoplasms: a pictorial atlas. Springer; 2015.

13. Hruban RH, Pitman MB, Klimstra DS, editors. Tumors of the pancreas. Washington, DC: Armed Forces Institue of Pathology; 2007.

14. Paiella S, Malleo G, Maggino L, et al. Pancreatectomy with para-aortic lymph node dissection for pancreatic head adenocarcinoma: pattern of nodal metastasis spread and analysis of prognostic factors. J Gastrointest Surg 2015;19:1610–20.

15. Kosmahl M, Pauser U, Anlauf M, et al. Pancreatic ductal adenocarcinomas with cystic features: neither rare nor uniform. Mod Pathol 2005;18: 1157–64.

16. Luchini C, Nottegar A, Solmi M, et al. Prognostic implications of extra-nodal extension in node-positive squamous cell carcinoma of the vulva: a systematic review and meta-analysis. Surg Oncol 2016;25(1):60–5.

17. Veronese N, Luchini C, Nottegar A, et al. Prognostic impact and implications of extra-nodal extension in lymph-node positive thyroid cancers: a systematic review and meta-analysis. J Surg Oncol 2015;112: 828–33.

18. Veronese N, Nottegar A, Pea A, et al. Prognostic impact and implications of extra-capsular lymph node involvement in colorectal cancer: a systematic review with meta-analysis. Ann Oncol 2016;27:42–8.

19. Luchini C, Veronese N, Pea A, et al. Extra-nodal extension in N1-adenocarcinoma of pancreas and papilla of Vater: a systematic review and meta-analysis of its prognostic significance. Eur J Gastroenterol Hepatol 2016;28:205–9.

20. Luttges J, Schemm S, Vogel I, et al. The grade of pancreatic ductal carcinoma is an independent prognostic factor and is superior to the immunohistochemical assessment of proliferation. J Pathol 2000;191:154–61.

21. Adsay NV, Bandyyopadhyay S, Basturk O, et al. Chronic pancreatitis or pancreatic ductal adenocarcinoma? Semin Diagn Pathol 2004;21:268–76.

22. Raman SP, Salaria SN, Hruban RH, et al. Groove pancreatitis: spectrum of imaging findings and radiology-pathology correlation. Am J Roentgenol 2013;201:29–39.

23. Brosens LA, Leguit RJ, Vleggaar FP, et al. EUS-guided FNA cytology diagnosis of paraduodenal pancreatitis (groove pancreatitis) with numerous giant cells: conservative management allowed by cytological and radiological correlation. Cytopathology 2015;26:122–5.

24. Frulloni L, Lunardi C, Simone R, et al. Identification of a novel antibody associated with autoimmune pancreatitis. N Engl J Med 2009;361: 2135–42.

25. Buscarini E, Frulloni L, De Lisi S, et al. Autoimmune pancreatitis: a challenging diagnostic puzzle for clinicians. Dig Liver Dis 2010;42(2):92–8.

26. Omiyale AO. Autoimmune pancreatitis. Gland Surg 2016;5:318–26.

27. Pitman MB, Deshpande V. Endoscopic ultrasound-guided fine needle aspiration cytology of the pancreas: a morphological and multimodal approach to the diagnosis of solid and cystic mass lesions. Cytopathology 2007;18:331–47.

28. Robins DB, Katz RL, Evans DB, et al. Fine needle aspiration of the pancreas. In quest of accuracy. Acta Cytol 1995;39:1–10.

29. Moll R, Lowe A, Laufer J, et al. Cytokeratin 20 in human carcinomas. A new histodiagnostic marker detected by monoclonal antibodies. Am J Pathol 1992;140:427–47.

30. Nagata K, Horinouchi M, Saitou M, et al. Mucin expression profile in pancreatic cancer and the precursor lesions. J Hepatobiliary Pancreat Surg 2007;14:243–54.

31. Terada T, Ohta T, Sasaki M, et al. Expression of MUC apomucins in normal pancreas and pancreatic tumours. J Pathol 1996;180:160–5.

32. Sessa F, Bonato M, Frigerio B, et al. Ductal cancers of the pancreas frequently express markers of gastrointestinal epithelial cells. Gastroenterology 1990;98:1655–65.

33. Ohike N, Kosmahl M, Klöppel G. Mixed acinar-endocrine carcinoma of the pancreas. A clinicopathological study and comparison with acinar-cell carcinoma. Virchows Arch 2004;445:231–5.

34. Scardoni M, Vittoria E, Volante M, et al. Mixed adenoneuroendocrine carcinomas of the gastrointestinal tract: targeted next-generation sequencing suggests a monoclonal origin of the two components. Neuroendocrinology 2014;100:310–6.

35. Cao D, Maitra A, Saavedra JA, et al. Expression of novel markers of pancreatic ductal adenocarcinoma in pancreatic nonductal neoplasms: additional evidence of different genetic pathways. Mod Pathol 2005;18:752–61.

36. Karanjawala ZE, Illei PB, Ashfaq R, et al. New markers of pancreatic cancer identified through differential gene expression analyses: claudin 18 and annexin A8. Am J Surg Pathol 2008;32: 188–96.

37. Borazanci E, Millis SZ, Korn R, et al. Adenosquamous carcinoma of the pancreas: molecular characterization of 23 patients along with a literature review. World J Gastrointest Oncol 2015;7:132–40.

38. Hameed O, Xu H, Saddeghi S, et al. Hepatoid carcinoma of the pancreas: a case report and literature review of a heterogeneous group of tumors. Am J Surg Pathol 2007;31:146–52.

39. Lukas Z, Dvorak K, Kroupova I, et al. Immunohistochemical and genetic analysis of osteoclastic giant cell tumor of the pancreas. Pancreas 2006;32: 325–9.

40. Jones S, Zhang X, Parsons DW, et al. Core signaling pathways in human pancreatic cancers revealed by global genomic analyses. Science 2008;321: 1801–6.

41. Almoguera C, Shibata D, Forrester K, et al. Most human carcinomas of the exocrine pancreas contain mutant c-K-ras genes. Cell 1988;53:549–54.

42. Luchini C, Veronese N, Solmi M, et al. Prognostic role and implications of mutation status of tumor suppressor gene ARID1A in cancer: a systematic review and meta-analysis. Oncotarget 2015;6: 39088–97.

43. Luchini C, Capelli P, Fassan M, et al. Next-generation histopathologic diagnosis: a lesson from a hepatic carcinosarcoma. J Clin Oncol 2014;32:e63–6.

44. Kardon DE, Thompson LD, Przygodzki RM, et al. Adenosquamous carcinoma of the pancreas: a clinicopathologic series of 25 cases. Mod Pathol 2001;14:443–51.

45. Nakata B, Wang YQ, Yashiro M, et al. Negative hMSH2 protein expression in pancreatic carcinoma may predict a better prognosis of patients. Oncol Rep 2003;10:997–1000.

46. Hoorens A, Prenzel K, Lemoine NR, et al. Undifferentiated carcinoma of the pancreas: analysis of intermediate filament profile and Ki-ras mutations provides evidence of a ductal origin. J Pathol 1998;185:53–60.

47. Sano M, Homma T, Hayashi E, et al. Clinicopathological characteristics of anaplastic carcinoma of the pancreas with rhabdoid features. Virchows Arch 2014;465:531–8.

# Pathology of Pancreatic Cancer Precursor Lesions

Michaël Noë, MD*, Lodewijk A.A. Brosens, MD, PhD

## KEYWORDS

- Pancreatic ductal adenocarcinoma • Precursor lesions • Carcinogenesis • Histopathology
- Molecular pathology • Intraductal papillary mucinous neoplasm
- Pancreatic intraepithelial neoplasia • Mucinous cystic neoplasm

## Key points

- Pancreatic cancer develops from 3 well-established precursor lesions: pancreatic intraepithelial neoplasia (PanIN), intraductal papillary mucinous neoplasm (IPMN), and mucinous cystic neoplasm (MCN).

- PanINs are the most common precursor lesion of pancreatic ductal adenocarcinoma (PDAC) and are by definition less than 0.5 cm in diameter.

- PanINs are characterized by cuboid to columnar cells with gastric foveolar differentiation and varying degrees of cytologic and architectural atypia.

- IPMNs are most often located in the proximal pancreas and are by definition greater than or equal to 1.0 cm in diameter.

- IPMNs are classified as main-duct type IPMNs, branch-duct type IPMNs, or mixed type IPMNs, and are further subclassified according to the predominant direction of differentiation as gastric, intestinal, pancreatobiliary, or oncocytic.

- Evidence is accumulating for the existence of 2 distinct pathways in the evolution of IPMN into pancreatic adenocarcinoma.

- Intraductal tubulopapillary neoplasm is considered a variant of IPMN, with a high prevalence of *PIK3CA* mutations.

- MCNs almost exclusively occur in female patients, are mainly located in the pancreatic body and tail, do not communicate with the pancreatic duct system, and are characterized by ovarian-type stroma.

- Recently, new guidelines were formulated for reporting pancreatic precursor lesions, improving reproducibility by encouraging a 2-tiered grading system for dysplasia.

## ABSTRACT

To better understand pancreatic ductal adenocarcinoma (PDAC) and improve its prognosis, it is essential to understand its origins. This article describes the pathology of the 3 well-established pancreatic cancer precursor lesions: pancreatic intraepithelial neoplasia, intraductal papillary mucinous neoplasm, and mucinous cystic neoplasm. Each of these precursor lesions has unique clinical findings, gross and microscopic features, and molecular aberrations. This article focuses on histopathologic diagnostic criteria and reporting guidelines. The genetics of these lesions are briefly discussed. Early detection and adequate treatment of pancreatic cancer precursor lesions has the potential to prevent pancreatic cancer and improve the prognosis of PDAC.

Disclosure: The authors have nothing to disclose.
Department of Pathology, University Medical Center Utrecht, Utrecht, The Netherlands
* Corresponding author.
E-mail address: m.p.m.noe@umcutrecht.nl

Surgical Pathology 9 (2016) 561–580
http://dx.doi.org/10.1016/j.path.2016.05.004
1875-9181/16/$ – see front matter © 2016 Elsevier Inc. All rights reserved.

## OVERVIEW

Noninvasive precursor lesions in the pancreas have been recognized for more than a century.[1] They have the ability to progress to pancreatic ductal adenocarcinoma (PDAC). However, it was not until 1999 that an international consensus meeting formed the basis for the current classification and definition of these precursor lesions.[2] Since then, multiple consensus meetings have been organized, updating the classification system with new insights.[3,4] Three precursor lesions are recognized: pancreatic intraepithelial neoplasia (PanIN), intraductal papillary mucinous neoplasm (IPMN), and mucinous cystic neoplasm (MCN). All of these meet the criteria for precursor lesion, as defined by a consensus conference, sponsored by the National Cancer Institute.[5] These precursors show a unique multistep morphologic and genetic progression to invasive carcinoma.

## PANCREATIC INTRAEPITHELIAL NEOPLASIA

### CLINICAL FEATURES

PanIN is the most common precursor lesion of PDAC. These lesions were first described a century ago by Hulst.[1] Both men and women are equally affected and the incidence tends to increase with age.[6–8] PanINs can be found in 82% of pancreata with invasive carcinoma, in 60% of pancreata with chronic pancreatitis, and in 16% of normal pancreata.[7] PanINs occur multifocally in patients with a family history of pancreatic adenocarcinoma.[9,10] Because of their small size (by definition <0.5 cm), these lesions cannot be seen on noninvasive abdominal imaging and they are not associated with clinical signs or symptoms. However, lobular atrophy and fibrosis can be clues for their presence. PanINs are typically found incidentally in resections or biopsy specimens.[6,11,12]

### PATHOLOGIC FEATURES

PanINs are noninvasive, microscopic, epithelial neoplasms and by definition involve pancreatic ducts less than 0.5 cm in diameter.[2–4] PanINs are characterized by cuboid to columnar cells with varying amounts of apical cytoplasmic mucin and varying degrees of cytologic and architectural atypia. PanINs almost always show gastric foveolar differentiation.[4]

Hruban and colleagues[2] described the generally accepted PanIN scheme to classify these lesions in 2001. Three grades are discriminated in this scheme, based on the degree of epithelial atypia: PanIN-1, PanIN-2, and PanIN-3. PanIN-1 lesions are characterized by minimal nuclear atypia, inconspicuous nucleoli, and absent mitotic figures and can be further subdivided into flat (PanIN-1A) and micropapillary (PanIN-1B) types. Moderate nuclear atypia, pseudostratification, loss of polarity, hyperchromasia, and rare mitotic figures are features of PanIN-2. PanIN-3 lesions have marked atypia; contain (atypical) mitotic figures; show loss of polarity; and have a papillary, micropapillary, or occasional flat architecture (Fig. 1). Cribriform structures, necrosis, and tufting of epithelial cells in the lumen may be present. PanIN-3 is almost exclusively found in association with invasive PDAC.[6,7] This feature is so striking that, in pancreata without a PDAC, a PanIN-3 lesion may serve as a surrogate marker for invasion elsewhere.[7,13] Another pitfall is the extension of an infiltrating carcinoma in pancreatic ducts (ie, ductal cancerization) mimicking a PanIN-3 lesion. The close proximity of an invasive carcinoma to a ductal lesion, the abrupt transition from highly atypical epithelium to normal ductal epithelium, luminal obstruction, and ductal destruction are clues to consider ductal cancerization.[2,3,14]

The clinical significance of PanIN-1 and PanIN-2 has been questioned by studies, because these lesions show little progression to PDAC.[7,15] Grading the lesions also showed poor interobserver agreement.[16] For these reasons, the latest consensus meeting advised the use of a 2-tiered grading system with low-grade PanIN (formerly PanIN-1A, PanIN-1B, and PanIN-2) and high-grade PanIN (formerly PanIN-3). Moreover, the presence of PanIN lesions of any grade at the surgical margin of pancreata resected for invasive PDAC does not influence patient prognosis and additional surgery is not required.[17]

PanINs show an increased expression of MUC 1 (Mucin 1) and MUC5AC (Mucin 5AC) in higher grades of dysplasia.[18–21] The opposite is seen for MUC6 (Mucin 6), showing reduced expression in higher grades of dysplasia.[19,22]

### MOLECULAR FEATURES

The early lesions with minimal cytologic atypia were not originally regarded as neoplastic, but instead were designated as hyperplasia or metaplasia.[23] After finding *KRAS* mutations, these lesions were considered neoplastic and the term pancreatic intraepithelial neoplasia was proposed.[2,13,24–27] It has been established that progression from low-grade PanIN to high-grade PanIN requires accumulation of genetic

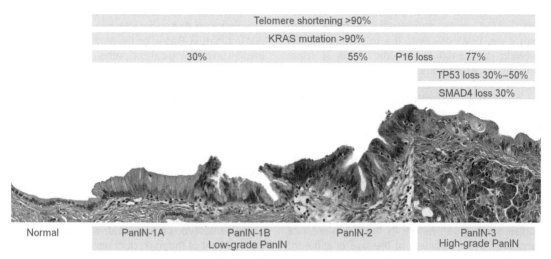

Telomere shortening >90%

KRAS mutation >90%

30%                                   55%        P16 loss        77%

TP53 loss 30%–50%

SMAD4 loss 30%

| Normal | PanIN-1A | PanIN-1B | PanIN-2 | PanIN-3 |
| | | Low-grade PanIN | | High-grade PanIN |

*Fig. 1.* The progression of PanIN is associated with an increase in cellular atypia and accumulation of genetic mutations. PanIN-1 shows minimal nuclear atypia. PanIN-1A has a flat growth pattern, whereas PanIN-1B shows formation of micropapillae. PanIN-2 shows loss of cellular polarity. PanIN-1 and PanIN-2 are both grouped as low-grade PanIN. PanIN-3 or high-grade PanIN has the most severe nuclear and architectural atypia. The PanIN-3 lesion shown here is the variant with a flat architecture.

alterations, starting with an activating *KRAS* mutations and telomere shortening, followed by *CDKN2A* mutations and later *P53* and *SMAD4* mutations (see **Fig. 1**).[21,28–31] Genetic features of PanIN are discussed (see Hosoda W, Wood L: Molecular Genetics of Pancreatic Neoplasms, in this issue).

## PanIN Key Points

- Microscopic lesion: involves by definition pancreatic ducts less than 0.5 cm in diameter

- Incidence increases with age

- Occurs multifocally in patients with family history of pancreatic cancer

- High-grade PanIN is almost exclusively seen in association with invasive carcinoma

## INTRADUCTAL PAPILLARY MUCINOUS NEOPLASM

### CLINICAL FEATURES

The first description of intraductal mucinous neoplasms of the pancreas probably dates back to 1936.[32,33] Until 1994, these tumors were described under various names, each emphasizing a different morphologic feature of the tumor.

In 1994, all these entities were grouped together under the term IPMN, as proposed by Morohoshi and colleagues.[34,35]

Initially, IPMN was considered a disease of older men, often with a history of cigarette smoking. However, a meta-analysis showed that there are geographic differences in the gender of patients with IPMN. The male/female ratios of main-duct type and branch-duct type IPMNs in Asia are 3 and 1.8, respectively. However, in the United States, these ratios are 1.1 and 0.76, and in Europe 1.5 and 0.66, respectively.[36] The mean age of patients at time of diagnosis is 60 to 66 years, irrespective of geographic location.[37–41] There is a lag time of 3 to 6 years before patients with noninvasive IPMN develop PDAC.[37–41]

IPMNs are seen most frequently in patients with a family history of pancreatic cancer, Peutz-Jeghers syndrome, familial adenomatous polyposis, Lynch syndrome, Carney complex, and McCune-Albright syndrome.[10,42–48] Because IPMNs are detectable with medical imaging techniques, these lesions can serve as a target for a screening test for the early detection of pancreatic neoplasia.[10]

IPMNs are mucin-producing, epithelial neoplasms with an intraductal proliferation of dysplastic cells that usually form papillae. This process leads to cystic dilatation of the pancreatic ducts. Although most people diagnosed with IPMN are asymptomatic, some patients experience nonspecific symptoms, including vague abdominal pain, weight loss, nausea, jaundice, (recent-onset) diabetes, or steator-rhea.[49] Mild acute pancreatitis is more often seen if the IPMN involves the main duct. IPMN involving only small pancreatic ducts is most likely to be asymptomatic.[37,40,50–52] On endoscopy, a classic patulous papilla extruding mucus can be seen in 25% of patients with IPMN. It is also called a fish eye or fish mouth and is virtually diagnostic for the presence of an IPMN (Fig. 2).[53,54]

IPMNs were thought to be rare pancreatic tumors, but the current widespread use of high-quality, cross-sectional abdominal imaging techniques has shown that pancreatic cysts and IPMNs are common. However, epidemiologic studies show great variety in the prevalence of pancreatic cysts because of the use of different imaging techniques and different study populations.[55–64] If only cysts larger than 0.5 cm in patients imaged for other indications than pancreatic disorder and without a history of pancreatic disorder are considered, the prevalence is 10% to 21%.[56,57] A different study in a younger and partially healthy population scanned at a center for preventive medicine showed a much lower prevalence of 2.4%.[65] However, not all pancreatic cysts are IPMNs. About a third of resected asymptomatic pancreatic cysts seem to be IPMN.[52,66]

IPMNs are most frequently located in the proximal pancreas (the pancreatic head and the processus uncinatus). Based on the pancreatic ducts they involve on radiological and pathologic examination, IPMNs are classified as main-duct type IPMNs, branch-duct type IPMNs, or mixed type IPMNs, if the main duct and the branch ducts are both involved.[67] However, there is considerable discrepancy between the radiological and the histopathologic assessment of the involved ducts. Studies have shown that the main duct often shows some degree of involvement, even in IPMNs that were classic branch-duct type IPMNs by radiological imaging.[68] Fritz and colleagues[69] showed that 29% of the IPMNs that were considered as branch-duct type on preoperative imaging showed involvement of the main duct histologically. These branch-duct type IPMNs with minimal involvement of the main duct were very similar to pure branch-duct type IPMNs with regard to clinicopathologic features as well as clinical outcome.[68]

A compilation of 3568 resected IPMNs from 20 studies showed that invasive carcinoma was present in 43.6% of main-duct type IPMNs, in 45.3% of mixed type IPMNs, and in 16.6% of branch-duct type IPMNs.[70] The limited percentage of cancer in the resected pancreata shows the clinical problem of overtreatment of IPMNs and, in

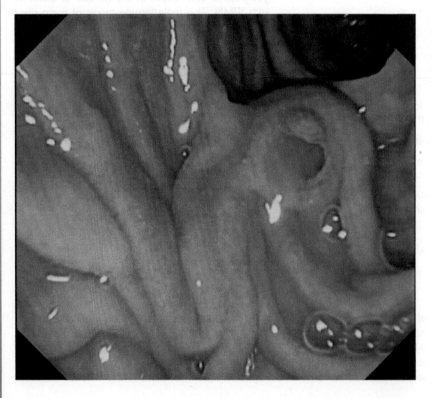

Fig. 2. A classic patulous papilla extruding mucus, also called fish eye or fish mouth, as seen on endoscopy in a patient with an IPMN.

particular, of the branch-duct type IPMNs. Several guidelines have been proposed for clinical management of IPMNs but the quality of evidence supporting most recommendations is low (Table 1).[70–75]

## PATHOLOGIC FEATURES

IPMNs have been defined in consensus meetings as "grossly visible, predominantly papillary or rarely flat, noninvasive mucin-producing epithelial neoplasm arising in the main pancreatic duct or branch ducts."[3] By definition, IPMNs are at least 1.0 cm in diameter.[2–4]

As for PanIN, a consensus meeting recently recommended to grade the IPMNs with a 2-tiered grading system. The former IPMN with low-grade dysplasia and IPMN with intermediate-grade dysplasia become IPMN, low grade. The former

IPMN with high-grade dysplasia becomes IPMN, high grade.[4]

IPMNs can be subtyped by their direction of differentiation as gastric, intestinal, pancreatobiliary, or oncocytic.[76]

- Gastric-type IPMN is characterized by cells that resemble the foveolar epithelium of the stomach with a single layer of cells with basally oriented nuclei and abundant mucinous cytoplasm. This epithelium can show a flat, papillary, or tubular/ductal growth pattern (Fig. 3). This subtype is rarely associated with high-grade dysplasia compared with other subtypes.[77] However, when high-grade dysplasia is present, the architecture becomes complex and the cuboidal cells with enlarged nuclei become mucin depleted, features that

**Table 1**
A brief overview of the most important current guidelines for the management of IPMNs

| Sendai Guidelines, 2006[71] | Updated Sendai Guidelines, 2012[70] | American Gastroenterological Association Guidelines, 2015[72] |
|---|---|---|
| Guideline for all cysts originating from the pancreatic duct system, suspected to be IPMN Criteria: <br> • Pancreatic fluid cytology with high-grade dysplasia or carcinoma <br> • Presence of a mural nodule <br> • Symptoms <br> • Main pancreatic duct diameter >0.6 cm <br> • Branch duct diameter >3.0 cm | Guideline for all cysts originating from the pancreatic duct system, suspected to be IPMN High-risk stigmata: <br> • Obstructive jaundice in a patient with a cystic lesion of the head of the pancreas <br> • Enhancing solid component within cyst <br> • Main pancreatic duct size ≥1.0 cm Worrisome features: <br> • Pancreatitis <br> • Main pancreatic duct size 0.5–0.9 cm <br> • Cyst size ≥3.0 cm <br> • Thickened enhanced cyst walls <br> • Nonenhanced mural nodules <br> • Abrupt change in the main pancreatic duct caliber with distal pancreatic atrophy <br> • Lymphadenopathy | Guideline for asymptomatic cysts from branch ducts, suspected to be IPMN: High-risk features: <br> • Cyst size ≥3.0 cm <br> • Dilated main pancreatic duct <br> • Presence of a solid component |
| If at least 1 criterion is present, consider resection | • If at least 1 high-risk stigma is present: consider resection <br> • If no high-risk stigmata are present, but at least 1 worrisome feature is present, consider EUS with FNA <br> In patients with positive cytology or concerning features on EUS (definite mural nodule, main duct features suspicious for involvement), consider resection | If at least 2 high-risk features are present: consider EUS with FNA In patients with positive cytology or concerning features on EUS (definite mural nodule, main duct features suspicious for involvement), consider resection |

Abbreviations: EUS, endoscopic ultrasonography; FNA, fine-needle aspiration.

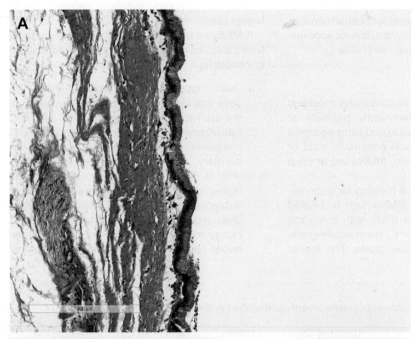

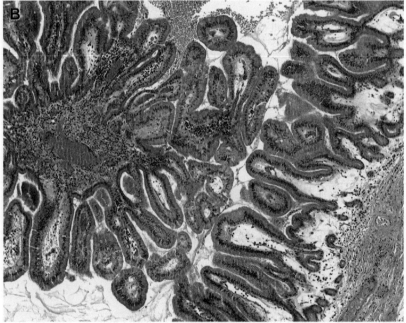

*Fig. 3.* Gastric-type IPMN. (*A*) Gastric-type IPMN with a flat architecture and a single layer of gastric foveolar-type epithelium. (*B*) Gastric-type IPMN with a villous architecture.

are very similar to pancreatobiliary-type IPMN.[78] Some investigators consider these features as different grades of dysplasia, whereas others consider them as different subtypes of IPMN.[79,80] Gastric-type IPMNs typically involve the branch ducts.[81]

- The pancreatobiliary-type IPMN is lined by cells with nuclei with marked variation in size and shape; these nuclei have irregular contours and prominent nucleoli and are most likely to progress to an invasive tubular carcinoma (**Fig. 4**).[81]

- The intestinal-type IPMN is morphologically similar to a colonic villous adenoma. The nuclei of the cells are hyperchromatic, elongated, show some degree of pseudostratification, and contain variable amounts of intracellular mucin. The papillae are typically long and

*Fig. 3. (continued)*. (*C*) Gastric-type IPMN with basal tubular/ductal growth. When tubular growth is extensive, these lesions have previously been designated as intraductal tubular adenoma, pyloric gland type, pyloric gland adenoma, or intraductal tubular adenoma (see Fig. 8). (*D*) IPMN with low-grade and high-grade dysplasia. Some investigators consider this as different subtypes of IPMN (ie, gastric-type IPMN and pancreatobiliary-type IPMN, respectively) whereas others consider this as different grades of dysplasia of gastric-type IPMN.

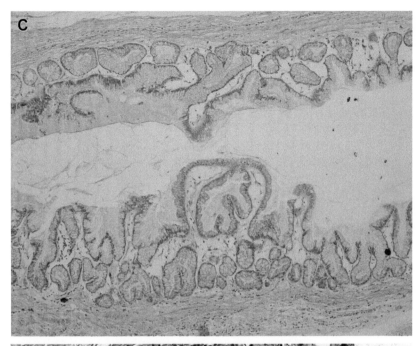

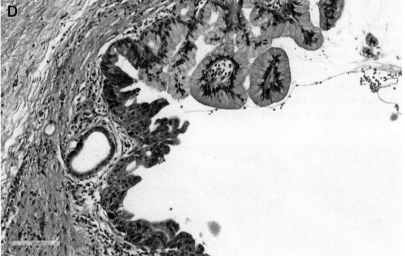

occasionally branching. This subtype most frequently involves the main duct (Fig. 5).[81]

- Oncocytic-type IPMN is a rare entity, characterized by cells with abundant eosinophilic cytoplasm, caused by the accumulation of mitochondria. The nuclei of these oncocytic cells contain a single, prominent, eccentric nucleolus. The growth pattern of these oncocytic-type IPMNs is distinctive, consisting of arborizing papillae, lined by 1 to 5 layers of cuboidal cells. A specific feature is the punched-out spaces in the epithelium (Fig. 6).

The 2010 World Health Organization classification of tumors of the digestive system provided an immunohistochemical aid for subtyping these IPMNs based on mucin stains. However, several studies have shown that some IPMNs are unclassifiable because of their uncharacteristic morphology and immunophenotype.[82–86] Mixed epithelial differentiation makes subtyping impossible in 25% of cases. For these reasons and because of the moderate interobserver agreement for morphologic subtyping of pancreatic IPMNs, subtyping of IPMNs has a poor reproducibility.[87] Studies have reported differences in prognosis

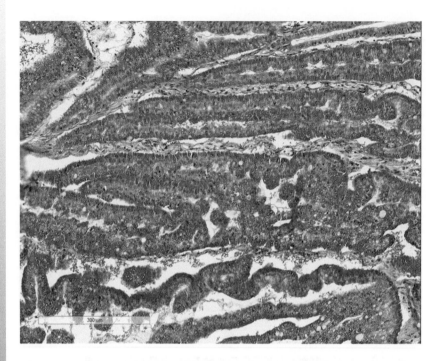

*Fig. 4.* Pancreatobiliary-type IPMN lined by cells with marked atypia and prominent nucleoli.

between the various subtypes of IPMNs, despite the poor reproducibility, which suggests that associations between histologic type and prognosis may be even stronger than reported.[77,81,83,87–90] A recent meta-analysis reviewed 14 studies and showed that the pancreatobiliary-type IPMN is associated with the most aggressive behavior and gastric-type IPMN has the lowest risk of invasive carcinoma.[81]

## MOLECULAR FEATURES

Whole-exome sequencing of IPMNs revealed an average of 26 mutated genes per IPMN.[91] *KRAS*

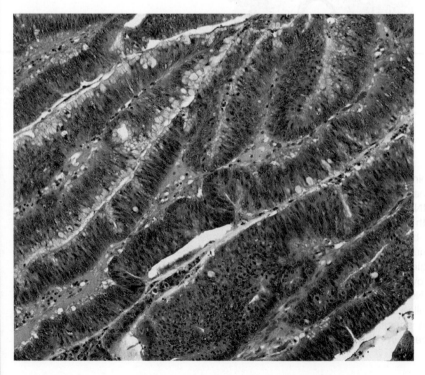

*Fig. 5.* Intestinal-type IPMN with high-grade dysplasia composed of papillae lined by cells with elongated nuclei and some degree of pseudostratification reminiscent of a colonic villous adenoma. Note the scattered goblet cells.

*Fig.    6.* Oncocytic-type IPMN, composed of cells with abundant eosinophilic cytoplasm, reflecting the accumulation of mitochondria.

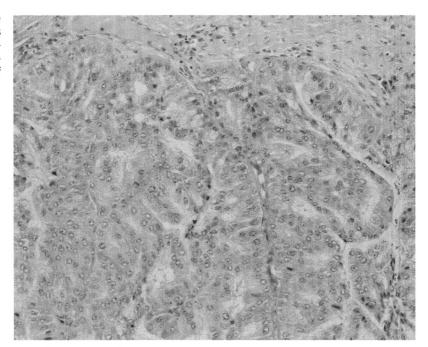

and *GNAS* are the most frequently mutated genes in 50% to 80% and 40% to 60% of IPMNs, respectively.[91,92] Moreover, *RNF43*, an E3 ubiquitin–protein ligase acting as a negative regulator of the Wnt-signaling pathway, is also frequently mutated in IPMN.[91] In addition, P53 and SMAD4 mutations can be found in high-grade dysplasia. Genetic features of IPMN are discussed (see Hosoda W, Wood L: Molecular Genetics of Pancreatic Neoplasms, in this issue).

Evidence is accumulating for the existence of 2 distinct molecular progression pathways in IPMN[20,93]:

- Pancreatobiliary-type IPMN is highly associated with tubular carcinoma, which has a mutation profile resembling conventional pancreatic adenocarcinoma including *KRAS* mutations.[93–95] *GNAS* mutations are less common in this presumed pathway.
- Intestinal-type IPMNs and associated colloid carcinomas typically harbor *GNAS* mutations, which is another similarity between intestinal-type IPMN and colonic villous adenomas.[96]

These different pathways are also reflected in a different immunophenotype with colloid carcinomas being MUC1 negative (0%) and MUC2 positive (100%), whereas tubular carcinomas are typically MUC1 positive (63%) and MUC2 negative (1%).[20] Colloid carcinomas have a less aggressive

behavior and a better prognosis than tubular carcinomas.[83,84] In gastric-type IPMNs, *KRAS* and *GNAS* mutations are identified equally. This finding suggests that gastric-type IPMNs are a heterogenic group of early lesions with a similar morphologic appearance, but, on a molecular level, are already committed to one of the 2 progression pathways.[93]

**IPMN Key Points**

- Macroscopic lesion: involves by definition pancreatic ducts greater than or equal to 1.0 cm in diameter

- Main-duct type and mixed type IPMN harbor higher risk for invasive carcinoma than branch-duct type IPMN

- Can become the target for a screening test for pancreatic cancer

- Two pathways toward invasive cancer may exist:

   o Pancreatobiliary-type IPMN (*KRAS* mutated) is associated with tubular carcinoma

   o Intestinal-type IPMN (*GNAS* mutated) is associated with colloid carcinoma

## DIFFERENTIAL DIAGNOSIS: PANCREATIC INTRAEPITHELIAL NEOPLASIA VERSUS INTRADUCTAL PAPILLARY MUCINOUS NEOPLASM

By definition, PanINs are smaller than 0.5 cm and IPMNs are at least 1.0 cm, which means that there is an indeterminate range between PanIN and IPMN for intraductal neoplastic precursor lesions with a diameter of greater than or equal to 0.5 cm and less than 1.0 cm. These lesions can be either large PanINs or small IPMNs. Differentiation of the epithelium toward intestinal-type, pancreatobiliary-type, or oncocytic-type epithelium or a mutation specific for IPMN (such as *GNAS* mutation) are clues for an IPMN.[4,76] If these clues are present, these lesions can be called incipient IPMN. However, small, gastric-type lesions, without features of an IPMN, should be documented descriptively.[4]

Initially, PanINs were defined as lesions arising from the ductules or small ducts, whereas IPMNs involve the main pancreatic duct or its major branches.[2,97,98] However, several case reports suggested that some PanINs arise from larger ducts, including the main duct.[11,97,99] Some of these PanINs may cause obstruction and retrograde dilatation of the duct, causing it to expand beyond the 1.0 cm cutoff. To address these large and main duct PanINs, the 2004 consensus guidelines defined diagnostic criteria, apart from the size criteria, to distinguish PanINs from IPMNs[3]:

- Papillae in PanIN are not as tall and complex as those in IPMN
- Abundant luminal mucin production is a feature of IPMN
- MUC2 expression is a specific, but insensitive, marker of an IPMN and is generally not present in PanIN

## INTRADUCTAL TUBULOPAPILLARY NEOPLASM

### CLINICAL FEATURES

Intraductal tubulopapillary neoplasms (ITPNs) are rare intraductal neoplasms of the pancreas. They occur equally in men and women. Symptoms are nonspecific and include abdominal pain, diabetes, vomiting, and weight loss. About 50% of these neoplasms involve the head of the pancreas, 30% diffusely involve the pancreas,[100] 15% are localized in the tail of the pancreas,[101] and 40% of cases harbor an associated invasive carcinoma. With a 5-year survival of more than

30%, prognosis of an ITPN-associated invasive tumor is significantly better than the prognosis of conventional PDAC. Recurrence or metastasis to lymph nodes or to the liver is seen in about a third of cases. Even these patients sometimes experience a protracted clinical course over more than 2 years, which is unusual for conventional PDAC.[100]

### PATHOLOGIC FEATURES

ITPN is characterized by densely packed tubules that frequently lie back to back, forming large sheets. Tubulopapillary growth is sometimes seen. The cells are cuboidal with modest amounts of eosinophilic cytoplasm and do not contain apparent mucin. There is moderate nuclear atypia and increased mitotic activity (Fig. 7). Extracellular mucin production is not prominent and cyst formation is less evident than in IPMN. Comedolike necrosis is sometimes present.[102]

In contrast with IPMN, immunohistochemistry for MUC5AC is typically negative in ITPNs.[28,102] MUC1 and MUC6 are positive in 100% and 60% of cases, respectively.[102] Because of similar morphology and shared positivity for MUC6 with gastric and duodenal pyloric gland adenomas, ITPNs have previously been described as intraductal, tubular adenomas, pyloric gland type.[103,104]

Pitfalls in diagnostic pathology of ITPN:

- ITPN should be differentiated from gastric-type IPMN with extensive tubular growth (Fig. 8). In the past, intraductal lesions with extensive tubular growth were distinguished from IPMN and designated as intraductal tubular adenoma, pyloric gland type or pyloric gland adenoma.[103–111] Later, this entity was renamed intraductal tubular adenoma (ITA) and intraductal tubular carcinoma (ITC), depending on the degree of dysplasia. Further studies showed that ITAs were more related to gastric-type IPMNs and ITCs were a different entity, with a different immunoprofile and different molecular changes, now known as ITPN.[112]
- Occasionally, acinar cell carcinomas have a component of intraductal polypoid growth.[113] When this intraductal growth becomes predominant, acinar cell carcinoma can mimic other intraductal neoplasms, such as ITPNs (Fig. 9). The architecture of both tumors can be very similar with sheets of back-to-back acinar structures. The presence of PAS+, diastase-resistant, apical, eosinophilic zymogen granules; intraluminal concretions;

Fig. 7. Intraductal tubulo-papillary neoplasm with features of both tubular and papillary growth.

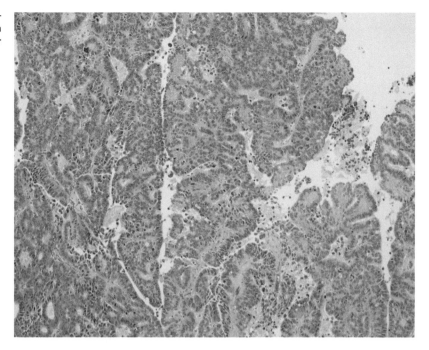

and prominent, central nucleoli are helpful features to distinguish acinar cell carcinomas from ITPNs[114] (see Fig. 9). Moreover, on immunohistochemistry, acinar cell carcinomas are positive for trypsin, chymotrypsin, and BCL10, and negative for CK19. ITPNs are negative for trypsin, chymotrypsin, and BCL10, but positive for CK19.[115]

## MOLECULAR FEATURES

ITPNs also differ from IPMNs on a molecular level. KRAS and GNAS mutations, frequently found in IPMNs, are found in only 7% and 0% of ITPNs, respectively.[116–119] However, PIK3CA mutations are frequently seen in ITPNs (21%–27%).[116,120] As a component of the mammalian target of rapamycin

Fig. 8. An intraductal, low-grade neoplasm, formerly known as an intraductal tubular adenoma (ITA), now better classified as a gastric-type IPMN with an extensive tubular/ductal growth pattern.

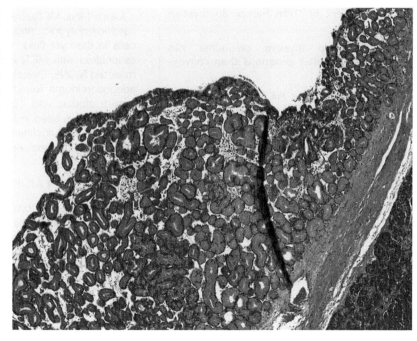

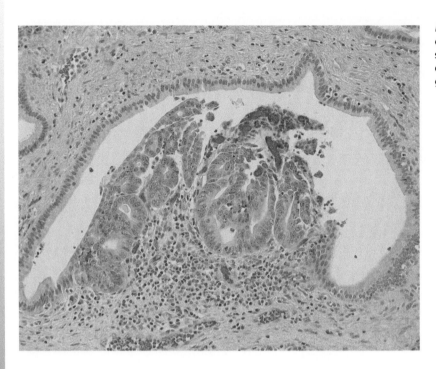

**Fig. 9.** Intraductal growth of an acinar cell carcinoma showing acinar structures composed of cells with single, large, central nucleoli.

(mTOR) pathway, *PIK3CA* is a potentially targetable mutation, because multiple drugs (like temsirolimus and everolimus) targeting the mTOR pathway have been tested and approved for clinical use.[121,122]

> ### *ITPN Key Points*
>
> - Forty percent of ITPNs harbor an invasive carcinoma
>
> - ITPN-associated invasive carcinoma has significantly better prognosis than conventional PDAC
>
> - ITPN frequently has *PIK3CA* mutation, but rarely *KRAS* and *GNAS* mutation

## MUCINOUS CYSTIC NEOPLASMS

### CLINICAL FEATURES

MCNs are almost exclusively seen in perimenopausal women. Only a few rare examples are documented in men.[123] This finding is in accordance with their counterparts in the hepatobiliary tree, mesentery, and retroperitoneum, and with the mixed epithelial and stromal tumor of the kidney, which are also more prevalent in women.[124–127] It has been hypothesized that pancreatic MCN develops from endodermal immature stroma, stimulated by female hormones.[128,129] MCNs are mainly located in the pancreatic body and tail and do not communicate with the pancreatic duct system.[130,131] The mean age of presentation of patients with a noninvasive MCN is 44 years. The mean age of presentation of patients with an MCN with associated adenocarcinoma is 55 years.[131]

Patients frequently present with nonspecific symptoms such as mild abdominal pain but some present with pancreatitis.[131]

Like IPMNs, MCNs frequently have high levels of carcinoembryonic antigen and mucinous epithelial cells in the cyst fluid.[132,133] An adenocarcinoma associated with MCN is found in 3% to 36% of resected MCNs. Overall, the mean percentage of adenocarcinoma found in 1096 resected MCNs from 9 studies was 16%,[128,130,131,134–139] which is less than is seen in main-duct type and mixed type IPMNs. Guidelines recommend resection of each MCN, irrespective of size.[70,71]

### PATHOLOGIC FEATURES

MCNs are lined by columnar cells with abundant apical mucin. Dysplastic change of the epithelial lining is graded in a 2-tiered system, as recommended by the latest consensus meeting. The former MCN with low-grade dysplasia and MCN with intermediate-grade dysplasia are now both classified as MCN, low grade.[4] Two distinct features that distinguish this tumor from an IPMN are the presence of characteristic ovarian-type stroma and lack of communication with the pancreatic duct system[70,101] (**Fig. 10**). When an MCN evolves into an invasive carcinoma, this is typically a tubular adenocarcinoma. MCNs rarely evolve into a colloid carcinoma, although an early study showed focal staining for CDX2 indicating intestinal differentiation in 51% of MCNs.[137,140] MCNs with malignant, sarcomatous stroma have been reported but are more likely spindle cell carcinomas rather than true mesenchymal neoplasms.[141–144]

Ovarian-type stroma may be only focally present or not obvious because of fibrosis or hypocellularity.[128,136] Sometimes, nests of epithelioid cells are seen in the stroma, suggesting luteinization. Rarely, a corpus luteum can be seen in the stroma. The cells of the ovarian-type stroma frequently express progesterone and estrogen receptor, inhibin, caldesmon, alfa-SMA, and desmin.[124,135]

## MOLECULAR FEATURES

Whole-exome sequencing of the MCNs showed on average 16.0 ± 7.6 nonsynonymous somatic mutations and few loss of heterozygosity events compared with IPMNs,[91] which could explain the lower frequency of progression to an invasive carcinoma in MCNs, because there is a correlation between aneuploidy and a poor prognosis.[145] Only 1 region on chromosome 17q, containing the gene *RNF43*, was lost in more than 1 tumor. In 3 MCNs, intragenic mutations were found in

the *RNF43* gene. Further analysis showed mutations in the 4 main pancreatic cancer genes *KRAS*, *CDKN2A*, *P53*, and *SMAD4*.[91] Genetic features of MCN are discussed (see Hosoda W, Wood L: Molecular Genetics of Pancreatic Neoplasms, in this issue).

> ### MCN Key Points
>
> - MCN is almost exclusively seen in perimenopausal women
> - Most often located in the body and tail of the pancreas
> - MCNs do not communicate with the pancreatic duct system
> - Mucinous epithelium is surrounded by cellular ovarian-type stroma

## SUMMARY

In the last 2 decades, a morphologic classification of precursor lesions to invasive adenocarcinoma of the pancreas has been established. Three precursor lesions are distinguished: PanIN, IPMN, and MCN. Each of these lesions has its own clinicopathologic manifestations. PanIN is the most

*Fig. 10.* MCN with mucinous epithelium with low-grade dysplasia and characteristic ovarian-type stroma.

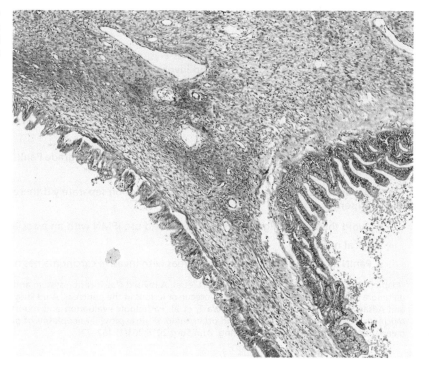

**Box 1**
**Practical recommendations of the Verona consensus meeting and the Baltimore consensus meeting**

*Grossing*

- Rule out invasive carcinoma by extensive (if not complete) sampling

- Sample tissue between IPMN and invasive carcinoma to assess concomitance or association of both lesions

*Reporting*

- Invasive tumor (if present):
  - Size:
    - Use the largest diameter of invasion and document the exact size (to enable staging and substaging)
    - Avoid the term minimally invasive
    - The term indeterminate/suspicious for invasion is acceptable in rare cases
  - Document distance between IPMN and invasive carcinoma to assess concomitance or association of both lesions
- Precursor lesion:
  - Differentiation PanIN versus IPMN:
    - The size of the affected duct is based on a cross-sectional measurement (from basement membrane to basement membrane)[3]
    - Use a description of the lesion, if the lesion affects ducts with a diameter of greater than or equal to 0.5 cm and less than 1.0 cm and has no features of IPMN (like *GNAS* mutation, intestinal differentiation, pancreatobiliary differentiation or oncocytic differentiation), because the lesion can be a large PanIN or a small IPMN
  - Consider intraductal spread of invasive carcinoma (cancerization) instead of high-grade PanIN or IPMN, high grade:
    - The close proximity of an invasive carcinoma to a ductal lesion
    - The abrupt transition from highly atypical epithelium to normal ductal epithelium
    - Luminal obstruction
    - Ductal destruction
  - Ducts:
    - Document main duct diameter and involvement, if possible
  - Subtype:
    - Document the subtype of the IPMN (gastric, intestinal, pancreatobiliary, oncocytic, mixed) if possible
  - Grade:
    - Use a 2-tiered system (terminology: low-grade PanIN; high-grade PanIN; IPMN, low grade; IPMN, high grade; MCN, low grade; MCN, high grade)
    - Document the highest grade of the precursor lesion separately if there is also an invasive tumor present
    - Avoid the term malignant IPMN, but instead use IPMN with an associated adenocarcinoma
  - Surgical margins:
    - PanIN at a margin of a resected pancreas with invasive carcinoma has no prognostic implications

*Adapted from* Basturk O, Hong S-M, Wood LD, et al. A revised classification system and recommendations from the Baltimore consensus meeting for neoplastic precursor lesions in the pancreas. Am J Surg Pathol 2015;39(12):1730–41; and Adsay V, Mino-Kenudson M, Furukawa T, et al. Pathologic evaluation and reporting of intraductal papillary mucinous neoplasms of the pancreas and other tumoral intraepithelial neoplasms of pancreatobiliary tract: recommendations of Verona consensus meeting. Ann Surg 2016;263(1):162–77.

prevalent precursor lesion, but is microscopic and not reliably detectable on imaging. IPMN is a macroscopic, cystic lesion, detectable on imaging and may therefore serve as a target for screening and prevention of pancreatic cancer. In addition, MCN is almost always found in the pancreatic body and tail of perimenopausal women. When detected in an early stage without associated adenocarcinoma, resection of IPMN and MCN is curative. However, because of the lack of biomarkers for high-risk lesions, selection of patients who benefit from resection is difficult. Further high-quality clinical and molecular studies are essential to improve clinical decision making in the management of these precursor lesions (Box 1).[73–75]

## ACKNOWLEDGMENTS

L.A.A. Brosens is funded by a Career Development Grant from the Dutch Digestive Foundation (CDG 14-02). The authors thank Dr Jeanin van Hooft for generously providing the endoscopic picture of a bulging ampulla of Vater with extruding thick mucin in a patient with an IPMN. We also thank Prof. Dr Ralph Hruban for generously providing the histopathologic picture of an acinar cell carcinoma with intraductal growth.

## REFERENCES

1. Hulst SPL. Zur Kenntnis der Genese des Adenokarzinoms und Karzinoms des Pankreas. Virchows Arch (B) 1905;180(2):288–316.
2. Hruban RH, Adsay NV, Albores-Saavedra J, et al. Pancreatic intraepithelial neoplasia: a new nomenclature and classification system for pancreatic duct lesions. Am J Surg Pathol 2001;25(5):579–86.
3. Hruban RH, Takaori K, Klimstra DS, et al. An illustrated consensus on the classification of pancreatic intraepithelial neoplasia and intraductal papillary mucinous neoplasms. Am J Surg Pathol 2004;28(8):977–87.
4. Basturk O, Hong S-M, Wood LD, et al. A revised classification system and recommendations from the Baltimore consensus meeting for neoplastic precursor lesions in the pancreas. Am J Surg Pathol 2015;39(12):1730–41.
5. Berman JJ, Albores-Saavedra J, Bostwick D, et al. Precancer: a conceptual working definition – results of a Consensus Conference. Cancer Detect Prev 2006;30(5):387–94.
6. Cubilla AL, Fitzgerald PJ. Morphological lesions associated with human primary invasive nonendocrine pancreas cancer. Cancer Res 1976;36(7 Pt 2):2690–8.
7. Andea A, Sarkar F, Adsay VN. Clinicopathological correlates of pancreatic intraepithelial neoplasia: a comparative analysis of 82 cases with and 152 cases without pancreatic ductal adenocarcinoma. Mod Pathol 2003;16(10):996–1006.
8. Recavarren C, Labow DM, Liang J, et al. Histologic characteristics of pancreatic intraepithelial neoplasia associated with different pancreatic lesions. Hum Pathol 2011;42(1):18–24.
9. Brune K, Abe T, Canto M, et al. Multifocal neoplastic precursor lesions associated with lobular atrophy of the pancreas in patients having a strong family history of pancreatic cancer. Am J Surg Pathol 2006;30(9):1067–76.
10. Shi C, Klein AP, Goggins M, et al. Increased prevalence of precursor lesions in familial pancreatic cancer patients. Clin Cancer Res 2009;15(24):7737–43.
11. Takaori K, Matsusue S, Fujikawa T, et al. Carcinoma in situ of the pancreas associated with localized fibrosis: a clue to early detection of neoplastic lesions arising from pancreatic ducts. Pancreas 1998;17(1):102–5.
12. Detlefsen S, Sipos B, Feyerabend B, et al. Pancreatic fibrosis associated with age and ductal papillary hyperplasia. Virchows Arch 2005;447(5):800–5.
13. Brat DJ, Lillemoe KD, Yeo CJ, et al. Progression of pancreatic intraductal neoplasias to infiltrating adenocarcinoma of the pancreas. Am J Surg Pathol 1998;22(2):163–9.
14. Ban S, Shimizu Y, Ogawa F, et al. Reevaluation of "cancerization of the duct" by pancreatic cancers. Mod Pathol 2007;20:276.
15. Konstantinidis IT, Vinuela EF, Tang LH, et al. Incidentally discovered pancreatic intraepithelial neoplasia: what is its clinical significance? Ann Surg Oncol 2013;20(11):3643–7.
16. Longnecker DS, Adsay NV, Fernandez-del Castillo C, et al. Histopathological diagnosis of pancreatic intraepithelial neoplasia and intraductal papillary-mucinous neoplasms: interobserver agreement. Pancreas 2005;31(4):344–9.
17. Matthaei H, Hong S-M, Mayo SC, et al. Presence of pancreatic intraepithelial neoplasia in the pancreatic transection margin does not influence outcome in patients with R0 resected pancreatic cancer. Ann Surg Oncol 2011;18(12):3493–9.
18. Maitra A, Adsay NV, Argani P, et al. Multicomponent analysis of the pancreatic adenocarcinoma progression model using a pancreatic intraepithelial neoplasia tissue microarray. Mod Pathol 2003;16(9):902–12.
19. Nagata K, Horinouchi M, Saitou M, et al. Mucin expression profile in pancreatic cancer and the precursor lesions. J Hepatobiliary Pancreat Surg 2007;14(3):243–54.

20. Adsay NV, Merati K, Andea A, et al. The dichotomy in the preinvasive neoplasia to invasive carcinoma sequence in the pancreas: differential expression of MUC1 and MUC2 supports the existence of two separate pathways of carcinogenesis. Mod Pathol 2002;15(10):1087–95.

21. Moriya T, Kimura W, Semba S, et al. Biological similarities and differences between pancreatic intraepithelial neoplasias and intraductal papillary mucinous neoplasms. Int J Gastrointest Cancer 2005;35(2):111–9.

22. Basturk O, Khayyata S, Klimstra DS, et al. Preferential expression of MUC6 in oncocytic and pancreatobiliary types of intraductal papillary neoplasms highlights a pyloropancreatic pathway, distinct from the intestinal pathway, in pancreatic carcinogenesis. Am J Surg Pathol 2010;34(3): 364–70.

23. Kozuka S, Sassa R, Taki T, et al. Relation of pancreatic duct hyperplasia to carcinoma. Cancer 1979; 43(4):1418–28.

24. Klimstra DS, Longnecker DS. K-ras mutations in pancreatic ductal proliferative lesions. Am J Pathol 1994;145(6):1547–50.

25. Lemoine NR, Jain S, Hughes CM, et al. Ki-ras oncogene activation in preinvasive pancreatic cancer. Gastroenterology 1992;102(1):230–6.

26. Yanagisawa A, Ohtake K, Ohashi K, et al. Frequent c-Ki-ras oncogene activation in mucous cell hyperplasias of pancreas suffering from chronic inflammation. Cancer Res 1993;53(5): 953–6.

27. DiGiuseppe JA, Hruban RH, Offerhaus GJ, et al. Detection of K-ras mutations in mucinous pancreatic duct hyperplasia from a patient with a family history of pancreatic carcinoma. Am J Pathol 1994;144(5):889–95.

28. Lüttges J, Galehdari H, Bröcker V, et al. Allelic loss is often the first hit in the biallelic inactivation of the p53 and DPC4 genes during pancreatic carcinogenesis. Am J Pathol 2001;158(5):1677–83.

29. van Heek NT, Meeker AK, Kern SE, et al. Telomere shortening is nearly universal in pancreatic intraepithelial neoplasia. Am J Pathol 2002;161(5): 1541–7.

30. Moskaluk CA, Hruban RH, Kern SE. p16 and K-ras gene mutations in the intraductal precursors of human pancreatic adenocarcinoma. Cancer Res 1997;57(11):2140–3.

31. Brosens LAA, Hackeng WM, Offerhaus GJ, et al. Pancreatic adenocarcinoma pathology: changing "landscape." J Gastrointest Oncol 2015;6(4): 358–74.

32. Werner J, Fritz S, Büchler MW. Intraductal papillary mucinous neoplasms of the pancreas–a surgical disease. Nat Rev Gastroenterol Hepatol 2012; 9(5):253–9.

33. Habán G. Papillomatose und Carcinom des Gangsystems der Bauchspeicheldrüse. Virchows Arch Path Anat 1936;297(1):207–20.

34. Sessa F, Solcia E, Capella C, et al. Intraductal papillary-mucinous tumours represent a distinct group of pancreatic neoplasms: an investigation of tumour cell differentiation and K-ras, p53 and c-erbB-2 abnormalities in 26 patients. Virchows Arch 1994;425(4):357–67.

35. Morohoshi T, Kanda M, Asanuma K, et al. Intraductal papillary neoplasms of the pancreas. A clinicopathologic study of six patients. Cancer 1989; 64(6):1329–35.

36. Ingkakul T, Warshaw AL, Fernández-Del Castillo C. Epidemiology of intraductal papillary mucinous neoplasms of the pancreas: sex differences between 3 geographic regions. Pancreas 2011; 40(5):779–80.

37. Salvia R, Fernández-del Castillo C, Bassi C, et al. Main-duct intraductal papillary mucinous neoplasms of the pancreas: clinical predictors of malignancy and long-term survival following resection. Ann Surg 2004;239(5):678–85, [discussion: 685–7].

38. Chari ST, Yadav D, Smyrk TC, et al. Study of recurrence after surgical resection of intraductal papillary mucinous neoplasm of the pancreas. Gastroenterology 2002;123(5):1500–7.

39. Ingkakul T, Sadakari Y, Ienaga J, et al. Predictors of the presence of concomitant invasive ductal carcinoma in intraductal papillary mucinous neoplasm of the pancreas. Ann Surg 2010;251(1):70–5.

40. Sohn TA, Yeo CJ, Cameron JL, et al. Intraductal papillary mucinous neoplasms of the pancreas: an updated experience. Ann Surg 2004;239(6): 788–97, [discussion: 797–9].

41. Crippa S, Fernández-Del Castillo C, Salvia R, et al. Mucin-producing neoplasms of the pancreas: an analysis of distinguishing clinical and epidemiologic characteristics. Clin Gastroenterol Hepatol 2010;8(2):213–9.

42. Maire F, Hammel P, Terris B, et al. Intraductal papillary and mucinous pancreatic tumour: a new extracolonic tumour in familial adenomatous polyposis. Gut 2002;51(3):446–9.

43. Gaujoux S, Tissier F, Ragazzon B, et al. Pancreatic ductal and acinar cell neoplasms in Carney complex: a possible new association. J Clin Endocrinol Metab 2011;96(11):E1888–95.

44. Gaujoux S, Chanson P, Bertherat J, et al. Hepatopancreato-biliary lesions are present in both Carney complex and McCune Albright syndrome: comments on P. Salpea and C. Stratakis. Mol Cell Endocrinol 2014;382(1):344–5.

45. Salpea P, Horvath A, London E, et al. Deletions of the PRKAR1A locus at 17q24.2-q24.3 in Carney complex: genotype-phenotype correlations and

implications for genetic testing. J Clin Endocrinol Metab 2014;99(1):E183–8.

46. Su GH, Hruban RH, Bansal RK, et al. Germline and somatic mutations of the STK11/LKB1 Peutz-Jeghers gene in pancreatic and biliary cancers. Am J Pathol 1999;154(6):1835–40.

47. Poley JW, Kluijt I, Gouma DJ, et al. The yield of first-time endoscopic ultrasonography in screening individuals at a high risk of developing pancreatic cancer. Am J Gastroenterol 2009;104(9):2175–81.

48. Sparr JA, Bandipalliam P, Redston MS, et al. Intraductal papillary mucinous neoplasm of the pancreas with loss of mismatch repair in a patient with Lynch syndrome. Am J Surg Pathol 2009;33(2):309–12.

49. Ferrone CR, Correa-Gallego C, Warshaw AL, et al. Current trends in pancreatic cystic neoplasms. Arch Surg 2009;144(5):448–54.

50. Traverso LW, Peralta EA, Ryan JA Jr, et al. Intraductal neoplasms of the pancreas. Am J Surg 1998; 175(5):426–32.

51. Klöppel G. Clinicopathologic view of intraductal papillary-mucinous tumor of the pancreas. Hepatogastroenterology 1998;45(24):1981–5.

52. Fernández-del Castillo C, Targarona J, Thayer SP, et al. Incidental pancreatic cysts: clinicopathologic characteristics and comparison with symptomatic patients. Arch Surg 2003;138(4):427–33, [discussion: 433–4].

53. Tanaka M, Kobayashi K, Mizumoto K, et al. Clinical aspects of intraductal papillary mucinous neoplasm of the pancreas. J Gastroenterol 2005;40(7):669–75.

54. Yamaguchi K, Tanaka M. Mucin-hypersecreting tumor of the pancreas with mucin extrusion through an enlarged papilla. Am J Gastroenterol 1991; 86(7):835–9.

55. Zhang X-M, Mitchell DG, Dohke M, et al. Pancreatic cysts: depiction on single-shot fast spin-echo MR images. Radiology 2002;223(2):547–53.

56. Matsubara S, Tada M, Akahane M, et al. Incidental pancreatic cysts found by magnetic resonance imaging and their relationship with pancreatic cancer. Pancreas 2012;41(8):1241–6.

57. Moris M, Bridges MD, Pooley RA, et al. Association between advances in high-resolution cross-section imaging technologies and increase in prevalence of pancreatic cysts from 2005 to 2014. Clin Gastroenterol Hepatol 2016;14(4):585–93.e3.

58. Lee KS, Sekhar A, Rofsky NM, et al. Prevalence of incidental pancreatic cysts in the adult population on MR imaging. Am J Gastroenterol 2010;105(9): 2079–84.

59. Kimura W, Nagai H, Kuroda A, et al. Analysis of small cystic lesions of the pancreas. Int J Pancreatol 1995;18(3):197–206.

60. Spinelli KS, Fromwiller TE, Daniel RA, et al. Cystic pancreatic neoplasms: observe or operate. Ann Surg 2004;239(5):651–7, [discussion: 657–9].

61. Ikeda M, Sato T, Morozumi A, et al. Morphologic changes in the pancreas detected by screening ultrasonography in a mass survey, with special reference to main duct dilatation, cyst formation, and calcification. Pancreas 1994;9(4):508–12.

62. Lee SH, Shin CM, Park JK, et al. Outcomes of cystic lesions in the pancreas after extended follow-up. Dig Dis Sci 2007;52(10):2653–9.

63. Edirimanne S, Connor SJ. Incidental pancreatic cystic lesions. World J Surg 2008;32(9):2028–37.

64. Girometti R, Intini S, Brondani G, et al. Incidental pancreatic cysts on 3D turbo spin echo magnetic resonance cholangiopancreatography: prevalence and relation with clinical and imaging features. Abdom Imaging 2011;36(2):196–205.

65. de Jong K, Nio CY, Hermans JJ, et al. High prevalence of pancreatic cysts detected by screening magnetic resonance imaging examinations. Clin Gastroenterol Hepatol 2010;8(9):806–11.

66. Goh BKP, Tan Y-M, Cheow P-C, et al. Cystic lesions of the pancreas: an appraisal of an aggressive resectional policy adopted at a single institution during 15 years. Am J Surg 2006; 192(2):148–54.

67. Nagai K, Doi R, Kida A, et al. Intraductal papillary mucinous neoplasms of the pancreas: clinicopathologic characteristics and long-term follow-up after resection. World J Surg 2008;32(2):271–8, [discussion: 279–80].

68. Sahora K, Fernández-del Castillo C, Dong F, et al. Not all mixed-type intraductal papillary mucinous neoplasms behave like main-duct lesions: implications of minimal involvement of the main pancreatic duct. Surgery 2014;156(3):611–21.

69. Fritz S, Klauss M, Bergmann F, et al. Pancreatic main-duct involvement in branch-duct IPMNs: an underestimated risk. Ann Surg 2014;260(5): 848–55, [discussion: 855–6].

70. Tanaka M, Fernández-del Castillo C, Adsay V, et al. International consensus guidelines 2012 for the management of IPMN and MCN of the pancreas. Pancreatology 2012;12(3):183–97.

71. Tanaka M, Chari S, Adsay V, et al. International consensus guidelines for management of intraductal papillary mucinous neoplasms and mucinous cystic neoplasms of the pancreas. Pancreatology 2006;6(1–2):17–32.

72. Vege SS, Ziring B, Jain R, et al, Clinical Guidelines Committee, American Gastroenterology Association. American Gastroenterological Association Institute guideline on the diagnosis and management of asymptomatic neoplastic pancreatic cysts. Gastroenterology 2015;148(4):819–22, [quiz: 12–3].

73. Moayyedi P, Weinberg DS, Schünemann H, et al. Management of pancreatic cysts in an evidence-based world. Gastroenterology 2015;148(4):692–5.

74. Canto MI, Hruban RH. Managing pancreatic cysts: less is more? Gastroenterology 2015;148(4): 688–91.

75. Lennon AM, Ahuja N, Wolfgang CL. AGA guidelines for the management of pancreatic cysts. Gastroenterology 2015;149(3):825.

76. Furukawa T, Klöppel G, Volkan Adsay N, et al. Classification of types of intraductal papillary-mucinous neoplasm of the pancreas: a consensus study. Virchows Arch 2005;447(5):794–9.

77. Furukawa T, Hatori T, Fujita I, et al. Prognostic relevance of morphological types of intraductal papillary mucinous neoplasms of the pancreas. Gut 2011;60(4):509–16.

78. Adsay NV, Merati K, Basturk O, et al. Pathologically and biologically distinct types of epithelium in intraductal papillary mucinous neoplasms: delineation of an "intestinal" pathway of carcinogenesis in the pancreas. Am J Surg Pathol 2004; 28(7):839–48.

79. Adsay NV, Conlon KC, Zee SY, et al. Intraductal papillary-mucinous neoplasms of the pancreas: an analysis of in situ and invasive carcinomas in 28 patients. Cancer 2002;94(1):62–77.

80. Ban S, Naitoh Y, Mino-Kenudson M, et al. Intraductal papillary mucinous neoplasm (IPMN) of the pancreas: its histopathologic difference between 2 major types. Am J Surg Pathol 2006;30(12): 1561–9.

81. Koh YX, Zheng HL, Chok A-Y, et al. Systematic review and meta-analysis of the spectrum and outcomes of different histologic subtypes of noninvasive and invasive intraductal papillary mucinous neoplasms. Surgery 2015;157(3):496–509.

82. Tsutsumi K, Sato N, Cui L, et al. Expression of claudin-4 (CLDN4) mRNA in intraductal papillary mucinous neoplasms of the pancreas. Mod Pathol 2011;24(4):533–41.

83. Nakata K, Ohuchida K, Aishima S, et al. Invasive carcinoma derived from intestinal-type intraductal papillary mucinous neoplasm is associated with minimal invasion, colloid carcinoma, and less invasive behavior, leading to a better prognosis. Pancreas 2011;40(4):581–7.

84. Sadakari Y, Ohuchida K, Nakata K, et al. Invasive carcinoma derived from the nonintestinal type intraductal papillary mucinous neoplasm of the pancreas has a poorer prognosis than that derived from the intestinal type. Surgery 2010;147(6): 812–7.

85. Yonezawa S, Higashi M, Yamada N, et al. Significance of mucin expression in pancreatobiliary neoplasms. J Hepatobiliary Pancreat Sci 2010;17(2): 108–24.

86. Kobayashi M, Fujinaga Y, Ota H. Reappraisal of the immunophenotype of pancreatic intraductal papillary mucinous neoplasms (IPMNs)–gastric pyloric and small intestinal immunophenotype expression in gastric and intestinal type IPMNs–. Acta Histochem Cytochem 2014;47(2): 45–57.

87. Schaberg KB, DiMaio MA, Longacre TA. Intraductal papillary mucinous neoplasms often contain epithelium from multiple subtypes and/or are unclassifiable. Am J Surg Pathol 2016; 40(1):44–50.

88. Mino-Kenudson M, Fernández-del Castillo C, Baba Y, et al. Prognosis of invasive intraductal papillary mucinous neoplasm depends on histological and precursor epithelial subtypes. Gut 2011; 60(12):1712–20.

89. Distler M, Kersting S, Niedergethmann M, et al. Pathohistological subtype predicts survival in patients with intraductal papillary mucinous neoplasm (IPMN) of the pancreas. Ann Surg 2013;258(2): 324–30.

90. Kim J, Jang K-T, Mo Park S, et al. Prognostic relevance of pathologic subtypes and minimal invasion in intraductal papillary mucinous neoplasms of the pancreas. Tumour Biol 2011;32(3):535–42.

91. Wu J, Jiao Y, Dal Molin M, et al. Whole-exome sequencing of neoplastic cysts of the pancreas reveals recurrent mutations in components of ubiquitin-dependent pathways. Proc Natl Acad Sci U S A 2011;108(52):21188–93.

92. Wu J, Matthaei H, Maitra A, et al. Recurrent GNAS mutations define an unexpected pathway for pancreatic cyst development. Sci Transl Med 2011;3(92):92ra66.

93. Tan MC, Basturk O, Brannon AR, et al. GNAS and KRAS mutations define separate progression pathways in intraductal papillary mucinous neoplasm-associated carcinoma. J Am Coll Surg 2015; 220(5):845–54.e1.

94. Dal Molin M, Matthaei H, Wu J, et al. Clinicopathological correlates of activating GNAS mutations in intraductal papillary mucinous neoplasm (IPMN) of the pancreas. Ann Surg Oncol 2013;20(12): 3802–8.

95. Hosoda W, Sasaki E, Murakami Y, et al. GNAS mutation is a frequent event in pancreatic intraductal papillary mucinous neoplasms and associated adenocarcinomas. Virchows Arch 2015;466(6): 665–74.

96. Yamada M, Sekine S, Ogawa R, et al. Frequent activating GNAS mutations in villous adenoma of the colorectum. J Pathol 2012;228(1):113–8.

97. Takaori K. Dilemma in classifications of possible precursors of pancreatic cancer involving the main pancreatic duct: PanIN or IPMN? J Gastroenterol 2003;38(3):311–3.

98. Takaori K. Current understanding of precursors to pancreatic cancer. J Hepatobiliary Pancreat Surg 2007;14(3):217–23.

99. Kogire M, Tokuhara K, Itoh D, et al. Atypical ductal hyperplasia of the pancreas associated with a stricture of the main pancreatic duct. J Gastroenterol 2003;38(3):295–7.

100. Klimstra DS, Adsay NV, Dhall D, et al. Intraductal tubular carcinoma of the pancreas: clinicopathologic and immunohistochemical analysis of 18 cases, [abstract]. Mod Pathol 2007;20:285.

101. Bosman FT, Carneiro F, Hruban RH, et al, editors. WHO classification of tumours of the digestive system. Lyon: IARC; 2010. p. 312.

102. Yamaguchi H, Shimizu M, Ban S, et al. Intraductal tubulopapillary neoplasms of the pancreas distinct from pancreatic intraepithelial neoplasia and intraductal papillary mucinous neoplasms. Am J Surg Pathol 2009;33(8):1164–72.

103. Bakotic BW, Robinson MJ, Sturm PD, et al. Pyloric gland adenoma of the main pancreatic duct. Am J Surg Pathol 1999;23(2):227–31.

104. Albores-Saavedra J, Sheahan K, O'Riain C, et al. Intraductal tubular adenoma, pyloric type, of the pancreas: additional observations on a new type of pancreatic neoplasm. Am J Surg Pathol 2004; 28(2):233–8.

105. Kato N, Akiyama S, Motoyama T. Pyloric gland-type tubular adenoma superimposed on intraductal papillary mucinous tumor of the pancreas. Pyloric gland adenoma of the pancreas. Virchows Arch 2002;440(2):205–8.

106. Chetty R, Serra S. Intraductal tubular adenoma (pyloric gland-type) of the pancreas: a reappraisal and possible relationship with gastric-type intraductal papillary mucinous neoplasm. Histopathology 2009;55(3):270–6.

107. Nakayama Y, Inoue H, Hamada Y, et al. Intraductal tubular adenoma of the pancreas, pyloric gland type: a clinicopathologic and immunohistochemical study of 6 cases. Am J Surg Pathol 2005; 29(5):607–16.

108. Fukatsu H, Kawamoto H, Tsutsumi K, et al. Intraductal tubular adenoma, pyloric gland-type, of the pancreas. Endoscopy 2007;39(Suppl 1):E88–9.

109. Itatsu K, Sano T, Hiraoka N, et al. Intraductal tubular carcinoma in an adenoma of the main pancreatic duct of the pancreas head. J Gastroenterol 2006;41(7):702–5.

110. Nagaike K, Chijiiwa K, Hiyoshi M, et al. Main-duct intraductal papillary mucinous adenoma of the pancreas with a large mural nodule. Int J Clin Oncol 2007;12(5):388–91.

111. Amaris J. Intraductal mucinous papillary tumor and pyloric gland adenoma of the pancreas. Gastrointest Endosc 2002;56(3):441–4.

112. Chang X, Jiang Y, Li J, et al. Intraductal tubular adenomas (pyloric gland-type) of the pancreas: clinicopathologic features are similar to gastric-type intraductal papillary mucinous neoplasms and different from intraductal tubulopapillary neoplasms. Diagn Pathol 2014;9:172.

113. Ban D, Shimada K, Sekine S, et al. Pancreatic ducts as an important route of tumor extension for acinar cell carcinoma of the pancreas. Am J Surg Pathol 2010;34(7):1025–36.

114. Basturk O, Zamboni G, Klimstra DS, et al. Intraductal and papillary variants of acinar cell carcinomas: a new addition to the challenging differential diagnosis of intraductal neoplasms. Am J Surg Pathol 2007;31(3):363–70.

115. Hosoda W, Sasaki E, Murakami Y, et al. BCL10 as a useful marker for pancreatic acinar cell carcinoma, especially using endoscopic ultrasound cytology specimens. Pathol Int 2013;63(3):176–82.

116. Yamaguchi H, Kuboki Y, Hatori T, et al. The discrete nature and distinguishing molecular features of pancreatic intraductal tubulopapillary neoplasms and intraductal papillary mucinous neoplasms of the gastric type, pyloric gland variant. J Pathol 2013;231(3):335–41.

117. Amato E, Molin MD, Mafficini A, et al. Targeted next-generation sequencing of cancer genes dissects the molecular profiles of intraductal papillary neoplasms of the pancreas. J Pathol 2014;233(3): 217–27.

118. Xiao HD, Yamaguchi H, Dias-Santagata D, et al. Molecular characteristics and biological behaviours of the oncocytic and pancreatobiliary subtypes of intraductal papillary mucinous neoplasms. J Pathol 2011;224(4):508–16.

119. Matsubara A, Sekine S, Kushima R, et al. Frequent GNAS and KRAS mutations in pyloric gland adenoma of the stomach and duodenum. J Pathol 2013;229(4):579–87.

120. Yamaguchi H, Kuboki Y, Hatori T, et al. Somatic mutations in PIK3CA and activation of AKT in intraductal tubulopapillary neoplasms of the pancreas. Am J Surg Pathol 2011;35(12):1812–7.

121. Hudes G, Carducci M, Tomczak P, et al. Temsirolimus, interferon alfa, or both for advanced renal-cell carcinoma. N Engl J Med 2007;356(22):2271–81.

122. Motzer RJ, Escudier B, Oudard S, et al. Efficacy of everolimus in advanced renal cell carcinoma: a double-blind, randomised, placebo-controlled phase III trial. Lancet 2008;372(9637):449–56.

123. Fallahzadeh MK, Zibari GB, Wellman G, et al. Mucinous cystic neoplasm of pancreas in a male patient: a case report and review of the literature. J La State Med Soc 2014;166(2):67–9.

124. Shiono S, Suda K, Nobukawa B, et al. Pancreatic, hepatic, splenic, and mesenteric mucinous cystic neoplasms (MCN) are lumped together as extra ovarian MCN. Pathol Int 2006;56(2):71–7.

125. Adsay NV, Eble JN, Srigley JR, et al. Mixed epithelial and stromal tumor of the kidney. Am J Surg Pathol 2000;24(7):958–70.

126. Buritica C, Serrano M, Zuluaga A, et al. Mixed epithelial and stromal tumour of the kidney with luteinised ovarian stroma. J Clin Pathol 2007; 60(1):98–100.

127. Matsubara M, Shiozawa T, Tachibana R, et al. Primary retroperitoneal mucinous cystadenoma of borderline malignancy: a case report and review of the literature. Int J Gynecol Pathol 2005;24(3): 218–23.

128. Zamboni G, Scarpa A, Bogina G, et al. Mucinous cystic tumors of the pancreas: clinicopathological features, prognosis, and relationship to other mucinous cystic tumors. Am J Surg Pathol 1999; 23(4):410–22.

129. Ridder GJ, Maschek H, Flemming P, et al. Ovarian-like stroma in an invasive mucinous cystadenocarcinoma of the pancreas positive for inhibin. A hint concerning its possible histogenesis. Virchows Arch 1998;432(5):451–4.

130. Yamao K, Yanagisawa A, Takahashi K, et al. Clinicopathological features and prognosis of mucinous cystic neoplasm with ovarian-type stroma: a multi-institutional study of the Japan pancreas society. Pancreas 2011;40(1):67–71.

131. Crippa S, Salvia R, Warshaw AL, et al. Mucinous cystic neoplasm of the pancreas is not an aggressive entity: lessons from 163 resected patients. Ann Surg 2008;247(4):571–9.

132. Park WG-U, Mascarenhas R, Palaez-Luna M, et al. Diagnostic performance of cyst fluid carcinoembryonic antigen and amylase in histologically confirmed pancreatic cysts. Pancreas 2011;40(1): 42–5.

133. Cizginer S, Turner BG, Turner B, et al. Cyst fluid carcinoembryonic antigen is an accurate diagnostic marker of pancreatic mucinous cysts. Pancreas 2011;40(7):1024–8.

134. Thompson LD, Becker RC, Przygodzki RM, et al. Mucinous cystic neoplasm (mucinous cystadenocarcinoma of low-grade malignant potential) of the pancreas: a clinicopathologic study of 130 cases. Am J Surg Pathol 1999;23(1):1–16.

135. Izumo A, Yamaguchi K, Eguchi T, et al. Mucinous cystic tumor of the pancreas: immunohistochemical assessment of "ovarian-type stroma". Oncol Rep 2003;10(3):515–25.

136. Reddy RP, Smyrk TC, Zapiach M, et al. Pancreatic mucinous cystic neoplasm defined by ovarian stroma: demographics, clinical features, and prevalence of cancer. Clin Gastroenterol Hepatol 2004; 2(11):1026–31.

137. Baker ML, Seeley ES, Pai R, et al. Invasive mucinous cystic neoplasms of the pancreas. Exp Mol Pathol 2012;93(3):345–9.

138. Jang K-T, Park SM, Basturk O, et al. Clinicopathologic characteristics of 29 invasive carcinomas arising in 178 pancreatic mucinous cystic neoplasms with ovarian-type stroma: implications for management and prognosis. Am J Surg Pathol 2015;39(2):179–87.

139. Kosmahl M, Pauser U, Peters K, et al. Cystic neoplasms of the pancreas and tumor-like lesions with cystic features: a review of 418 cases and a classification proposal. Virchows Arch 2004; 445(2):168–78.

140. Seidel G, Zahurak M, Iacobuzio-Donahue C, et al. Almost all infiltrating colloid carcinomas of the pancreas and periampullary region arise from in situ papillary neoplasms: a study of 39 cases. Am J Surg Pathol 2002;26(1):56–63.

141. Bakker RFR, Stoot JHMB, Blok P, et al. Primary retroperitoneal mucinous cystadenoma with sarcoma-like mural nodule: a case report and review of the literature. Virchows Arch 2007;451(4):853–7.

142. Hirano H, Morita K, Tachibana S, et al. Undifferentiated carcinoma with osteoclast-like giant cells arising in a mucinous cystic neoplasm of the pancreas. Pathol Int 2008;58(6):383–9.

143. van den Berg W, Tascilar M, Offerhaus GJ, et al. Pancreatic mucinous cystic neoplasms with sarcomatous stroma: molecular evidence for monoclonal origin with subsequent divergence of the epithelial and sarcomatous components. Mod Pathol 2000; 13(1):86–91.

144. Fukushima N, Zamboni G. Mucinous cystic neoplasms of the pancreas: update on the surgical pathology and molecular genetics. Semin Diagn Pathol 2014;31(6):467–74.

145. Southern JF, Warshaw AL, Lewandrowski KB. DNA ploidy analysis of mucinous cystic tumors of the pancreas. Correlation of aneuploidy with malignancy and poor prognosis. Cancer 1996;77(1):58–62.

# Nonductal Pancreatic Cancers

Sun-Young Jun, MD, PhD[a], Seung-Mo Hong, MD, PhD[b],*

## KEYWORDS

- Pancreas • Solid pseudopapillary • Acinar • Pancreatoblastoma

## Key points

- Nonductal pancreatic neoplasms share common features of cellular tumors with little intervening stroma and show abnormal beta-catenin expression.

- Pancreatoblastomas are the most common tumors with acinar differentiation in childhood, whereas acinar cell carcinomas are the most frequent tumors in adults.

- For differential diagnoses of nonductal pancreatic neoplasms, identifying characteristic histologic features, such as pseudopapillae, acinar architecture with single prominent nucleoli, or squamoid nests, is important.

- Acinar cell (trypsin/chymotrypsin/B-Cell Leukemia/Lymphoma 10 [BCL10]) or neuroendocrine (synaptophysin/chromogranin) markers and E-cadherin are helpful for differential diagnosis of nonductal pancreatic neoplasms and pancreatic neuroendocrine tumors.

## ABSTRACT

Nonductal pancreatic neoplasms, including solid pseudopapillary neoplasms, acinar cell carcinomas, and pancreatoblastomas, are uncommon. These entities share overlapping gross, microscopic, and immunohistochemical features, such as well-demarcated solid neoplasms, monotonous cellular tumor cells with little intervening stroma, and abnormal beta-catenin expression. Each tumor also has unique clinicopathologic characteristics with diverse clinical behavior. To differentiate nonductal pancreatic neoplasms, identification of histologic findings, such as pseudopapillae, acinar cell features, and squamoid corpuscles, is important. Immunostainings for acinar cell or neuroendocrine markers are helpful for differential diagnosis. This article describes the clinicopathologic and immunohistochemical features of nonductal pancreatic cancers.

## OVERVIEW

The pancreas is mainly composed of 3 types of epithelial cells: enzyme-producing acinar cells (85%), hormone-producing endocrine cells (3% to 5%), and ductal cells (up to 3%).[1] In general, the most common epithelial neoplasm arises from the most common normal epithelial component in an organ. However, in the pancreas, the most prevalent tumors are not acinar cell carcinomas (ACCs) but ductal adenocarcinomas.[2] Because pancreatic neuroendocrine tumors (PanNETs) are discussed elsewhere in this issue (see Salaria SN, Shi C: Pancreatic Neuroendocrine Tumors, in this issue), they are not discussed here. Excluding PanNETs, nonductal pancreatic tumors comprise less than 5% of pancreatic neoplasms.[2] This article discusses existing knowledge of these uncommon nonductal pancreatic neoplasms, including solid pseudopapillary neoplasms (SPNs), ACCs, and pancreatoblastomas (PBs).

Disclosure: This study was supported by a grant (1320200) from the National R&D Program for Cancer Control, Ministry of Health & Welfare, Republic of Korea.
[a] Department of Pathology, Incheon St. Mary's Hospital, The Catholic University of Korea, 56, Dongsu-ro, Bupyeong-gu, Incheon 403-720, Republic of Korea; [b] Department of Pathology, Asan Medical Center, University of Ulsan College of Medicine, 88, Olympic-ro 43-gil, Songpa-gu, Seoul 138-736, Republic of Korea
* Corresponding author.
*E-mail address:* smhong28@gmail.com

surgpath.theclinics.com

## SOLID PSEUDOPAPILLARY NEOPLASM

SPNs are low-grade carcinomas characterized by a solid growth pattern and pseudopapillary formation by poorly cohesive monomorphic epithelial tumors cells with occasional degenerative cystic changes.[3] SPNs are rare, accounting for 1% to 3% of all exocrine pancreatic neoplasms and only 5% of cystic neoplasms.[4] These tumors occur predominantly in young women, with a male to female ratio of 1:9 and a mean patient age of 29 years.[5–7] Forty percent of SPNs are incidentally found without specific symptoms.[5,6] Clinical features for symptomatic patients are usually nonspecific and include abdominal pain and a palpable mass.[5]

### GROSS FEATURES

SPNs are well-demarcated or partially encapsulated large single masses with an average size of 8 to 10 cm.[4,8] The tumors occur more frequently in the body or tail of the pancreas than in the head.[5–7] SPNs have variable appearances, including purely solid, mixed solid and cystic, and pure cystic (Fig. 1). Most cases are mixed solid and cystic tumors.[3] Small tumors tend to be purely solid, but as tumor size increases they are more likely to be cystic because of the development of degenerative cystic changes.[3] Gross features of completely cystic degenerative SPNs are similar to those of pseudocysts.[8] The cut surface shows variable colors, such as yellow, tan, red-tan, brown, and gray, based on the presence and proportions of accompanying hemorrhagic necrosis and degeneration.[4,8] Calcification is present in approximately 33% of SPN cases.[9,10]

### MICROSCOPIC FEATURES

At scanning-power magnification, SPNs show variable growth patterns in combination with solid, pseudopapillary, and pseudocystic structures (Fig. 2A). Although the tumors are well demarcated from normal pancreatic parenchyma and are even found partially encapsulated on gross examinations, tumor cells have been found to have infiltrative borders with surrounding normal pancreatic parenchyma microscopically (Fig. 2B).[11] In solid

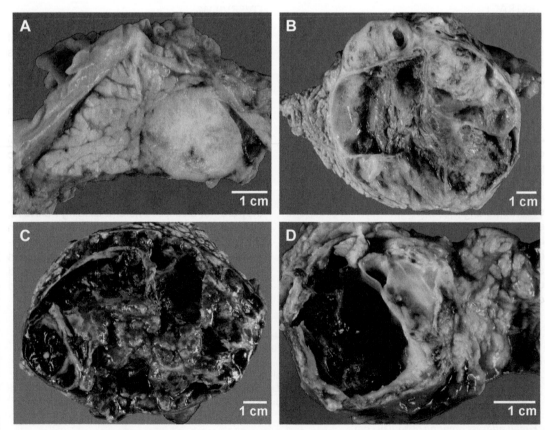

Fig. 1. Solid-pseudopapillary neoplasm showing variable gross appearances of (A) pure solid, (B, C) mixed solid and cystic, and (D) pure cystic tumor.

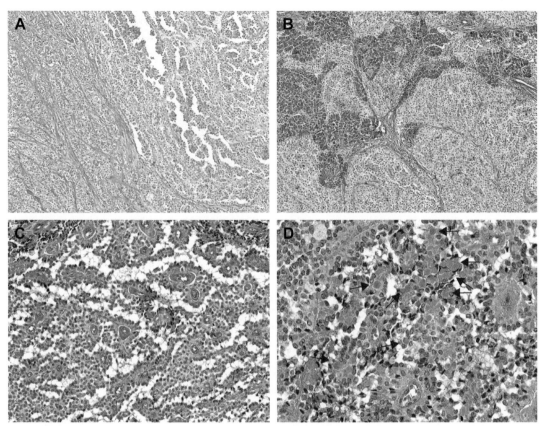

Fig. 2. Solid pseudopapillary neoplasm. (A) Area of mixed solid and pseudopapillary structures and sometimes (B) infiltrating border with normal pancreatic parenchyma are seen. Tumor cells show (C) characteristic features of pseudopapillae, (D) eosinophilic hyaline globules (arrows), and round to oval nuclei with occasional nuclear grooves (H&E, original magnification A and B ×100; C ×200; D ×400).

areas, the tumors consist of sheets of monomorphic polygonal tumor cells mixed with abundant capillary-sized blood vessels.[3] Tumor cells do not form glandular architectures and are generally poorly cohesive.[8] Tumor cells that drop away from thin-walled vessels are frequently noted, especially in areas distant from the capillary-sized vessels. Remaining tumor cells cover blood vessels, resulting in the characteristic features of pseudopapillae (Fig. 2C).[12–14] Tumor cells have round to oval nuclei with occasional nuclear grooves and indistinct nucleoli. Mitotic figures are rare. Occasional eosinophilic hyaline globules (Fig. 2D), which are stained with periodic acid-Schiff (PAS) staining and are resistant to diastase treatment, are noted in the cytoplasm of tumor cells.[15] The tumor cells have either eosinophilic or vacuolated clear cytoplasm (Fig. 3A).[16,17] Nuclear pleomorphism or prominent atypical multinucleated giant cells are observed in 7% to 13% of SPNs (Fig. 3B).[18,19] Such features are commonly observed in elderly patients but are not associated with recurrent or aggressive clinical

behavior and are therefore considered degenerative changes rather than malignant features.[18,19] Other degenerative changes include clustering of foamy macrophages and cholesterol crystals.[4] In general, the stromal component of these tumors is scanty, but some cases show fibrous, hyalinized, or myxoid stroma.[4] Metastatic SPNs show similar histologic features of monomorphic tumor cells with primary SPNs.[3] However, additional atypical features, including nuclear pleomorphism, tumor necrosis, increased mitosis/Ki-67 labeling index, and foci of sarcomatoid transformation, are noted in metastatic tumors.[20,21]

More than 90% of SPNs show abnormal nuclear and cytoplasmic beta-catenin labeling (Fig. 3C).[22–24] Loss of membranous E-cadherin labeling or nuclear and cytoplasmic beta-catenin labeling coupled with loss of membranous E-cadherin labeling[24,25] is also consistently observed in these tumors (Fig. 3D).[12,13] Markers for alpha1-antitrypsin, CD10, CD56, neuron-specific enolase, progesterone receptors, and vimentin are also consistently positive in SPNs.[8] SPNs are focally

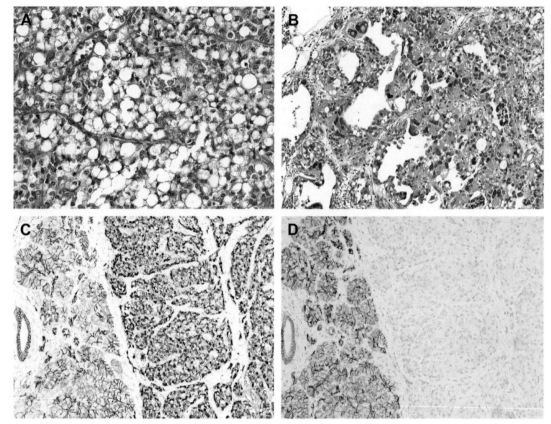

*Fig. 3.* Solid pseudopapillary neoplasm. Tumor cells can show (*A*) cytoplasmic vacuolization (H&E) and (*B*) pleomorphic nuclei (H&E). Immunohistochemically, tumor cells present (*C*) abnormal nuclear and cytoplasmic beta-catenin labeling and (*D*) loss of membranous E-cadherin expression the in right half, whereas normal ductal and acinar cells in the left half show (*C*) membranous beta-catenin labeling and (*D*) intact membranous E-cadherin labeling (original magnification *A, B* ×400; *C, D*, ×200).

positive for synaptophysin but consistently negative for chromogranin labeling.[4,8,24,26,27]

## DIFFERENTIAL DIAGNOSES

Other nonductal pancreatic neoplasms with solid and cellular appearance, including PanNETs, ACCs, and PBs, should be included as differential diagnoses from SPNs.[2] SPNs have histologic features that overlap considerably with those of PanNETs, including monomorphic tumor cells with round to oval nuclei. Suggestive histologic features of SPNs include the area of pseudopapillae and accumulation of foamy histiocytes.[3] SPNs show abnormal nuclear and cytoplasmic beta-catenin labeling in association with loss of membranous E-cadherin labeling and variable labeling with synaptophysin, but they are consistently negative for chromogranin labeling. In contrast, PanNETs diffusely and strongly express the neuroendocrine markers synaptophysin and chromogranin.[3] Because completely cystic degeneration of SPNs shares similar gross and histologic features with pseudocysts, careful gross examination and collection of a sufficient number of additional sections for identifying residual tumor cells from remaining tissue is warranted.[8]

> **Key Features**
> OF SOLID PSEUDOPAPILLARY
> NEOPLASMS
>
> - Well-demarcated or partially encapsulated large single mass
> - Variably mixed solid and cystic portion
> - Increased cellularity
> - Sheets of monomorphic polygonal tumor cells
> - Pseudopapillary structure
> - Nuclear and cytoplasmic beta-catenin labeling

## MOLECULAR PATHOLOGY

Because the molecular genetics of pancreas neoplasms are discussed elsewhere in this issue (see Wood L, Hosoda W: Molecular Genetics of Pancreatic Neoplasms, in this issue), this article only briefly touches on the key molecular features of such tumors. Almost all SPNs harbor activating somatic mutations in the CTNNB1 gene, which encodes beta-catenin. These mutations lead to abnormal nuclear and cytoplasmic localization of beta-catenin.[22,23,28] In addition to activation of the Wnt/beta-catenin, Hedgehog and androgen receptor signaling pathways and epithelial-mesenchymal transition-related genes have been reported in SPNs.[29] However, mutation of KRAS, TP53, CDKN2A/p16, and SMAD4, which are classically observed in ductal adenocarcinomas, are not identified in SPNs.[28]

## PROGNOSIS

After surgical resection, patients with SPNs have a 5-year survival rate of 95%.[5,30,31] Despite favorable prognosis, 10% to 15% of patients have local invasion or distant metastases to the liver or peritoneum.[20,30] Perineural or lymphovascular invasion, invasion to peripancreatic soft tissue or an adjacent organ, capsular invasion, lymph node or distant metastasis, and increased solid proportion are highly associated with recurrence.[5,32]

## ACINAR CELL CARCINOMA

ACCs are composed of epithelial cells that bear a morphologic resemblance to acinar cells and produce pancreatic exocrine enzymes.[33] ACCs account for approximately 1% to 2% of adult and 15% of pediatric exocrine pancreatic neoplasms.[8,33,34] The mean age of the patients is 59 years, and men are more frequently affected than women (male to female ratio, 2:1).[33,35] Patients usually present with nonspecific symptoms such as abdominal pain, weight loss, nausea, and diarrhea. In contrast with ductal adenocarcinomas, patients rarely present with jaundice.[33] Patients with metastatic disease show symptoms caused by lipase hypersecretion, including subcutaneous fat necrosis, polyarthralgia, and eosinophilia.[33,35] Occasional increase of serum alpha fetoprotein (AFP) levels is observed, especially in younger patients.[8,34,36] Most ACCs occur sporadically; however, a few cases are reported in patients with hereditary nonpolyposis colorectal cancer syndrome (Lynch syndrome) or familial adenomatous polyposis (FAP).[34,35,37,38]

## GROSS FEATURES

ACCs can be observed in any part of the pancreas, but are most commonly noted in the pancreatic head.[33,35] Most ACCs are well-circumscribed, bulky, solitary masses with an average diameter of 8 to 11 cm.[33,35] The cut surface is usually pink to tan, soft, and fleshy (Fig. 4A). Hemorrhage, necrosis, and cystic changes can be observed. Infiltration into adjacent structures through the capsule is present in about 50% of ACC cases.[35] Some cases show polypoid tumor growth in the dilated pancreatic ducts,[39–42] which may be related to less infiltrative clinicopathologic characteristics.[41]

## MICROSCOPIC FEATURES

At scanning-power magnification, ACCs are cellular tumors with scant fibrous stroma.[2] ACCs have several different structural patterns, including acinar (Fig. 4B), solid (Fig. 4C), cribriform, trabecular, and glandular (Fig. 4D) patterns. The most common pattern is acinar, which is characterized by the arrangement of tumor cells into acinar units with basally located nuclei and moderate amounts of granular eosinophilic apical cytoplasm containing minute lumens. The solid pattern is characterized by large sheets of cells without evident luminal formation. Less common patterns include glandular, cribriform, and trabecular patterns. A mixture of these structural patterns is often found within an individual tumor.[8] These growth patterns are also common in PanNETs; therefore, PanNETs are included as a differential diagnosis with ACCs.

At higher-power magnification, tumor cells contain fairly uniform nuclei. Large, central, single, prominent nucleoli are characteristic and can provide an important clue for the diagnosis in cases with a solid growth pattern.[8] Marked nuclear pleomorphism is uncommonly observed (Fig. 5A).[35] Cytoplasm varies from eosinophilic to amphophilic, is finely granular, and contains abundant zymogen granules. In some cases, cytoplasmic granularity is not well developed.

Uncommonly, ACCs show morphologic variations, including oncocytic (Fig. 5B), clear cell (Fig. 5C), signet ring cell (Fig. 5D), and spindle cell features.[35] Oncocytic features are characterized by abundant eosinophilic granular cytoplasm with single, prominent nucleoli. Clear cell features show clear cytoplasm. Signet ring cell features are characterized by peripheral nuclear displacement by abundant granular cytoplasm. A rare malignant cystic lesion (acinar cell cystadenocarcinoma) also exists.[43]

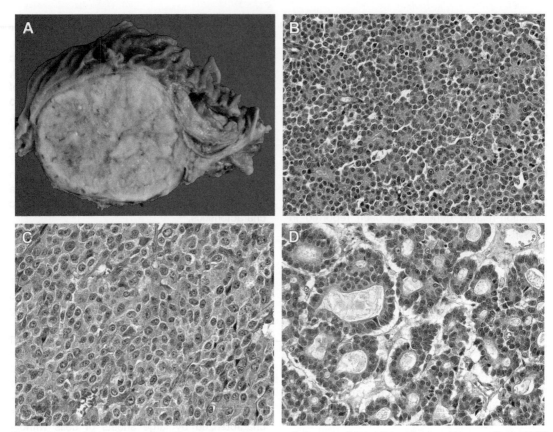

*Fig. 4.* Acinar cell carcinoma. (*A*) Gross features show a well-circumscribed solid, soft mass. Tumor cells show (*B*) acinar, (*C*) solid, and (*D*) glandular patterns. Tumor cells contain fairly uniform round to oval nuclei with single prominent nucleoli (H&E, original magnification *B–D*, ×400).

Special stains are needed to show the presence of enzymatic production in some cases, and zymogen granules are positive for PAS staining and resistant after diastase digestion. Immunohistochemical staining is much more specific and sensitive for pancreatic exocrine enzymes, including trypsin, chymotrypsin, lipase, and BCL10.[44] Trypsin and chymotrypsin have a 95% sensitivity to detect acinar differentiation (Fig. 6A).[8,44] BCL10 antibody (clone 331.3) recognizes the carboxy terminal of carboxyl ester lipase and is highly specific and sensitive for ACCs (Fig. 6B).[35,45,46] Pancreatic and duodenal homeobox (Pdx1),[47] pancreatic stone protein, pancreatic secretory trypsin inhibitor, and phospholipase A2 are also commonly expressed in ACCs.[44,47,48] Of these acinar markers, trypsin, chymotrypsin, and BCL10 are reliable markers.[35] ACCs commonly contain focal endocrine differentiation. Identifying the neuroendocrine component is difficult with routine hematoxylin-eosin slides. As such, immunohistochemical staining for the neuroendocrine markers synaptophysin and chromogranin is mandatory.[34]

## MIXED ACINAR CELL CARCINOMAS

Mixed ACCs are defined by the presence of significant (>25%) portions of other tumor components, including PanNETs and ductal adenocarcinomas, with ACCs.[33] For example, mixed acinar-neuroendocrine carcinomas are classified when both neuroendocrine (>25% of the neoplastic cells) and acinar (>25%) components are substantial parts of the tumor.[33,49] Similarly, mixed acinar-ductal carcinoma is categorized when the tumor has ACC (>25%) and ductal adenocarcinoma (>25%) as parts of the tumor volume.[33,49] Mixed acinar-neuroendocrine-ductal carcinomas are carcinomas containing ACC, ductal adenocarcinoma, and PanNET components.[33]

## DIFFERENTIAL DIAGNOSES

Other nonductal pancreatic neoplasms with solid and cellular appearances, including PanNETs, PBs, and SPNs, should be included as differential diagnoses with ACCs.[2]

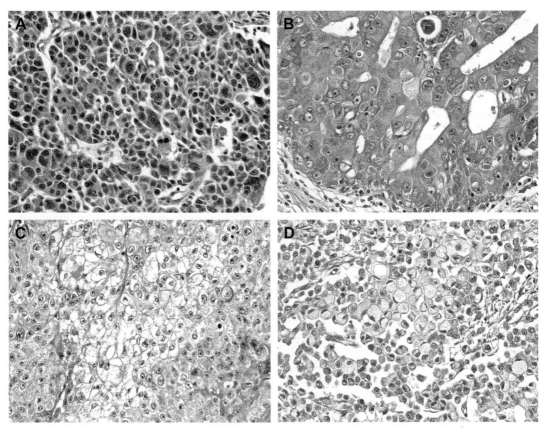

*Fig. 5.* Acinar cell carcinoma. Rarely, acinar cell carcinomas show (*A*) marked nuclear pleomorphism, and (*B*) oncocytic, (*C*) clear cell, and (*D*) signet ring cell features (H&E, original magnification *A–D* ×400).

PanNETs have overlapping structural patterns with ACCs, including trabecular, solid, and acinar patterns, and cytologic features such as monomorphic nuclei and eosinophilic or amphophilic cytoplasm. Histologic features suggestive of ACCs include large tumor size with diameter greater than 6 cm, diffuse necrosis, basally located nuclei, single prominent nucleoli, eosinophilic cytoplasm, and high mitotic count (>10/10 high-power fields).[3,35]

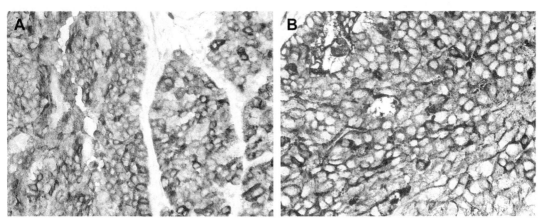

*Fig. 6.* Acinar cell carcinoma. Tumor cells show diffuse cytoplasmic labeling for (*A*) trypsin and (*B*) BCL10 (original magnification *A, B* ×400).

**Key Features**
OF ACINAR CELL CARCINOMAS

- Well-circumscribed, solid pancreatic head mass

- Cellular tumors with scant fibrous stroma

- Predominant acinar or solid patterns

- Tumor cells with fairly uniform nuclei and large, central, and single prominent nucleoli

- Diffusely positive for the acinar cell markers trypsin, chymotrypsin, and BCL10

## MOLECULAR PATHOLOGY

Half of ACCs show loss of heterozygosity (LOH) on chromosome 11p.[50,51] Alterations in the APC/beta-catenin pathway, either an activating CTNNB1 mutation or a truncating APC mutation, are observed in up to 25% of ACCs.[50,52,53] Similarly, abnormal nuclear and cytoplasmic beta-catenin labeling is reported in up to 20% of ACCs.[35,54] TP53 mutations are present in 17% to 23% of ACCs,[53,54] and corresponding abnormal nuclear p53 expression is noted in 27% of ACCs.[35] DPC4/SMAD4 mutations are reported in up to 17% of ACCs.[50,53–56]

## PROGNOSIS

ACCs are highly aggressive neoplasms.[33] Patient outcomes are better than for stage-matched ductal adenocarcinomas but worse than for PanNETs.[57,58] All mixed ACCs are clinically aggressive, similar to pure ACCs.[35] The most important prognostic factor is stage.[33,35] Most often, metastatic disease is found in regional lymph nodes and the liver.[8] The median survival for all patients is 18 to 19 months,[59] and it is common for patients with distant metastases to survive for 2 to 3 years.[8] ACCs occurring in young patients (<20 years old) seem to have a better prognosis.[33]

## PANCREATOBLASTOMA

PBs are carcinomas with multilineage differentiation (most commonly acinar differentiation with distinctive squamoid nests or corpuscles, and less commonly endocrine and ductal differentiation).[60] PBs show a bimodal age distribution pattern, with one peak in childhood (first decade of life) and the second peak in late adulthood.[60] After PB was first reported by Becker[61] in 1957, fewer than 200 PB cases in children and fewer than 50 cases in adults have been reported in the English literature.[62–64] The median age of patients with PB is 4 years (range, 1 month to 17 years) for children and 37 years (range, 18–78 years) for adults.[8,64,65] In both children and adults, a slight male predominance is observed.[65,66] Presenting symptoms are usually nonspecific and include abdominal pain, weight loss, jaundice, and palpable abdominal mass.[64] Like ACCs, PBs can cause an increased serum AFP level. Although most PBs occur sporadically, some cases present in patients with Beckwith-Wiedemann syndrome, which is characterized by abnormal body growth, including hemihypertrophy, exomphalos, macroglossia, and gigantism.[67] A single case of adult PB was reported in a patient with FAP.[68]

## GROSS FEATURES

Most PBs are well-circumscribed, bulky, solitary, masses with an average diameter of 11 cm.[60] The tumors occur in the head and tail of the pancreas with equal frequencies.[8] The cut surface is usually yellow, tan, or gray, and soft and fleshy (Fig. 7A). Most tumors are partially encapsulated and lobulated with prominent necrosis.[60] Rarely, the tumors are cystic, especially in cases arising in patients with Beckwith-Wiedemann syndrome.[69,70] Hemorrhage, necrosis, and calcifications are also frequently observed in PBs.[71]

## MICROSCOPIC FEATURES

At scanning-power magnification, PBs consist of large, highly cellular lobules separated by dense fibrous stroma (Fig. 7B).[8] The lobules often produce an appearance of darker and lighter staining cells.[8] The darker staining cells form sheets or nests of small epithelial cells with acinar differentiation, which show round nuclei and prominent central nucleoli with scanty amphophilic cytoplasm.[8,60] The lighter-staining cells usually form circumscribed nests and contain larger nuclei and more abundant eosinophilic cytoplasm.[8] These cells are called squamoid nests or squamoid corpuscles and are a diagnostic clue for PB. Squamoid nests show variable appearances, from large islands of plump epithelioid cells to whorled nests of spindled cells (Fig. 7C).[60] Occasional keratinization of squamoid nests is also reported.[72] Often, clear nuclei are noted only in tumor cells of squamoid nests, which are reactive for biotin.[73] Neuroendocrine components are usually dispersed diffusely among the acinar cells but are often arranged with solid nests or trabecular architecture.[3] Neuroendocrine cells have round

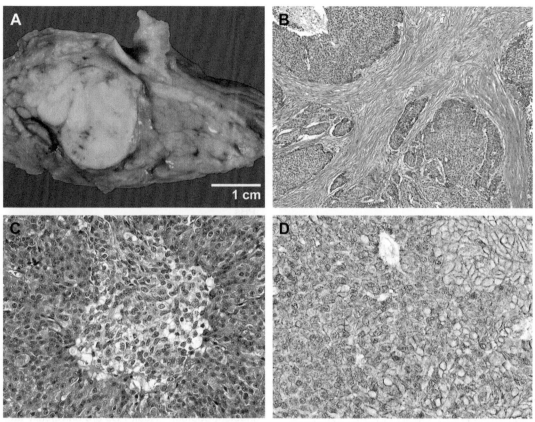

**Fig. 7.** Pancreatoblastoma. (*A*) Grossly, a well-circumscribed, lobulated, solid, soft mass is seen. (*B*) A geographic lobulated tumor is separated by fibrous stroma. (*C*) A well-circumscribed squamoid nest surrounded by tumor cells shows (*D*) patchy abnormal beta-catenin labeling in sheetlike pattern, whereas other surrounding tumor cells show membranous beta-catenin labeling ([B] H&E, ×100; [C] H&E, ×400; [D] beta-catenin, ×400).

to oval nuclei with typical salt-and-pepper patterned chromatin. Ductal components present focally in most cases.[3] Rarely, cases have mucinous glands and are positive for mucicarmine staining.[3] Fibrous stroma divides lobules in PBs, and the cellularity of spindle cells in the stroma varies from acellular to hypercellular.[3] The stroma is usually more hypercellular in pediatric tumors than in adult tumors.[60] Some heterologous components, such as cartilage and bone, are also present.

Similar to ACCs, zymogen granules in tumor cells with acinar cell differentiation are positive for PAS staining and resistant after diastase treatment. Because PBs are carcinomas with multilineage differentiation and contain tumor cells with predominantly acinar differentiation and less common endocrine and ductal differentiation, the tumor cells show variable immunoreactivity based on their differentiation lineage. All PB components are diffusely labeled by epithelial membranous antigen and special cytokeratin subclasses, including cytokeratin 8, 18, and 19.[74] PBs express

markers of acinar, endocrine, and ductal differentiation. Because the predominant component of PBs is acinar cell differentiation, they show immunoreactivity for pancreatic exocrine enzymes, including trypsin and chymotrypsin in most cases, whereas lipase is less commonly expressed.[75] The neuroendocrine markers synaptophysin and chromogranin are labeled in variable proportions in 66% of PB cases.[75] Pdx1 labeling has been reported in acinar components but not in squamoid nests.[47] Aberrant cytoplasmic and nuclear beta-catenin labeling is reported in 75% of PBs.[68,76] Although abnormal labeling is patchy and limited to squamoid nests of sheetlike growth (**Fig. 7**D), tumor cells with acinar differentiation and stromal cells show normal membranous beta-catenin labeling.[3]

## DIFFERENTIAL DIAGNOSES

Other nonductal pancreatic neoplasms with solid and cellular appearance, such as PanNETs, ACCs, and SPNs, should be included as differential diagnoses with PBs.[2] Of these diseases, differentials with ACCs are extremely difficult, especially in the biopsy setting, because of the overlapping histologic features of PBs and ACCs. In children, most tumors with acinar differentiation are PBs, and thoroughly searching for identifying squamoid nests is important.[8] In adults, the frequency of ACCs is higher than that of PBs. Pathologists should reserve the diagnosis of PB for cases in which the classic histologic features of lobular tumors, geographic scanning-power view, predominant neuroendocrine and ductal differentiation, and characteristic squamoid nests are present.[8]

## Key Features
### OF PANCREATOBLASTOMAS

- Well-circumscribed, lobulated, solid mass
- Cellular geographic lobules are separated by fibrous stroma
- Tumor cells with predominantly acinar, less commonly neuroendocrine and ductal, differentiation
- Squamoid nests: large islands of plump epithelioid cells to whorled nests of spindled cells

## MOLECULAR PATHOLOGY

Recent whole-exome sequencing analysis showed fewer genome-wide mutations in PBs than in ACCs.[51] The most common genetic alteration is LOH of chromosome 11p, similar to ACCs.[51,68,77] Alterations in the beta-catenin/APC pathway have also been reported in 50% to 90% of PBs.[51,68,76] The most commonly involved gene is CTNNB1, which encodes beta-catenin. One patient with FAP showed biallelic APC inactivation.[68] SMAD4/DPC4 mutations are detected in a small portion of cases, but no KRAS mutations or abnormal p53 expressions have been detected in PBs.[68,78]

## PROGNOSIS

Metastasis is detected in approximately 50% of pediatric and adult patients with PB at the time of diagnosis.[64–66] The most commonly occurring metastatic sites for PBs, in order of decreasing frequency, are the liver, regional lymph nodes, lung, and peritoneum.[8,75] Outcome is more favorable in children than in adults.[65,66] One of the reasons for a more favorable prognosis in children is that pediatric PBs more often present with a nonmetastatic and well-encapsulated tumor and show an indolent course.[60] Adult PBs are universally fatal, with rapid progression in most cases.[66,75] Factors associated with better prognosis include surgical resection and localized disease.[64,66]

### Table 1
Differential diagnosis of nonductal pancreatic neoplasms

|  | Solid pseudopapillary neoplasms | Acinar cell carcinomas | Pancreatoblastomas |
|---|---|---|---|
| Age (y) | 29 | 59 | 4 (pediatric)/37 (adult) |
| Sex Predominance | Female (1:9) | Male (2:1) | Slightly male |
| Gross | Mixed solid and cystic portions | Solid | Solid |
| Microscopic | Solid growth Cellular tumors Sheets of monomorphic polygonal tumor cells Pseudopapillary structure Abundant degenerative changes | Cellular tumors with scant fibrous stroma Predominant acinar or solid patterns Tumor cells with fairly uniform nuclei Large, prominent nucleoli | Cellular geographic lobules separated by fibrous stroma Tumor cells with acinar, neuroendocrine, and ductal differentiation Squamoid nests |
| Immunohistochemical | Nuclear/cytoplasmic beta-catenin (>95%) CD10 (83%) Loss of membranous E-cadherin | Trypsin/chymotrypsin BCL10 (86%) Nuclear/cytoplasmic beta-catenin (13%) | Nuclear/cytoplasmic beta-catenin (75%) |
| CTNNB1 Mutation (%) | 95 | 25 | 55 |

## SUMMARY

Although they are uncommon, nonductal pancreatic cancers such as SPNs, ACCs, and PBs share overlapping gross, microscopic, immunohistochemical, and genetic features, including well-demarcated solid neoplasms, monotonous cellular tumor cells with little intervening stroma, and abnormal beta-catenin expression. Nonductal pancreatic cancers also have clinicopathologic characteristics that are different from those of more commonly encountered ductal adenocarcinomas. Understanding of these characteristic clinicopathologic features is useful for correct diagnosis and treatment of patients with nonductal pancreatic cancers (Table 1).

## REFERENCES

1. Klimstra DS, Hruban RH, Pitman MB. Pancreas. In: Mills SE, editor. Histology for pathologists. 4th edition. Philadelphia: Lippincott Williams & Wilkins; 2012. p. 777–816.

2. Klimstra DS, Pitman MB, Hruban RH. An algorithmic approach to the diagnosis of pancreatic neoplasms. Arch Pathol Lab Med 2009;133:454–64.

3. Hruban RH, Pitman MB, Klimstra DS. Tumors of the pancreas. 4th edition. Washington, DC: American Registry of Pathology; 2007.

4. Kloppel G, Hruban RH, Klimstra DS, et al. Solid-pseudopapillary neoplasm of the pancreas. In: Bosman FT, Carneiro F, Hruban RH, et al, editors. WHO classification of the tumors of the digestive system. 4th edition. Lyon (France): IARC Press; 2010. p. 327–30.

5. Kang CM, Choi SH, Kim SC, et al. Predicting recurrence of pancreatic solid pseudopapillary tumors after surgical resection: a multicenter analysis in Korea. Ann Surg 2014;260:348–55.

6. Kim CW, Han DJ, Kim J, et al. Solid pseudopapillary tumor of the pancreas: can malignancy be predicted? Surgery 2011;149:625–34.

7. Law JK, Ahmed A, Singh VK, et al. A systematic review of solid-pseudopapillary neoplasms: are these rare lesions? Pancreas 2014;43:331–7.

8. Klimstra DS. Nonductal neoplasms of the pancreas. Mod Pathol 2007;20(Suppl 1):S94–112.

9. Yamaguchi K, Hirakata R, Kitamura K. Papillary cystic neoplasm of the pancreas: radiological and pathological characteristics in 11 cases. Br J Surg 1990;77:1000–3.

10. Buetow PC, Buck JL, Pantongrag-Brown L, et al. Solid and papillary epithelial neoplasm of the pancreas: imaging-pathologic correlation on 56 cases. Radiology 1996;199:707–11.

11. Matsunou H, Konishi F, Yamamichi N, et al. Solid, infiltrating variety of papillary cystic neoplasm of the pancreas. Cancer 1990;65:2747–57.

12. Stommer P, Kraus J, Stolte M, et al. Solid and cystic pancreatic tumors. Clinical, histochemical, and electron microscopic features in ten cases. Cancer 1991;67:1635–41.

13. Lieber MR, Lack EE, Roberts JR Jr, et al. Solid and papillary epithelial neoplasm of the pancreas. An ultrastructural and immunocytochemical study of six cases. Am J Surg Pathol 1987;11:85–93.

14. Pettinato G, Manivel JC, Ravetto C, et al. Papillary cystic tumor of the pancreas. A clinicopathologic study of 20 cases with cytologic, immunohistochemical, ultrastructural, and flow cytometric observations, and a review of the literature. Am J Clin Pathol 1992;98:478–88.

15. Meriden Z, Shi C, Edil BH, et al. Hyaline globules in neuroendocrine and solid-pseudopapillary neoplasms of the pancreas: a clue to the diagnosis. Am J Surg Pathol 2011;35:981–8.

16. Albores-Saavedra J, Simpson KW, Bilello SJ. The clear cell variant of solid pseudopapillary tumor of the pancreas: a previously unrecognized pancreatic neoplasm. Am J Surg Pathol 2006;30:1237–42.

17. Goldstein J, Benharroch D, Sion-Vardy N, et al. Solid cystic and papillary tumor of the pancreas with oncocytic differentiation. J Surg Oncol 1994;56:63–7.

18. Kim SA, Kim MS, Kim MS, et al. Pleomorphic solid pseudopapillary neoplasm of the pancreas: degenerative change rather than high-grade malignant potential. Hum Pathol 2014;45:166–74.

19. Li L, Othman M, Rashid A, et al. Solid pseudopapillary neoplasm of the pancreas with prominent atypical multinucleated giant tumour cells. Histopathology 2013;62:465–71.

20. Tang LH, Aydin H, Brennan MF, et al. Clinically aggressive solid pseudopapillary tumors of the pancreas: a report of two cases with components of undifferentiated carcinoma and a comparative clinicopathologic analysis of 34 conventional cases. Am J Surg Pathol 2005;29:512–9.

21. Yang F, Yu X, Bao Y, et al. Prognostic value of Ki-67 in solid pseudopapillary tumor of the pancreas: Huashan experience and systematic review of the literature. Surgery 2015;159(4):1023–31.

22. Abraham SC, Klimstra DS, Wilentz RE, et al. Solid-pseudopapillary tumors of the pancreas are genetically distinct from pancreatic ductal adenocarcinomas and almost always harbor beta-catenin mutations. Am J Pathol 2002;160:1361–9.

23. Tanaka Y, Kato K, Notohara K, et al. Frequent beta-catenin mutation and cytoplasmic/nuclear accumulation in pancreatic solid-pseudopapillary neoplasm. Cancer Res 2001;61:8401–4.

24. Kim MJ, Jang SJ, Yu E. Loss of E-cadherin and cytoplasmic-nuclear expression of beta-catenin are the most useful immunoprofiles in the diagnosis of solid-pseudopapillary neoplasm of the pancreas. Hum Pathol 2008;39:251–8.

25. El-Bahrawy MA, Rowan A, Horncastle D, et al. E-cadherin/catenin complex status in solid pseudo-papillary tumor of the pancreas. Am J Surg Pathol 2008;32:1–7.

26. Notohara K, Hamazaki S, Tsukayama C, et al. Solid-pseudopapillary tumor of the pancreas: immunohis-tochemical localization of neuroendocrine markers and CD10. Am J Surg Pathol 2000;24:1361–71.

27. Martin RC, Klimstra DS, Brennan MF, et al. Solid-pseudopapillary tumor of the pancreas: a surgical enigma? Ann Surg Oncol 2002;9:35–40.

28. Wu J, Jiao Y, Dal Molin M, et al. Whole-exome sequencing of neoplastic cysts of the pancreas reveals recurrent mutations in components of ubiquitin-dependent pathways. Proc Natl Acad Sci U S A 2011;108:21188–93.

29. Park M, Kim M, Hwang D, et al. Characterization of gene expression and activated signaling pathways in solid-pseudopapillary neoplasm of pancreas. Mod Pathol 2014;27:580–93.

30. Reddy S, Cameron JL, Scudiere J, et al. Surgical management of solid-pseudopapillary neoplasms of the pancreas (Franz or Hamoudi tumors): a large single-institutional series. J Am Coll Surg 2009;208:950–9.

31. Papavramidis T, Papavramidis S. Solid pseudopapil-lary tumors of the pancreas: review of 718 patients reported in English literature. J Am Coll Surg 2005;200:965–72.

32. Hwang J, Kim DY, Kim SC, et al. Solid-pseudopapil-lary neoplasm of the pancreas in children: can we predict malignancy? J Pediatr Surg 2014;49:1730–3.

33. Klimstra DS, Hruban RH, Kloppel G, et al. Acinar cell neoplasms of the pancreas. In: Bosman FT, Carneiro F, Hruban RH, et al, editors. WHO classifi-cation of the tumors of the digestive system. 4th edi-tion. Lyon (France): IARC Press; 2010. p. 314–8.

34. La Rosa S, Sessa F, Capella C. Acinar cell carci-noma of the pancreas: overview of clinicopathologic features and insights into the molecular pathology. Front Med (Lausanne) 2015;2:41.

35. La Rosa S, Adsay V, Albarello L, et al. Clinicopatho-logic study of 62 acinar cell carcinomas of the pancreas: insights into the morphology and immu-nophenotype and search for prognostic markers. Am J Surg Pathol 2012;36:1782–95.

36. Cingolani N, Shaco-Levy R, Farruggio A, et al. Alpha-fetoprotein production by pancreatic tumors exhibiting acinar cell differentiation: study of five cases, one arising in a mediastinal teratoma. Hum Pathol 2000;31:938–44.

37. Karamurzin Y, Zeng Z, Stadler ZK, et al. Unusual DNA mismatch repair-deficient tumors in Lynch syndrome: a report of new cases and review of the literature. Hum Pathol 2012;43:1677–87.

38. Liu W, Shia J, Gonen M, et al. DNA mismatch repair abnormalities in acinar cell carcinoma of the pancreas: frequency and clinical significance. Pancreas 2014;43:1264–70.

39. Toll AD, Mitchell D, Yeo CJ, et al. Acinar cell carci-noma with prominent intraductal growth pattern: case report and review of the literature. Int J Surg Pathol 2011;19:795–9.

40. Basturk O, Zamboni G, Klimstra DS, et al. Intraduc-tal and papillary variants of acinar cell carcinomas: a new addition to the challenging differential diag-nosis of intraductal neoplasms. Am J Surg Pathol 2007;31:363–70.

41. Ban D, Shimada K, Sekine S, et al. Pancreatic ducts as an important route of tumor extension for acinar cell carcinoma of the pancreas. Am J Surg Pathol 2010;34:1025–36.

42. Fabre A, Sauvanet A, Flejou JF, et al. Intraductal acinar cell carcinoma of the pancreas. Virchows Arch 2001;438:312–5.

43. Colombo P, Arizzi C, Roncalli M. Acinar cell cystade-nocarcinoma of the pancreas: report of rare case and review of the literature. Hum Pathol 2004;35:1568–71.

44. Hoorens A, Lemoine NR, McLellan E, et al. Pancre-atic acinar cell carcinoma. An analysis of cell lineage markers, p53 expression, and Ki-ras mutation. Am J Pathol 1993;143:685–98.

45. La Rosa S, Franzi F, Marchet S, et al. The mono-clonal anti-BCL10 antibody (clone 331.1) is a sensi-tive and specific marker of pancreatic acinar cell carcinoma and pancreatic metaplasia. Virchows Arch 2009;454:133–42.

46. Hosoda W, Sasaki E, Murakami Y, et al. BCL10 as a useful marker for pancreatic acinar cell carcinoma, especially using endoscopic ultrasound cytology specimens. Pathol Int 2013;63:176–82.

47. Park JY, Hong SM, Klimstra DS, et al. Pdx1 expres-sion in pancreatic precursor lesions and neoplasms. Appl Immunohistochem Mol Morphol 2011;19:444–9.

48. Kuopio T, Ekfors TO, Nikkanen V, et al. Acinar cell carcinoma of the pancreas. Report of three cases. APMIS 1995;103:69–78.

49. Stelow EB, Shaco-Levy R, Bao F, et al. Pancreatic acinar cell carcinomas with prominent ductal differ-entiation: Mixed acinar ductal carcinoma and mixed acinar endocrine ductal carcinoma. Am J Surg Pathol 2010;34:510–8.

50. Abraham SC, Wu TT, Hruban RH, et al. Genetic and immunohistochemical analysis of pancreatic acinar cell carcinoma: frequent allelic loss on chromosome 11p and alterations in the APC/beta-catenin pathway. Am J Pathol 2002;160:953–62.

51. Jiao Y, Yonescu R, Offerhaus GJ, et al. Whole-exome sequencing of pancreatic neoplasms with acinar dif-ferentiation. J Pathol 2014;232:428–35.

52. Furlan D, Sahnane N, Bernasconi B, et al. APC alter-ations are frequently involved in the pathogenesis of

acinar cell carcinoma of the pancreas, mainly through gene loss and promoter hypermethylation. Virchows Arch 2014;464:553–64.

53. Chmielecki J, Hutchinson KE, Frampton GM, et al. Comprehensive genomic profiling of pancreatic acinar cell carcinomas identifies recurrent RAF fusions and frequent inactivation of DNA repair genes. Cancer Discov 2014;4:1398–405.

54. de Wilde RF, Ottenhof NA, Jansen M, et al. Analysis of LKB1 mutations and other molecular alterations in pancreatic acinar cell carcinoma. Mod Pathol 2011; 24:1229–36.

55. Moore PS, Orlandini S, Zamboni G, et al. Pancreatic tumours: molecular pathways implicated in ductal cancer are involved in ampullary but not in exocrine nonductal or endocrine tumorigenesis. Br J Cancer 2001;84:253–62.

56. Rigaud G, Moore PS, Zamboni G, et al. Allelotype of pancreatic acinar cell carcinoma. Int J Cancer 2000; 88:772–7.

57. Schmidt CM, Matos JM, Bentrem DJ, et al. Acinar cell carcinoma of the pancreas in the United States: prognostic factors and comparison to ductal adenocarcinoma. J Gastrointest Surg 2008; 12:2078–86.

58. Wisnoski NC, Townsend CM Jr, Nealon WH, et al. 672 patients with acinar cell carcinoma of the pancreas: a population-based comparison to pancreatic adeno-carcinoma. Surgery 2008;144:141–8.

59. Klimstra DS, Heffess CS, Oertel JE, et al. Acinar cell carcinoma of the pancreas. A clinicopathologic study of 28 cases. Am J Surg Pathol 1992;16: 815–37.

60. Morohoshi T, Hruban RH, Klimstra DS, et al. Pancreatoblastoma. In: Bosman FT, Carneiro F, Hruban RH, et al, editors. WHO classification of the tumors of the digestive system. Lyon (France): IARC Press; 2010. p. 319–21.

61. Becker WF. Pancreatoduodenectomy for carcinoma of the pancreas in an infant; report of a case. Ann Surg 1957;145:864–72.

62. Omiyale AO. Clinicopathological review of pancreatoblastoma in adults. Gland Surg 2015;4:322–8.

63. Zouros E, Manatakis DK, Delis SG, et al. Adult pancreatoblastoma: a case report and review of the literature. Oncol Lett 2015;9:2293–8.

64. Salman B, Brat G, Yoon YS, et al. The diagnosis and surgical treatment of pancreatoblastoma in adults: a case series and review of the literature. J Gastrointest Surg 2013;17:2153–61.

65. Bien E, Godzinski J, Dall'igna P, et al. Pancreatoblastoma: a report from the European Cooperative Study Group for Paediatric Rare Tumours (EXPeRT). Eur J Cancer 2011;47:2347–52.

66. Dhebri AR, Connor S, Campbell F, et al. Diagnosis, treatment and outcome of pancreatoblastoma. Pancreatology 2004;4:441–53.

67. Muguerza R, Rodriguez A, Formigo E, et al. Pancreatoblastoma associated with incomplete Beckwith-Wiedemann syndrome: case report and review of the literature. J Pediatr Surg 2005;40:1341–4.

68. Abraham SC, Wu TT, Klimstra DS, et al. Distinctive molecular genetic alterations in sporadic and familial adenomatous polyposis-associated pancreatoblastomas: frequent alterations in the APC/beta-catenin pathway and chromosome 11p. Am J Pathol 2001;159:1619–27.

69. Drut R, Jones MC. Congenital pancreatoblastoma in Beckwith-Wiedemann syndrome: an emerging association. Pediatr Pathol 1988;8:331–9.

70. Koh TH, Cooper JE, Newman CL, et al. Pancreatoblastoma in a neonate with Wiedemann-Beckwith syndrome. Eur J Pediatr 1986;145:435–8.

71. Kohda E, Iseki M, Ikawa H, et al. Pancreatoblastoma. Three original cases and review of the literature. Acta Radiol 2000;41:334–7.

72. Hammer ST, Owens SR. Pancreatoblastoma: a rare, adult pancreatic tumor with many faces. Arch Pathol Lab Med 2013;137:1224–6.

73. Tanaka Y, Ijiri R, Yamanaka S, et al. Pancreatoblastoma: optically clear nuclei in squamoid corpuscles are rich in biotin. Mod Pathol 1998;11:945–9.

74. Nishimata S, Kato K, Tanaka M, et al. Expression pattern of keratin subclasses in pancreatoblastoma with special emphasis on squamoid corpuscles. Pathol Int 2005;55:297–302.

75. Klimstra DS, Wenig BM, Adair CF, et al. Pancreatoblastoma. A clinicopathologic study and review of the literature. Am J Surg Pathol 1995;19:1371–89.

76. Tanaka Y, Kato K, Notohara K, et al. Significance of aberrant (cytoplasmic/nuclear) expression of beta-catenin in pancreatoblastoma. J Pathol 2003;199: 185–90.

77. Kerr NJ, Chun YH, Yun K, et al. Pancreatoblastoma is associated with chromosome 11p loss of heterozygosity and IGF2 overexpression. Med Pediatr Oncol 2002;39:52–4.

78. Hoorens A, Gebhard F, Kraft K, et al. Pancreatoblastoma in an adult: its separation from acinar cell carcinoma. Virchows Arch 1994;424:485–90.

# Pancreatic Neuroendocrine Tumors

Safia N. Salaria, MD, Chanjuan Shi, MD, PhD*

## KEYWORDS

- Well-differentiated pancreatic neuroendocrine tumor • Pancreatic neuroendocrine carcinoma
- Pathologic features • Morphologic variants • WHO classification • Differential diagnosis
- Prognosis • Ki67

## Key points

- Pancreatic neuroendocrine neoplasms are classified into well-differentiated pancreatic neuroendocrine tumor (PanNET) and pancreatic neuroendocrine carcinoma (NEC) with well-differentiated PanNET accounting for most neoplasms.

- Although most well-differentiated PanNETs are well-circumscribed and hypercellular lesions composed of uniform tumor cells showing salt-pepper chromatin and arranged in different patterns, a number of morphologic variants have been described.

- Several immunohistochemical markers can be used to differentiate pancreatic neuroendocrine neoplasms from other pancreatic primaries or metastatic carcinomas from other origins; however, there are no specific markers that can be used to differentiate pancreatic neuroendocrine neoplasms from neuroendocrine neoplasms of other sites.

- NECs are uniformly deadly, but well-differentiated PanNETs have variable prognosis. Ki67 is the only prognostic marker routinely used in clinical practice.

## ABSTRACT

Pancreatic neuroendocrine neoplasms include well-differentiated pancreatic neuroendocrine tumors (PanNETs) and neuroendocrine carcinomas (NECs) with well-differentiated PanNETs accounting for most cases. Other pancreatic primaries and metastatic carcinomas from other sites can mimic pancreatic neuroendocrine neoplasms. Immunohistochemical studies can be used to aid in the differential diagnosis. However, no specific markers are available to differentiate PanNETs from NETs of other sites. Although NECs are uniformly deadly, PanNETs have variable prognosis. Morphology alone cannot predict the tumor behavior. Although some pathologic features are associated with an aggressive course, Ki67 is the only prognostic molecular marker routinely used in clinical practice.

## OVERVIEW

Pancreatic neuroendocrine tumors (PanNETs) represent up to 2% of all pancreatic neoplasms. After pancreatic ductal adenocarcinoma they are the second most common primary pancreatic malignancy. There has been a gradual increase in incidence over the past 40 years, with annual incidence among the general population of less than 1 per 100,000 persons per year.[1–3] They are seen only slightly more frequently in men compared with women and in African American as compared with white individuals. Most occur sporadically in adults between the sixth and eighth decades;

Disclosure Statement: There is no conflict of interest for both authors.
Department of Pathology, Microbiology, and Immunology, Vanderbilt University Medical Center, 1161 21st Avenue South, C-3321 MCN, Nashville, TN 37232-2561, USA
* Corresponding author.
E-mail address: Chanjuan.Shi@vanderbilt.edu

Surgical Pathology 9 (2016) 595–617
http://dx.doi.org/10.1016/j.path.2016.05.006

**Table 1**
Hereditary syndromes associated with pancreatic neuroendocrine tumor (PanNET)

| Syndrome | Gene Involved | Clinical Presentations | Frequency of PanNET | Clinicopathologic Features |
|---|---|---|---|---|
| Multiple endocrine neoplasia, type 1 | MEN-1 | Hyperplasia/neoplasms in the parathyroid, pituitary, pancreas, and duodenum | Up to 100% | Nonfunctional or functional (insulinoma: most common functional tumor); gastrinoma (always in the duodenum) |
| von Hippel Lindau | VHL | Pheochromocytoma, hemangioblastoma, clear-cell renal cell carcinoma, pancreatic tumors (PanNETs and serous cystadenoma), and tumors of the middle ear and epididymis | 11%–17% | Nonfunctional only; can be clear-cell PanNETs (need to be differentiated from metastatic renal cell carcinoma or solid serous cystadenoma) |
| Neurofibromatosis type 1 | NF-1 | Café-au-lait macules, neurofibromas, skin-fold freckling, iris Lisch nodules, and bony dysplasia | Rare | Nonfunctional or functional; mostly ampullary somatostatinoma |
| Tuberous sclerosis | TSC1 TSC2 | Hamartomas, disabling neurologic disorders, and dermatologic findings | 2% | Nonfunctional or functional |

however, PanNETs associated with syndromes, for example, multiple endocrine neoplasia (MEN) 1 and Von Hippel Lindau (VHL), do occur in younger patients.[1] There are 4 well-established hereditary syndromes associated with PanNETs (Table 1 and further discussed in the article see Pittman ME, Brosens LA, Wood LD: Genetic Syndromes with Pancreatic Manifestations, in this issue).

PanNETs are classified as functional when associated with hormone secretion and a clinical syndrome (Table 2) or nonfunctioning. More than 50% of PanNETs are nonfunctional in contemporary studies.[4] PanNETs measuring smaller than 0.5 cm are referred to as pancreatic neuroendocrine microadenomas and are by definition nonfunctional.[5] They are more frequently encountered in the setting of MEN1.[6]

The 2010 World Health Organization (WHO) classification divides the tumors into 3 grades (Table 3): grade 1 and 2 are classified as well-differentiated neuroendocrine tumors (NETs), and grade 3 is regarded as neuroendocrine carcinoma (NEC). The latter is further classified as small-cell or large-cell neuroendocrine carcinoma.

**Table 2**
Four most common functional pancreatic neuroendocrine tumors

| Pancreatic Neuroendocrine Tumor | Incidence (million/y) | Hormone | Syndrome | Clinical Behavior |
|---|---|---|---|---|
| Insulinoma | 1–3 | Insulin | Vasomotor symptoms, low blood sugar, and reversal of symptoms by glucose administration | Indolent |
| Gastrinoma | 0.1 | Gastrin | Complicated and uncomplicated gastric/duodenal ulcers | Can be aggressive |
| VIPoma | 0.05–0.2 | VIP | Large-volume secretory diarrhea causing dehydration and electrolyte disturbances | Mostly aggressive |
| Glucagonoma | 0.01–0.1 | Glucagon | Glucose intolerance, weight loss, and necrolytic migratory erythema | Mostly aggressive |

Abbreviation: VIP, vasoactive intestinal polypeptide.

*Table 3*
**Classification of pancreatic neuroendocrine neoplasms**

| Pancreatic Neuroendocrine Tumor | WHO Tumor Grade | | Pathologic Features | Subtypes |
|---|---|---|---|---|
| Well-differentiated neuroendocrine tumor | Grade 1 | Ki67 ≤2% and Mitosis <2/10 HPF | Tumor necrosis or apoptosis can be present, but rare and not prominent | 1. Grade 1–2 tumors 2. Well-differentiated tumors with high Ki67 3. Poorly differentiated component in well-differentiated tumors |
| | Grade 2 | Ki67 = 3–20% and Mitosis = 2–20/10 HPF | | |
| Neuroendocrine carcinoma | Grade 3 | Ki67 >20% or Mitosis >20/10 HPF | Frequent and prominent tumor necrosis and apoptosis | 1. Large-cell neuroendocrine carcinoma 2. Small-cell carcinoma |

*Abbreviation:* HPF, high-power field.

## GROSS FEATURES

## WELL-DIFFERENTIATED PANCREATIC NEUROENDOCRINE TUMORS

Well-differentiated PanNETs account for most pancreatic neuroendocrine neoplasms. They can arise throughout the pancreas; the pancreatic head and tail are common locations for functional tumors. Nonfunctional tumors have a predilection for the pancreatic head.[7] The cut surface can be red, yellow, tan, and variegated and the consistency ranges from firm fibrotic tumors to soft (**Figs. 1** and **2**). Some tumors may have areas of hemorrhage.

Smaller tumors (≤2 cm) can be single, well circumscribed, and limited to the pancreatic parenchyma (see **Fig. 2**). In contrast, larger PanNETs (≥5 cm) tend to be multinodular with extension into the peripancreatic soft tissue or adjacent organs (see **Fig. 1**). Small cystic spaces are a rare feature of PanNETs and are often a consequence of degenerative changes in larger lesions (see **Fig. 1**). Approximately 10% of PanNETs are well-demarcated, unilocular cystic lesions that contains clear to straw-colored fluid (**Fig. 3**).[8]

## PANCREATIC NEUROENDOCRINE CARCINOMA

Pancreatic NECs are often large with a diameter of 4 cm on average. Although NECs tend to demonstrate peripheral fibrosis, unlike well-differentiated tumors, their borders are more infiltrative. Necrosis and hemorrhage are frequently noted findings in NECs (**Fig. 4**). For this reason, these tumors tend to have firm and soft consistencies within the same lesion.[9]

*Fig. 1.* Gross picture of a large well-differentiated NET with multinodular appearance and tan/variegated/fibrotic cut surface. The tumor invades the spleen.

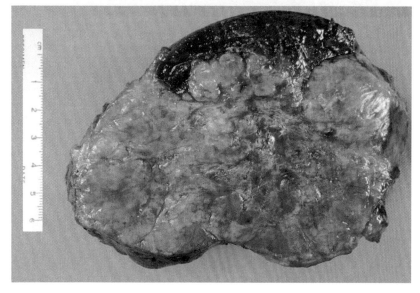

598

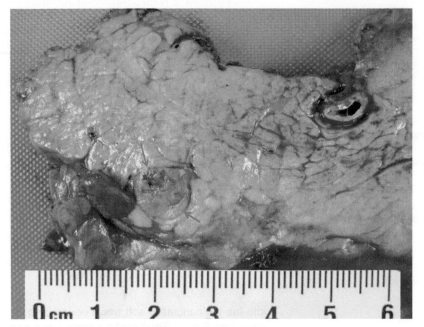

*Fig. 2.* Gross picture of a small well-differentiated NET with variegated and soft cut surface. The *arrows* are pointing to a small nodule of pancreatic neuroendocrine tumor. Note: the tumor is a single nodule that is well circumscribed.

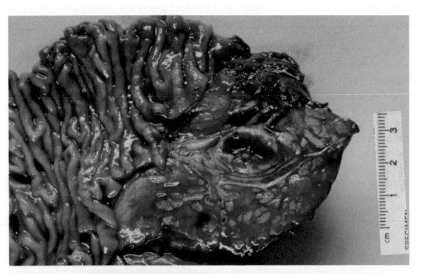

*Fig. 3.* Gross picture of a unilocular cystic NET that is well-defined from the background pancreas.

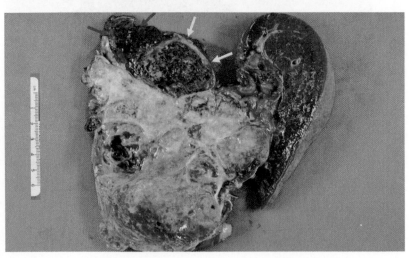

*Fig. 4.* Gross picture of a neuroendocrine carcinoma with variegated cut surface, focal hemorrhage (*red arrows*), and focal necrosis (*yellow arrows*). The tumor invades peripancreatic soft tissue.

*Fig. 5.* Microscopic picture of a small well-differentiated NET with a well-defined and pushing border (original magnification ×40).

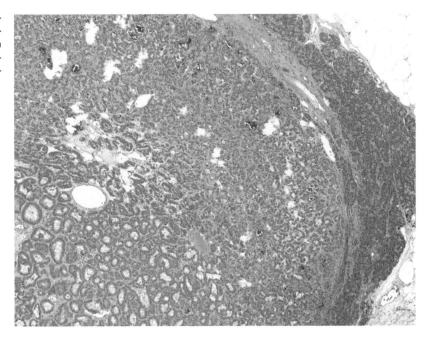

## MICROSCOPIC FEATURES

### WELL-DIFFERENTIATED PANCREATIC NEUROENDOCRINE TUMORS

The histomorphology of well-differentiated PanNETs is similar to that of NETs outside of the pancreas. The tumors are often delineated from the background pancreatic parenchyma by a fibrous pseudocapsule with a pushing border

(Fig. 5). Unlike pancreatic ductal adenocarcinoma, most PanNETs are hypercellular with minimal fibrous stroma, but tumors with abundant fibrous stroma (Fig. 6) or thick fibrous septa do exist (Fig. 7). Variable amount of hyalinized stroma may be seen in some PanNETs (Fig. 8).

Neoplastic cells are arranged as pseudoglands (Fig. 9), trabeculae (Fig. 10), organoids (Fig. 11), ribbons/festoons (Fig. 12), angiomatoid pattern (Fig. 13), nests (Fig. 14), rosettes (Fig. 15), acini

*Fig. 6.* Representative section of a well-differentiated NET with dense stromal fibrosis (original magnification ×200).

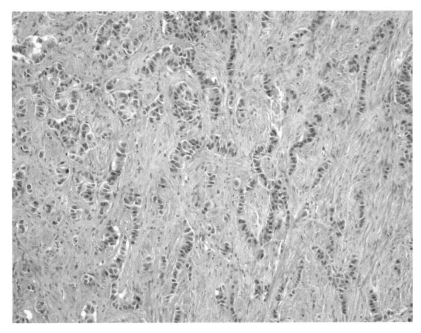

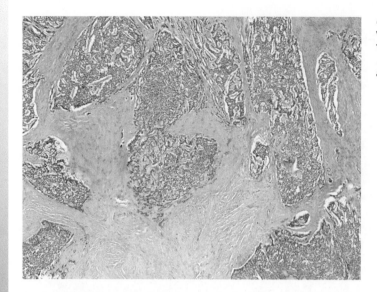

*Fig. 7.* Representative section of a well-differentiated NET with thick fibrotic septa (original magnification ×40). Tumors with thick fibrotic septa are frequently aggressive.

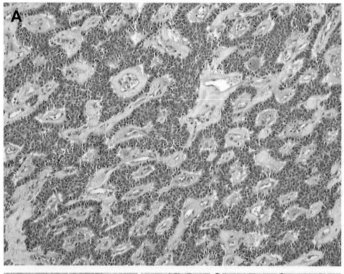

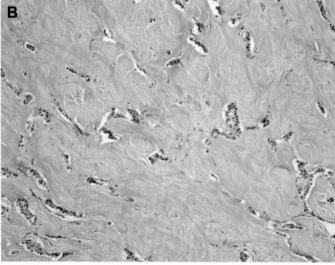

*Fig. 8.* Well-differentiated NETs with variable hyalinized stroma. (*A*) A NET with some hyalinized stroma (original magnification ×100); (*B*) A NET with abundant hyalinized stroma (original magnification ×200).

*Fig. 9.* A well-differentiated NET with neoplastic cells forming glandular structures (original magnification ×200).

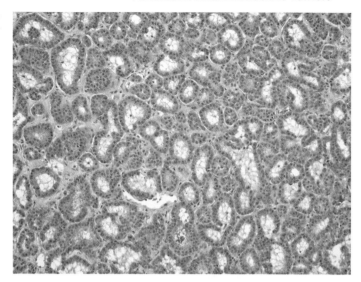

*Fig. 10.* A well-differentiated NET with neoplastic cells arranged in trabecular pattern (original magnification ×100).

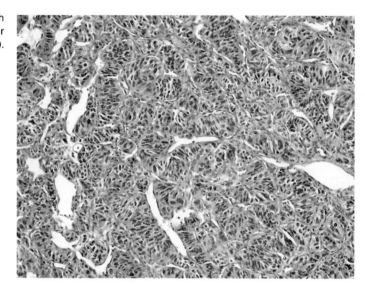

*Fig. 11.* A well-differentiated NET with neoplastic cells forming organoids (original magnification ×200).

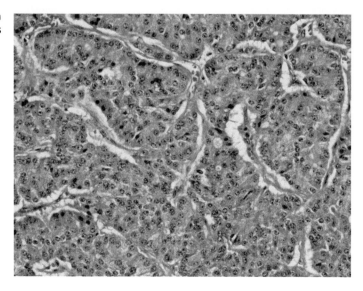

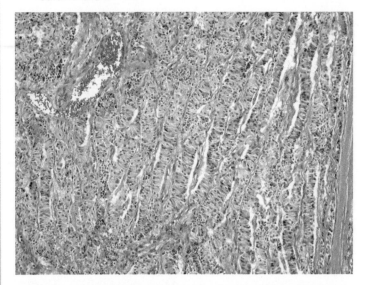

*Fig. 12.* A well-differentiated NET with neoplastic cells forming ribbons (original magnification ×100).

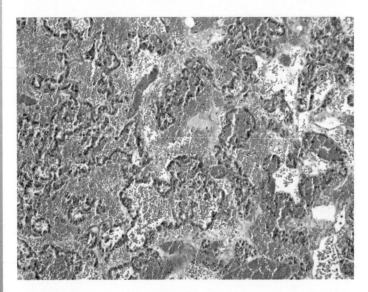

*Fig. 13.* A well-differentiated NET with an angiomatoid appearance (original magnification ×100).

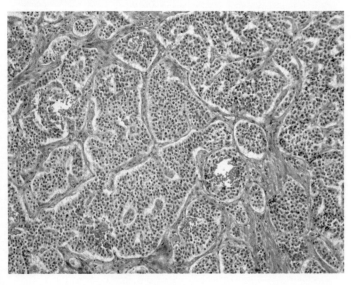

*Fig. 14.* A well-differentiated NET with neoplastic cells forming nests with different sizes (original magnification ×100).

*Fig. 15.* A well-differentiated NET with neoplastic cells forming rosettes (original magnification ×200).

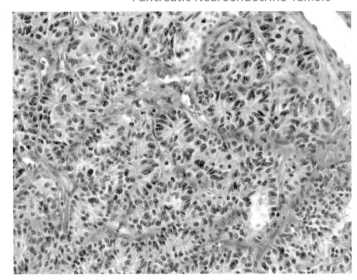

*Fig. 16.* A well-differentiated NET with neoplastic cells forming acini (original magnification ×100).

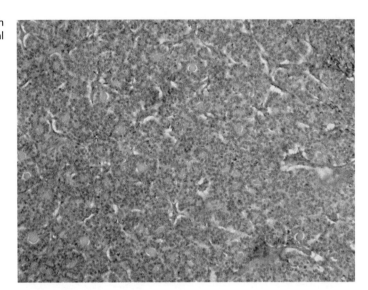

*Fig. 17.* A well-differentiated NET composed of sheets of neoplastic cells (original magnification ×100).

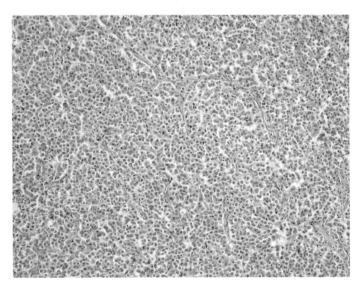

(Fig. 16), or sheets (Fig. 17). Multiple morphologies can be found in a single tumor (Fig. 18). The tumor cells have relatively uniform nuclear and cytoplasmic features. The polygonal cells have cytoplasm that is often finely granular and eosinophilic. The round/oval nucleus has characteristic coarse chromatin arranged in "salt-and-pepper" clumps (Fig. 19), but a prominent nucleolus can be seen in rare tumors (Fig. 20). Marked nuclear degenerative change can be seen in some tumors (Fig. 21), which is not associated with aggressive biology.

Occasionally neoplastic cells have a "rhabdoid-type" appearance (Fig. 22).

Functional and nonfunctional PanNETs share the same histomorphology with an exception of insulinoma. Amyloid deposits are frequently seen within the neoplastic cells or in the stroma of insulinomas (Fig. 23).[10] In addition to frequent multifocal PanNETs, patients with MEN1 always have multiple neuroendocrine microadenomas (Fig. 24) and multiple duodenal NETs (see Table 1). Of note, duodenal NETs often present as small

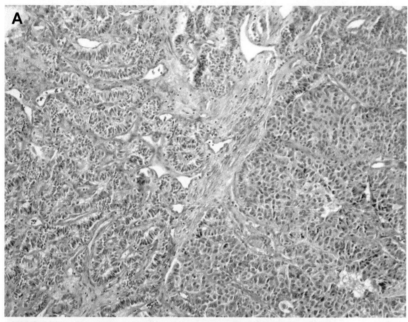

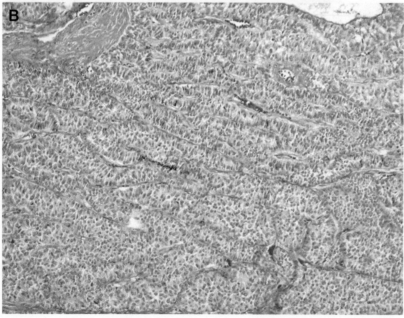

*Fig. 18.* A well-differentiated NET with neoplastic cells arranged in different patterns (original magnification ×100). (*A*) Neoplastic cells in rosette, trabecular, and organoid patterns; (*B*) Neoplastic cells in ribbons and organoids (original magnification ×100).

*Fig. 19.* Representative section of a well-differentiated NET composed of relatively uniform neoplastic cells with salt-pepper chromatin and moderate amount of cytoplasm (original magnification ×400).

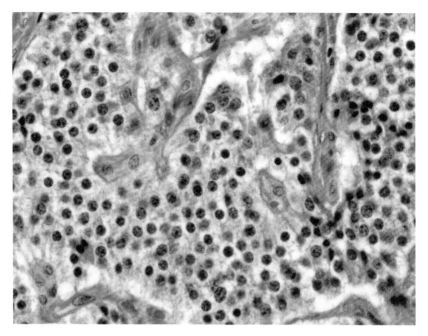

submucosal nodules; special care is needed not to miss the duodenal tumors when evaluating Whipple specimens from patients with MEN1. Most duodenal NETs in patients with MEN1 are gastrinoma.

A number of morphologic variants (Table 4) have been described, including PanNETs with dense stromal fibrosis and frequent expression of serotonin and intestinal markers (Figs. 25 and 26),[11–15] cystic PanNETs (Fig. 27), clear-cell variant (Fig. 28), and oncocytic variant (Fig. 29).[16–18]

## NEUROENDOCRINE CARCINOMAS

NECs are characterized by an ill-defined border and infiltrative growth pattern.[9] They are composed of neoplastic cells arranged in nests

*Fig. 20.* A well-differentiated NET with neoplastic cells showing a prominent nucleolus (original magnification ×200). Note: low-mid portion is an islet of Langerhans.

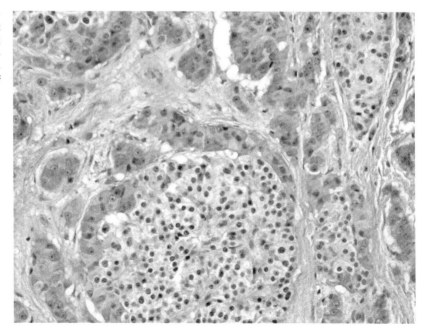

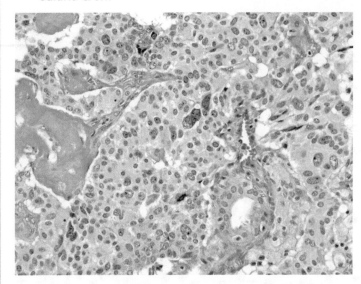

*Fig. 21.* A well-differentiated NET with some neoplastic cells showing marked nuclear atypia (original magnification ×200). The nuclear atypia is caused by a degenerative process. There is no increase in mitosis.

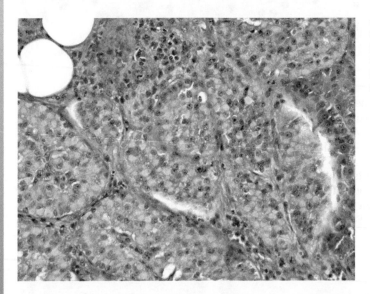

*Fig. 22.* A well-differentiated NET with neoplastic cells containing abundant pale cytoplasm and eccentric nuclei (original magnification ×200). This histology has been described as "rhabdoid feature".

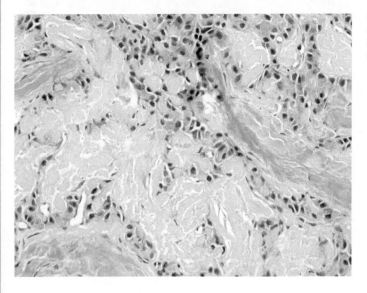

*Fig. 23.* An insulinoma with prominent intracellular and extracellular amyloid deposition (original magnification ×200).

*Fig. 24.* A cross section of pancreatectomy from a patient with MEN1 showing multiple neuroendocrine microadenomas (original magnification ×20). Note: one of the microadenomas has amyloid deposition.

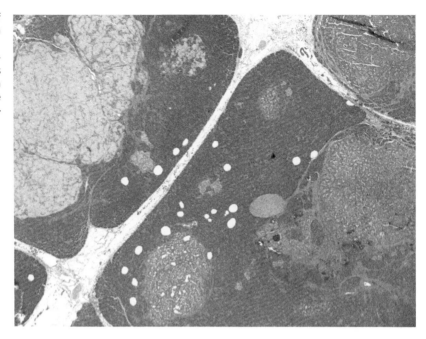

or sheets demonstrating abundant necrosis, brisk mitotic activity, and prominent apoptosis. Large-cell NECs are more common than small-cell carcinomas in the pancreas, which are exceptionally rare. The cells of large-cell NECs have moderate amounts of cytoplasm and ovoid nuclei with vesicular/coarse chromatin or prominent nucleoli (**Fig. 30**).[9] Small-cell carcinomas of the pancreas

**Table 4**
**Histomorphologic variants of pancreatic neuroendocrine tumors (PanNETs)**

| Variants | Clinical/Radiographic Features | Pathologic Features |
|---|---|---|
| PanNETs with dense stroma | 1. Frequently adjacent to a large pancreatic duct, causing duct stenosis and chronic pancreatitis<br>2. Distal pancreatic duct dilation or atrophy of distal pancreas radiographically | 1. Infiltrative growth pattern and dense stromal fibrosis<br>2. Tumor cells arranged in small nests or tubules and expressing serotonin and intestinal markers<br>3. Lymph node metastasis even when tumor size is <2 cm |
| Cystic PanNETs | 1. Frequently located in the body or tail<br>2. Cystic lesions of the pancreas with rim of enhancement with contrast radiographically | 1. Clear to straw-colored cystic fluid<br>2. Cyst lined by multiple layers of neoplastic cells<br>3. Less frequently associated with adverse pathologic features and often present at a lower stage. |
| Clear-cell PanNETs | Most are seen in patients with von Hippel Lindau syndrome, but can be also seen in general populations | 1. Neoplastic cells with clear cytoplasm arranged in nests, cords, festoons, and tubules<br>2. Can mimic clear-cell renal cell carcinoma |
| Oncocytic PanNETs | Tumors may be associated with a more aggressive behavior | 1. Neoplastic cells with abundant, finely granular, eosinophilic cytoplasm<br>2. Can mimic metastatic hepatocellular carcinoma, adrenal cortical carcinoma, and other neoplasms |

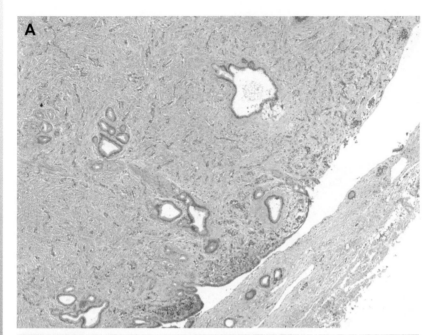

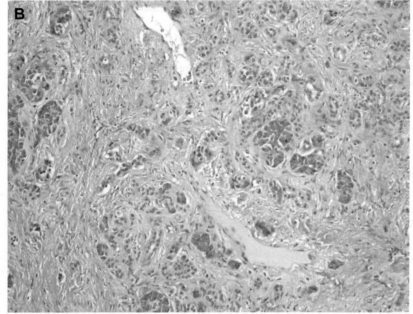

*Fig. 25.* A well-differentiated NET with dense stromal fibrosis. (*A*) The tumor is adjacent to a large pancreatic duct (original magnification ×40); (*B*) Small tumor nests infiltrate around acinar structures (original magnification ×100).

are composed of small to medium-sized cells with scant cytoplasm and nuclear molding (**Fig. 31**). Invasion of vessels and nerves is not uncommon at the time of diagnosis.

In some instances, NECs will demonstrate a proliferative (Ki67) index (≥20%) without distinct small-cell or large-cell histomorphologic features. These tumors maybe referred to as poorly differentiated NECs, WHO grade 3.

## DIFFERENTIAL DIAGNOSIS

## WELL-DIFFERENTIATED PANCREATIC NEUROENDOCRINE TUMORS

The differential diagnosis of PanNETs includes primary solid neoplasms of the pancreas including solid pseudopapillary neoplasms (SPNs), acinar cell carcinoma (ACC), mixed

*Fig. 26.* The tumor cells express CDX2 (*A*, original magnification ×100) and serotonin (*B*, original magnification ×100).

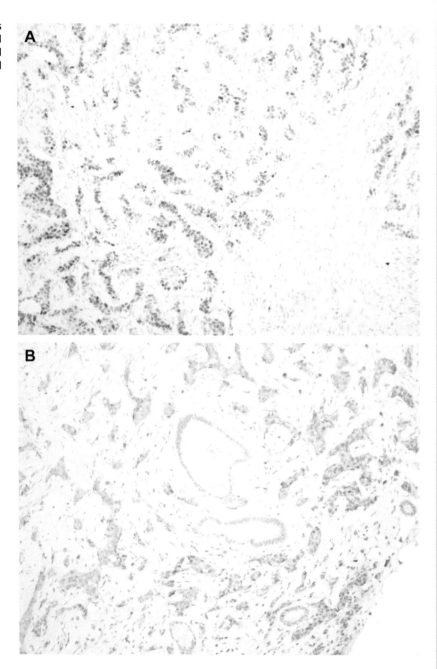

acinar-neuroendocrine carcinoma, and pancreatoblastoma being the most challenging (**Table 5**). Like PanNETs, these 4 neoplasms are characterized by hypercellularity and minimal fibrous stroma. Histomorphologic and immunohistochemical overlap exists between PanNETs and SPNs.[19,20] Hyaline globules can be seen in both neoplasms (**Fig. 32**). Cells with a single prominent nucleolus and expression of acinar markers are distinctive features of ACC and mixed acinar-neuroendocrine carcinomas.[21,22] To be classified as a true mixed acinar-neuroendocrine carcinoma, at least one-third of the neoplastic cells within the tumor must demonstrate neuroendocrine or acinar differentiation. Pancreatoblastoma is a tumor of the pediatric age group with squamoid corpuscles as a prominent and distinctive histologic feature.[23,24]

Occasionally, PanNETs with pseudoglandular morphologies and marked nuclear pleomorphism

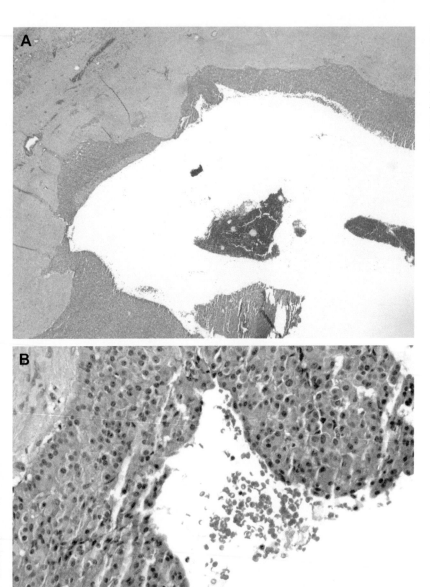

*Fig. 27.* Cystic pancreatic NET. (*A*) A cyst lined with several layers of neoplastic cells (original magnification ×20). (*B*) The neoplastic cells have typical features of NET (original magnification ×200).

can be mistaken for pancreatic ductal adenocarcinomas. In addition, clear-cell PanNETs, most frequently encountered in patients with VHL, can mimic clear-cell renal cell carcinoma.[17,25] Immunohistochemical stains for neuroendocrine markers can be helpful in such circumstances.

## NEUROENDOCRINE CARCINOMAS

Proliferative (Ki67) index is a useful tool in distinguishing well-differentiated PanNETs from NECs. In addition, the presence of more than 20 mitoses in 10 high-power fields (HPF) is most in keeping with a pancreatic NEC. Metastatic NECs to the pancreas from other primaries occasionally occur. Immunohistochemical stain for thyroid transcription factor 1 (TTF1) cannot differentiate pancreatic small-cell carcinoma from small-cell carcinoma of nonpancreatic origin, as both can express TTF1.

Primitive neuroectodermal tumors of the pancreas can show both histologic and immunohistochemical overlap (both tumors express CD99

*Fig. 28.* Clear-cell pancreatic NET composed of neoplastic cells with clear cytoplasm and salt-pepper chromatin (original magnification ×200).

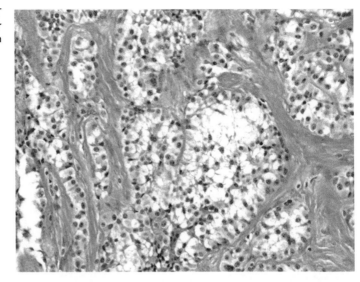

*Fig. 29.* Oncocytic cell pancreatic NET composed of neoplastic cells containing abundant eosinophilic cytoplasm (original magnification ×200).

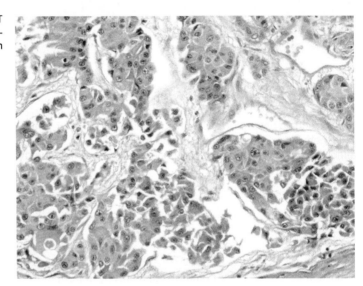

*Fig. 30.* NEC, large-cell NEC (original magnification ×200). The carcinoma cells have a moderate amount of cytoplasm, vesicular nuclei, and brisk mitoses.

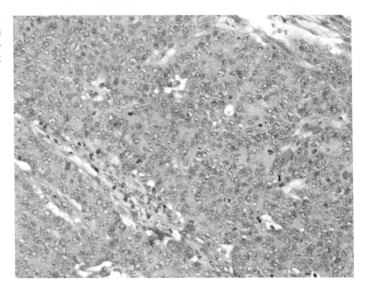

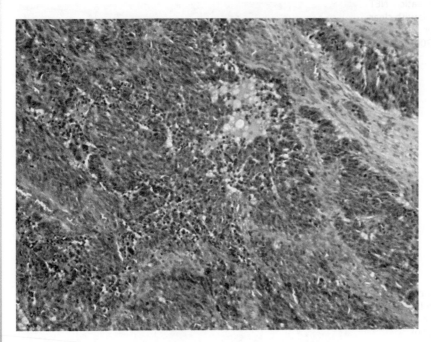

*Fig. 31.* NEC, small-cell carcinoma (original magnification ×100). The carcinoma cells have minimal cytoplasm and nuclear molding. There are brisk mitoses, prominent apoptosis, and focal tumor necrosis.

and cytokeratins). They are seen in young patients. Molecular testing for the 11:22 chromosomal translocation should be done in cases that are histologically nebulous.[26] Desmoplastic small round-cell tumors are also more common in younger patients; however, they can demonstrate endocrine differentiation. The characteristic desmoplastic stroma and positive labeling with desmin and WT-1, in addition to molecular study adjuncts can help facilitate the differentiation from pancreatic NECs.[27]

**Table 5**
**Differentiation of well-differentiated pancreatic neuroendocrine tumors from other hypercellular pancreatic neoplasms**

| Types | Pathologic Features | Immunohistochemical Stains |
|---|---|---|
| Pancreatic neuroendocrine tumors | Composed of relatively uniform cells with salt-pepper chromatin | Positive synaptophysin and chromogranin |
| Solid pseudopapillary neoplasms | 1. Fibrovascular cores lined by 3–4 layers of neoplastic cells with nuclear grooves<br>2. Frequent cystic degeneration<br>3. Presence of hyaline globules is not specific for solid pseudopapillary neoplasms | 1. Positive synaptophysin but negative chromogranin<br>2. Other specific markers: β-catenin nuclear accumulation with loss of E-cadherin and expression of CD10 |
| Acinar cell carcinoma | 1. Neoplastic cells with prominent nucleoli<br>2. Frequent mitosis | 1. Negative synaptophysin and chromogranin<br>2. Expression of acinar markers: trypsin, chymotrypsin, lipase, or BCL10 |
| Mixed neuroendocrine-acinar cell carcinoma | Both acinar cell and neuroendocrine carcinoma components | Tumors express both neuroendocrine and acinar cell markers |
| Pancreatoblastoma | Mixtures of acini, squamoid nests and less commonly endocrine or ductal features | Acinar cell markers in acini and nuclear/cytoplasmic expression of β-catenin in squamoid nests |

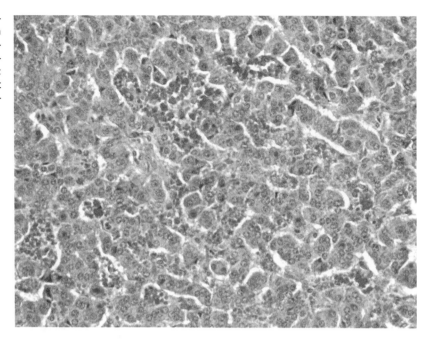

*Fig. 32.* A well-differentiated NET with abundant hyaline globules (original magnification ×200). Note: hyaline globules are not specific for solid pseudo-papillary neoplasm.

Poorly differentiated pancreatic ductal adenocarcinoma can occasionally be difficult to distinguish from pancreatic NECs. Oftentimes the former will demonstrate a focus of moderately to well-differentiated adenocarcinoma that can help distinguish it from NECs. Most importantly, a panel of neuroendocrine immunohistochemical markers should be performed to rule out a mixed adeno-neuroendocrine carcinoma. Mixed neuroendocrine-ACC have cancer cells with prominent nucleoli and frequent mitoses, which can mimic large-cell neuroendocrine carcinoma. Application of neuroendocrine and acinar cell markers can distinguish them from each other.

## DIAGNOSIS

### WELL-DIFFERENTIATED PANCREATIC NEUROENDOCRINE TUMORS

Immunohistochemical stains can be used to diagnose NETs. Synaptophysin is more sensitive and demonstrates diffuse labeling, whereas chromogranin, although more specific, tends to label in a focal and patchy distribution (**Fig. 33**).[28] There are no immunohistochemical markers specific for NETs of the pancreas. A subset of PanNETs express CDX2. Therefore, CDX2 cannot be used to differentiate PanNETs from other digestive NETs.[29] Although Islet 1 gene product, pancreatico-duodenal homeobox 1 gene product, and PAX8 are considered lineage markers for NETs of pancreatic origin, recent studies have

demonstrated their expression in NETs of extrapancreatic origin.[30–33]

Functioning PanNETs will label with specific peptides, for example, insulin and glucagon; however, it is important to understand that association with a clinical syndrome rather than labeling with specific peptides defines functionality in PanNETs.

The current WHO classification (2010) uses mitotic count and Ki67 labeling index in classifying PanNETs into 3 grades (see **Table 3**). The Ki67 index is to be based on counting hot spots: 500 to 2000 cells in the highest labeling regions within the tumor.[34,35] Mitoses should be counted in 50 HPFs. Discrepancies between mitotic count and Ki67 frequently occur.[36] In these instances, the higher grade should be used. As the Ki67 index is always indicative of the higher grade, there are strong data supporting the use of this marker in grading well-differentiated PanNETs.[35,36]

A small number of PanNETs have well-differentiated morphology, but a Ki67 index greater than 20% (see **Fig. 33**). The mitotic rate is always low in these tumors. Based on the WHO criteria, they would be classified as NEC. A number studies have demonstrated that this group of tumors is different from true NECs in multiple aspects, including prognosis and response to platinum-based therapy.[34,35] Such cases should be classified as well-differentiated PanNET with a high Ki67 index. Occasionally, well-differentiated PanNETs contain a morphologically apparent high-grade component (**Fig. 34**).

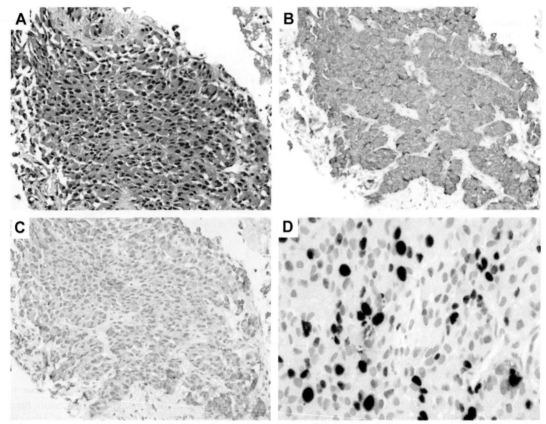

*Fig. 33.* A representative well-differentiated NET (*A*, original magnification ×100) with diffuse expression of synaptophysin (*B*, original magnification ×100), focal expression of chromogranin (*C*, original magnification ×100) and a Ki67 index of greater than 20% (*D*, original magnification ×200).

These tumors are distinct from NECs with a much better prognosis compared with NECs.[35]

## NEUROENDOCRINE CARCINOMAS

NECs, both small-cell and large-cell NECs, demonstrate a mitotic rate greater than 20 per 10 HPFs and a Ki67 index approaching 100%. These tumors show variable expression of neuroendocrine markers (synaptophysin and chromogranin). The documentation of these markers is more important in large-cell NECs than small-cell carcinoma. Although small-cell carcinoma can be diagnosed based on morphology, to diagnose large-cell NEC, at least one neuroendocrine marker is expressed by most of the neoplastic cells.

## PROGNOSIS

It is important to understand that all NETs of the pancreas, with the exception of neuroendocrine microadenomas, are considered to be malignant.

## WELL-DIFFERENTIATED PANCREATIC NEUROENDOCRINE TUMORS

The malignant behavior of PanNETs is unpredictable. Despite that, distant metastasis, tumor size, necrosis, mitotic rate, extension beyond the pancreas, and vascular and lymph node invasion are well documented as markers of adverse prognosis. Insulinomas have a more favorable prognosis than nonfunctional tumors, whereas other functional tumors can be aggressive. Although additional biomarkers may be associated with a poor prognosis, Ki67 is the only molecule that has been proven to be prognostic in large-scale studies.[36,37]

## NEUROENDOCRINE CARCINOMAS

Pancreatic NECs are highly aggressive malignancies with a mortality rate approaching 100%. These tumors are locally aggressive, spreading into the peripancreatic tissue and the duodenum. Metastases to distant organs and lymph nodes are common at initial diagnosis.

*Fig. 34.* A well-differentiated NET with poorly differentiated component. (*A*) Well-differentiated component with no mitosis (original magnification ×200); (*B*) Poorly differentiated component with tumor necrosis (original magnification ×200); (*C*) Poorly differentiated component with brisk mitoses and apoptotic bodies (original magnification ×400).

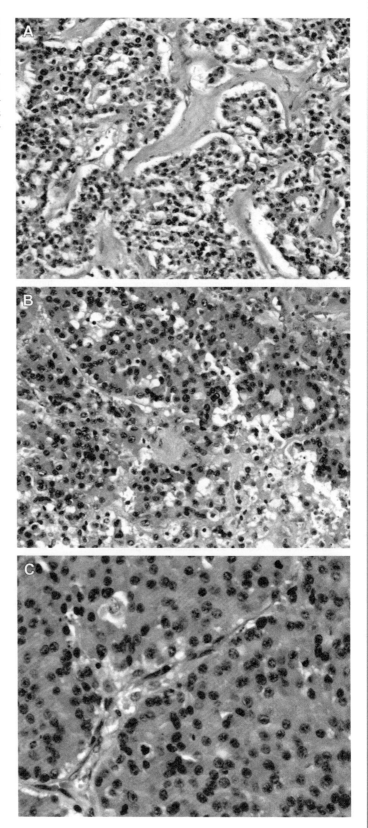

# REFERENCES

1. Fraenkel M, Kim MK, Faggiano A, et al. Epidemiology of gastroenteropancreatic neuroendocrine tumours. Best Pract Res Clin Gastroenterol 2012; 26:691–703.

2. Lawrence B, Gustafsson BI, Chan A, et al. The epidemiology of gastroenteropancreatic neuroendocrine tumors. Endocrinol Metab Clin North Am 2011; 40(1):1–18, vii.

3. Halfdanarson TR, Rubin J, Farnell MB, et al. Pancreatic endocrine neoplasms: epidemiology and prognosis of pancreatic endocrine tumors. Endocr Relat Cancer 2008;15:409–27.

4. Falconi M, Bartsch DK, Eriksson B, et al. ENETS consensus guidelines for the management of patients with digestive neuroendocrine neoplasms of the digestive system: well-differentiated pancreatic non-functioning tumors. Neuroendocrinology 2012;95:120–34.

5. Kimura W, Kuroda A, Morioka Y. Clinical pathology of endocrine tumors of the pancreas - analysis of autopsy cases. Dig Dis Sci 1991;36:933–42.

6. Kloppel G, Willemer S, Stamm B, et al. Pancreatic lesions and hormonal profile of pancreatic tumors in multiple endocrine neoplasia type-I - an immunocytochemical study of 9 patients. Cancer 1986;57: 1824–32.

7. Liu TH, Zhu Y, Cui QC, et al. Nonfunctioning pancreatic endocrine tumors - an immunohistochemical and electron-microscopic analysis of 26 cases. Pathol Res Pract 1992;188:191–8.

8. Singhi AD, Chu LC, Tatsas AD, et al. Cystic pancreatic neuroendocrine tumors: a clinicopathologic study. Am J Surg Pathol 2012;36:1666–73.

9. Basturk O, Tang L, Hruban RH, et al. Poorly differentiated neuroendocrine carcinomas of the pancreas: a clinicopathologic analysis of 44 cases. Am J Surg Pathol 2014;38:437–47.

10. Williams AJ, Coates PJ, Lowe DG, et al. Immunochemical investigation of insulinomas for islet amyloid polypeptide and insulin - evidence for differential synthesis and storage. Histopathology 1992; 21:215–23.

11. Shi C, Siegelman SS, Kawamoto S, et al. Pancreatic duct stenosis secondary to small endocrine neoplasms: a manifestation of serotonin production? Radiology 2010;257:107–14.

12. McCall CM, Shi C, Klein AP, et al. Serotonin expression in pancreatic neuroendocrine tumors correlates with a trabecular histologic pattern and large duct involvement. Hum Pathol 2012;43:1169–76.

13. Kawamoto S, Johnson PT, Shi C, et al. Pancreatic neuroendocrine tumor with cystlike changes: evaluation with MDCT. AJR Am J Roentgenol 2013;200: W283–90.

14. Salaria S, Means A, Revetta F, et al. Expression of CD24, a stem cell marker, in pancreatic and small intestinal neuroendocrine tumors. Am J Clin Pathol 2015;144:642–8.

15. Johnson A, Wright JP, Zhao ZG, et al. Cadherin 17 is frequently expressed by "sclerosing variant" pancreatic neuroendocrine tumor. Pancreas 2015; 44:347–8.

16. Volante M, La Rosa S, Castellano I, et al. Clinicopathological features of a series of 11 oncocytic endocrine tumours of the pancreas. Virchows Arch 2006;448:545–51.

17. Nunobe S, Fukushima N, Yachida S, et al. Clear cell endocrine tumor of the pancreas which is not associated with von Hippel-Lindau disease: report of a case. Surg Today 2003;33:470–4.

18. Capurso G, Festa S, Valente R, et al. Molecular pathology and genetics of pancreatic endocrine tumours. J Mol Endocrinol 2012;49:R37–50.

19. Abraham SC, Klimstra DS, Wilentz RE, et al. Solid-pseudopapillary tumors of the pancreas are genetically distinct from pancreatic ductal adenocarcinomas and almost always harbor beta-catenin mutations. Am J Pathol 2002;160:1361–9.

20. Hruban RH, Klimstra DS, Wilentz RE, et al. Solid-pseudopapillary tumors of the pancreas frequently harbor alterations in the APC/beta-catenin pathway. Lab Invest 2002;82:287a.

21. Klimstra DS, Heffess CS, Oertel JE, et al. Acinar cell-carcinoma of the pancreas - a clinicopathological study of 28 cases. Am J Surg Pathol 1992;16: 815–37.

22. Stelow EB, Shaco-Levy R, Bao F, et al. Pancreatic acinar cell carcinomas with prominent ductal differentiation: mixed acinar ductal carcinoma and mixed acinar endocrine ductal carcinoma. Am J Surg Pathol 2010;34:510–8.

23. Klimstra DS, Wenig BM, Adair CF, et al. Pancreatoblastoma. A clinicopathologic study and review of the literature. Am J Surg Pathol 1995;19:1371–89.

24. Salman B, Brat G, Yoon YS, et al. The diagnosis and surgical treatment of pancreatoblastoma in adults: a case series and review of the literature. J Gastrointest Surg 2013;17:2153–61.

25. Chambers TP, Fishman EK, Hruban RH. Pancreatic metastases from renal cell carcinoma in von Hippel-Lindau disease. Clin Imaging 1997;21:40–2.

26. Movahedi-Lankarani S, Hruban RH, Westra WH, et al. Primitive neuroectodermal tumors of the pancreas - a report of seven cases of a rare neoplasm. Am J Surg Pathol 2002;26:1040–7.

27. Bismar TA, Basturk C, Gerald WL, et al. Desmoplastic small cell tumor in the pancreas. Am J Surg Pathol 2004;28:808–12.

28. Lloyd RV, Mervak T, Schmidt K, et al. Immunohistochemical detection of chromogranin and

neuron-specific enolase in pancreatic endocrine neoplasms. Am J Surg Pathol 1984;8:607–14.

29. Saqi A, Alexis D, Remotti F, et al. Usefulness of CDX2 and TTF-1 in differentiating gastrointestinal from pulmonary carcinoids. Am J Clin Pathol 2005; 123:394–404.

30. Graham RP, Shrestha B, Caron BL, et al. Islet-1 is a sensitive but not entirely specific marker for pancreatic neuroendocrine neoplasms and their metastases. Am J Surg Pathol 2013;37:399–405.

31. Zhou XY, Dhall D, Moschiano E, et al. The immunohistochemical expression of islet 1 and PAX8 by rectal neuroendocrine tumors should be taken into account in the differential diagnosis of metastatic neuroendocrine tumors of unknown primary origin. Pancreas 2014;43:509.

32. Weissferdt A, Tang XM, Wistuba II, et al. Comparative immunohistochemical analysis of pulmonary and thymic neuroendocrine carcinomas using PAX8 and TTF-1. Mod Pathol 2013;26:1554–60.

33. Hermann G, Konukiewitz B, Schmitt A, et al. Hormonally defined pancreatic and duodenal neuroendocrine tumors differ in their transcription factor signatures: expression of ISL1, PDX1, NGN3 and CDX2. Virchows Arch 2011;459:S218.

34. Yang ZH, Tang LH, Klimstra DS. Effect of tumor heterogeneity on the assessment of Ki67 labeling index in well-differentiated neuroendocrine tumors metastatic to the liver: implications for prognostic stratification. Am J Surg Pathol 2011;35:853–60.

35. Tang LH, Gonen M, Hedvat C, et al. Objective quantification of the Ki67 proliferative index in neuroendocrine tumors of the gastroenteropancreatic system a comparison of digital image analysis with manual methods. Am J Surg Pathol 2012;36:1761–70.

36. McCall CM, Shi CJ, Cornish TC, et al. Grading of well-differentiated pancreatic neuroendocrine tumors is improved by the inclusion of both Ki67 proliferative index and mitotic rate. Am J Surg Pathol 2013;37:1671–7.

37. Basturk O, Yang ZH, Tang LH, et al. The high-grade (WHO G3) pancreatic neuroendocrine tumor category is morphologically and biologically heterogenous and includes both well differentiated and poorly differentiated neoplasms. Am J Surg Pathol 2015;39:683–90.

# Benign Tumors and Tumorlike Lesions of the Pancreas

Olca Basturk, MD*, Gokce Askan, MD

## KEYWORDS

- Benign • Serous • Lymphoepithelial • Squamoid • Epidermoid • Hamartoma • Inflammatory
- Pancreatitis

## ABSTRACT

The pancreas is a complex organ that may give rise to large number of neoplasms and non-neoplastic lesions. This article focuses on benign neoplasms, such as serous neoplasms, and tumorlike (pseudotumoral) lesions that may be mistaken for neoplasm not only by clinicians and radiologists, but also by pathologists. The family of pancreatic pseudotumors, by a loosely defined conception of that term, includes a variety of lesions including heterotopia, hamartoma, and lipomatous pseudohypertrophy. Autoimmune pancreatitis and paraduodenal ("groove") pancreatitis may also lead to pseudotumor formation. Knowledge of these entities will help in making an accurate diagnosis.

## OVERVIEW: SEROUS NEOPLASMS

Serous neoplasms of the pancreas are rare benign tumors accounting for approximately 1% of all pancreatic lesions. These tumors reveal a unique cytomorphology characterized by distinctive cuboidal epithelial cells with uniform round nuclei, dense, homogeneous chromatin, and a prominent epithelium-associated microvascular mesh-work.[1,2] They are generally regarded under the category of ductal-type tumors; however, they do not produce mucin despite their presumed ductal lineage, instead, they produce abundant glycogen.

Several morphologic variants of serous neoplasms have been described. These include microcystic and macrocystic (a.k.a. oligocystic) serous cystadenomas, solid serous adenoma, and von Hippel-Lindau (vHL)-associated serous cystic neoplasm. The microcystic serous cystic neoplasm consists of innumerable small, irregularly contoured tubular structures of variable shapes, the vast majority of which measure in sub-millimeters. The macrocystic (oligocystic) serous cystic neoplasms are predominantly or completely composed of fewer (typically <10) but much larger cysts, each measuring in centimeters. Although "serous cystadenoma (SCA)" and "serous cystic neoplasm (SCN)" terms technically refer to the microcystic variant, they are often used interchangeably for both microcystic and macrocystic variants. Solid serous adenoma is characterized by uniform, small, evenly shaped and sized nests or tubules with minimal or no lumen formation.[1] vHL-associated SCNs are often more a patchy transformation in the pancreas, although some may form a well-defined localized mass.[3-8]

## MICROCYSTIC AND MACROCYSTIC (OLIGOCYSTIC) SEROUS CYSTADENOMAS

Serous cystadenomas can occur at any age but are more common in elderly female patients.[1,7-21] They are often asymptomatic,[11,22,23] discovered incidentally, either sporadically or as part of vHL disease.[7,8,24-27] If the mass is located in the pancreatic head, it can obstruct the biliary tract.[25,28] Rarely, the lesions are multiple, specifically when associated with vHL.

A "honeycomb" appearance on computed tomography (CT) or MRI, associated with a central scar that may or may not be calcified, is

The authors have no conflict of interest to declare.
Memorial Sloan Kettering Cancer Center, New York, NY, USA
* Corresponding author. Department of Pathology, Memorial Sloan Kettering Cancer Center, 1275 York Avenue, New York, NY 10065.
E-mail address: basturko@mskcc.org

Surgical Pathology 9 (2016) 619–641
http://dx.doi.org/10.1016/j.path.2016.05.007

characteristic for *microcystic* variant.[16,17,22,29–31] However, the diagnosis is often not accomplished preoperatively by imaging studies. Similarly, the *macrocystic (oligocystic)* variant, especially if only a single cyst is evident,[32] radiographically simulates intraductal papillary mucinous neoplasms, mucinous cystic neoplasms, and pseudocysts.[16,19,30,33–35]

The fine-needle aspiration diagnosis of serous neoplasms has also proven to be unexpectedly challenging because of the very low aspirate cellularity, probably due to the cohesiveness and adhesion of the cells to the tissue.[1,36–38] The tumor cells are bland, cuboidal, and arranged in loose clusters or monolayers. The cytoplasm is usually cleared or vacuolated; however, the cells are frequently stripped of cytoplasm, showing only small, round nuclei with fine but dense, homogenous nuclear chromatin.[31,36,39]

The presurgical diagnosis of pancreatic cysts has traditionally relied on measuring cyst fluid amylase, as well as the tumor markers CA19 to 9 and carcinoembryonic antigen (CEA) to identify and distinguish the mucinous neoplasms from nonmucinous lesions, such as serous neoplasms.[40] However, the sensitivity and specificity of these markers are relatively low.[41] Recently, in an enzyme-linked immunosorbent assay analysis of cyst fluid and tumoral tissue, Yip-Schneider and colleagues[42] found that vascular endothelial growth factor-A (VEGF-A) was markedly elevated in SCNs when compared with pseudocysts, intraductal papillary mucinous neoplasms, mucinous cystic neoplasms, and pancreatic ductal adenocarcinoma. With a cutoff of 8500 pg/mL, VEGF-A had 100% sensitivity and 97% specificity as a marker of SCNs, making it a very promising biomarker for the diagnosis and distinction of SCNs from other pancreatic cysts, particularly when used in conjunction with CEA.[42]

Similarly, the identification of cyst-specific somatic mutations (involving *KRAS, GNAS, RNF43, CTNNB1,* and *VHL* genes) offers great promise in the presurgical diagnosis of pancreatic cysts. Recently, *KRAS* and *GNAS* mutations have been shown to have 96% sensitivity and 100% specificity for the differentiation of intraductal papillary mucinous neoplasm from SCN.[41] Molecular assays containing a 5-gene panel may be especially useful in the pretreatment diagnosis of SCNs because isolated *VHL* mutations have not been identified in intraductal papillary mucinous neoplasms and mucinous cystic neoplasms. However, it should be kept in mind that pancreatic neuroendocrine tumors may also be cystic and may harbor *VHL* deletions in up to 25% of sporadic cases.

These new developments seem to be very promising for the preoperative diagnosis (and thus possible conservative management) of SCNs; however, they need to be verified in larger-scale studies before they can be put into daily clinical management.

The mean diameter of SCNs is approximately 4 cm but now smaller lesions are found using improved imaging techniques.[1,9,10] They occur anywhere in the organ and appear as circumscribed and well-demarcated from the surrounding pancreas. *Microcystic* SCNs form partly encapsulated, lobulated masses composed of innumerable tiny cysts, which impart the highly distinctive and entity-defining spongelike appearance on sectioning (**Fig. 1**). Irregular central scars, frequently calcified, may be seen in the larger tumors. The fluid in the cysts is clear and watery, appearing colorless, yellow, or blood stained. Foci of hemorrhage can occur.[43] *Macrocystic (oligocystic)* SCNs, by definition, are composed of much larger cysts with fewer loculi and devoid of central fibrosis or calcification (**Fig. 2**).

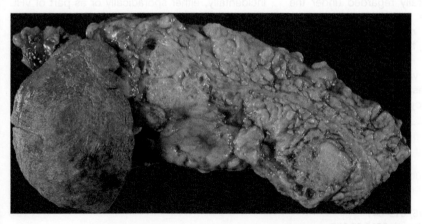

**Fig. 1.** Two *microcystic* serous cystadenomas are present in this distal pancreas. The neoplasms are well demarcated and composed of numerous small cysts, most of which measure in submillimeters.

*Fig. 2. Macrocystic (oligocystic) serous cystadenoma has either a singular locule or a few locules (as illustrated here) with a flattened lining.*

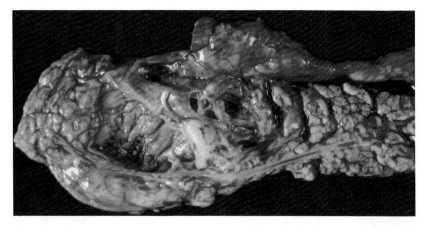

Microscopic examination of *microcystic* SCNs reveal back-to-back tubules of variable size and shape (**Fig. 3**), creating a characteristic *microcystic* pattern formed by cuboidal epithelium. Scattered larger (up to a centimeter in diameter), more irregular cysts lined by low cuboidal to flat cells may also be seen.[7,15,17,19–21,44] Dense stroma can occur in the lesions with these larger cysts. Some of the stroma may be hyalinized or myxoid. The tumor cells usually have abundant clear cytoplasm due to abundant glycogen (**Fig. 4**). Some cases reveal more oncocytoid cells with granular cytoplasm. Nuclei are small, round, compact, and uniform, with inconspicuous nucleoli. The presence of a capillary meshwork immediately adjacent to (almost within) the epithelium is highly characteristic,[45,46] and has been noted as a striking analogy with other clear-cell tumors arising in association with vHL, including renal cell carcinomas and hemangioblastomas.[45] Macrocystic (oligocystic) SCNs may be missing much of its lining, thus requiring multiple sections to find the epithelium. The lining of the cysts display the characteristic serous cytology (**Fig. 5**).

SCNs often show degenerative changes (hemorrhage, inflammation, and cholesterol clefts). Calcifications, tufting/micropapillae (**Fig. 6**), the presence of satellite nodules, and frequent intermixing of neuroendocrine cell proliferation in a pseudoinvasive pattern are also common.[1]

*Fig. 3. Microcystic serous cystadenoma is characterized by numerous small, irregular tubular structures of variable shapes. Note the hyalinized stroma at the center (H&E, ×20).*

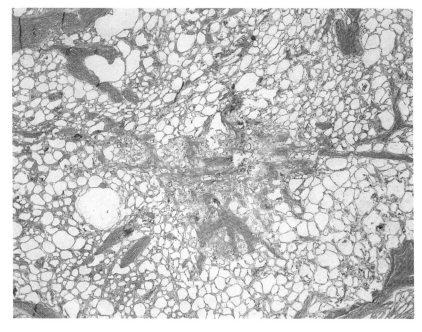

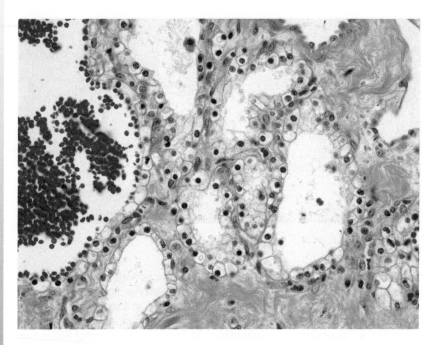

*Fig. 4.* The cysts of serous cystadenomas are lined by cuboidal cells, with round, central to slightly eccentric nuclei and clear cytoplasm (H&E, ×200).

Both histologically and immunophenotypically, these neoplasms appear to recapitulate centroacinar cells.[18,46–48] The glycogen-rich cytoplasm is typically periodic acid-Schiff positive, diastase sensitive, and reacts with broad-spectrum and low-molecular-weight keratins, EMA, and inhibin.[15,49] Ductal mucin markers (B72.3, CA19–9, CEA, and MUC1) are either negative or only focally positive, although MUC6 is usually positive.[49] Molecules implicated in clear-cell tumorigenesis (glucose uptake and transporter-1 [GLUT-1], hypoxia-inducible factor-1$\alpha$ [HIF-1$\alpha$], and carbonic anhydrase IX [CA-IX]) are also consistently expressed.[45]

At a molecular level, *VHL* gene allelic deletions (chromosome 3p) are detected in SCNs from

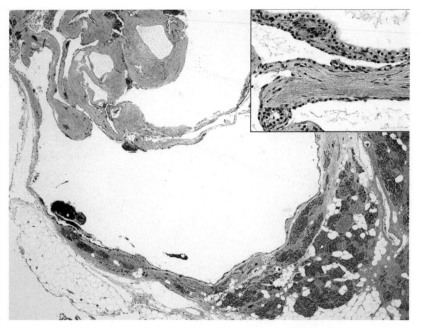

*Fig. 5.* Although the cysts are fewer and larger than in the *microcystic* serous cystadenoma, *macrocystic* (*oligocystic*) serous cystadenoma is also lined by the same cuboidal cells with clear cytoplasm (inset) (H&E, ×20; H&E, ×200).

*Fig. 6.* Although the lining epithelium is usually flat, prominent but stubby papillary projections might be seen in some serous cystadenomas (H&E, ×100).

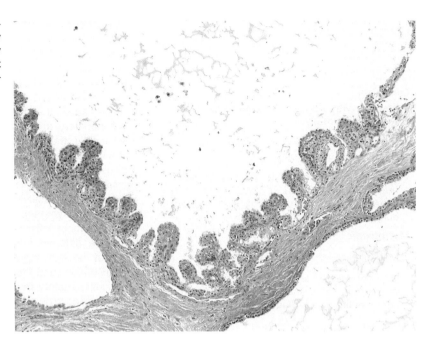

patients with vHL, providing molecular evidence of their neoplastic nature and integral association with vHL disease.[6-8] However, *VHL* gene alterations may also be detected in sporadic cases.[50] To date, the genetic alterations seen in pancreatic ductal adenocarcinoma (*TP53, KRAS, SMAD4,* and *p16/CDKN2A*), neuroendocrine tumors (*MEN1, DAXX,* and *ATRX*), and intraductal papillary mucinous neoplasms (*GNAS, RNF43, PIK3CA,* and *STK11/LKB1*) have not been reported in serous neoplasms.[41,50]

SCNs are very slow-growing tumors,[9,51] with an estimated doubling time of 12 years.[52] Therefore, if a definitive diagnosis can be accomplished, watchful waiting is a distinct option for smaller tumors.[9,11,14,25,44,52-54] For symptomatic cases and/or larger ones, surgical removal is still the treatment of choice.[44,55] More recently, radiofrequency ablation, ethanol, and chemotherapeutic agent injection have been proposed as options in the nonsurgical management of patients with limited disease.[56,57]

The 2010 World Health Organization (WHO) classification requires the presence of distant metastasis as the criterion for "malignancy" in SCN. Thus, many of the cases that had been reported as "malignant" based on "vascular invasion" would no longer qualify by the WHO classification.[58] Similarly, larger serous neoplasms (>11.0 cm) with inflammation and hemorrhage may show localized adhesion and/or penetration of neighboring organs, including lymph nodes,

spleen, stomach, and colon, which does not seem to be an indicator of malignant behavior. Even for serous neoplasms occurring in the liver, the possibility of synchronous independent tumors may have to be considered before concluding metastasis, especially considering there was no fatality related to this and no reported metastases to other remote sites.[1,9] Of note, there are isolated cases reported in which a cytologically obvious carcinoma arose within a microcystic serous cystadenoma ("carcinoma *ex* microcystic adenoma").[59] The biological behavior of these rare cases is yet to be defined.

## SOLID SEROUS ADENOMA

Solid serous tumors with uniform, small, evenly shaped and sized nests or tubules with minimal or no lumen formation have also been described. These typically lack central fibrosis and often misinterpreted radiologically as neuroendocrine tumors. Tumor cells reveal typical glycogen-laden clear cytoplasm and bland, round to oval hyperchromatic nuclei.[60-64] Distinguishing solid serous adenomas from other solid neoplasms, such as neuroendocrine tumors, or other clear-cell neoplasms, such as metastatic renal cell carcinoma, may be difficult; even more so in the setting of vHL, where both lesions may be concurrently present. Special studies and immunohistochemical analysis are helpful.[65]

## Key Features
### SEROUS CYSTIC NEOPLASM

*Clinical*

- Present with nonspecific symptoms or detected incidentally

- Have well-established association with von Hippel-Lindau syndrome

- Molecular assays containing a 5-gene panel (*KRAS, GNAS, RNF43, CTNNB1,* and *VHL* genes) may be useful in the pretreatment diagnosis

*Macroscopic*

- Medium-size lesion (mean size = 4 cm)

- Well-demarcated and spongelike appearance with innumerable small cysts, each measuring a few millimeters is diagnostic

- Central stellate scar common in *microcytic* variant

*Microscopic*

- Conglomerate of cysts lined by simple cuboidal epithelium

- Clear or eosinophilic cells with distinct cytoplasmic borders

- Small, round nuclei with dense, homogeneous chromatin

- Similar to vHL syndrome–associated other clear-cell tumors, a prominent epithelium-associated microvascular meshwork is present

## INFLAMMATORY MYOFIBROBLASTIC TUMOR

Inflammatory myofibroblastic tumor is a rare, especially in the pancreas, and distinctive entity.[66–69] The pancreatic head is affected most frequently by an ill-defined and firm mass causing obstructive jaundice. Therefore, patients are often suspected to suffer from pancreatic ductal adenocarcinoma.[70,71]

At low-power magnification, inflammatory myofibroblastic tumor has a relatively pushing border (**Fig. 7**). Fibroblasts and myofibroblasts, usually arranged in a storiform pattern, with moderate to marked inflammation composed of lymphocytes and plasma cells are characteristic (**Fig. 8**). Cytologic atypia and mitotic figures are rarely observed.

In approximately 50% of inflammatory myofibroblastic tumors, various gene aberrations, including the anaplastic lymphoma kinase (*ALK*) gene at chromosome 2p23, leading to aberrant

ALK expression in the myofibroblasts, have been identified.[72–75] These observations have led to the development of the concept of inflammatory myofibroblastic tumor as a clonal neoplastic lesion rather than a reactive process.[69] Of note, *ALK* gene abnormality is more often seen in children or young adults than in elderly people.[67]

Inflammatory myofibroblastic tumors share, at least focally, the morphologic appearance of the immunoglobulin (Ig)G4-related sclerosing disease (discussed separately in this issue, see autoimmune pancreatitis section), particularly at areas with prominent fibroblastic/myofibroblastic proliferation mingled with lymphocytes and plasma cells.[69,76] However, most inflammatory myofibroblastic tumors are different from IgG4-related lesions in terms of the ALK expression, low level of IgG4+ cell infiltration, and lack of obstructive phlebitis. Thus, inflammatory myofibroblastic tumor should be recognized to be a distinctive neoplastic entity.[69]

## Key Features
### INFLAMMATORY
### MYOFIBROBLASTIC TUMOR

- Composed of fibroblasts and myofibroblasts, usually arranged in a storiform pattern, with moderate to marked inflammation

- In half of inflammatory myofibroblastic tumors, various *ALK* gene abnormalities, leading to aberrant ALK expression in the myofibroblasts, have been identified

- ALK expression and low level of IgG4+ cell infiltration help distinguishing inflammatory myofibroblastic tumors from IgG4-related sclerosing disease

## LYMPHOEPITHELIAL CYST

Lymphoepithelial cyst is usually asymptomatic, with the lesion found incidentally on imaging studies performed for unrelated reasons or at autopsy.[77,78] In contrast to its salivary gland analogues, no autoimmune disorder is identified and there is no syndrome association. Association with human immunodeficiency virus also appears to be coincidental and exceedingly uncommon.[79]

It typically presents as a unilocular or multilocular cyst within, or protruding from, the pancreas. Imaging studies cannot consistently separate lymphoepithelial cyst from neoplastic mucinous cysts, such as intraductal pancreatic mucinous neoplasm or mucinous cystic neoplasm.[80] Fine-needle aspiration can support the diagnosis of a

*Fig.* 7. Inflammatory myofibroblastic tumor with well-defined margins (H&E, ×100).

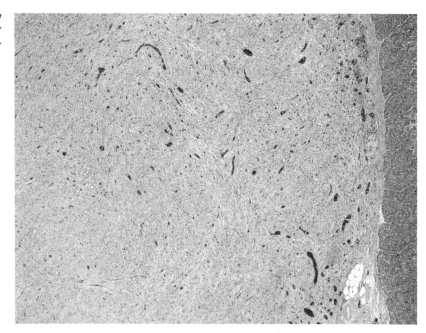

lymphoepithelial cyst when squamous cells, amorphous keratinaceous debris, cholesterol clefts, and/or lymphocytes are present.[81] However, fine-needle aspiration may be inconclusive. Using cyst fluid CEA as a discriminating test has its limitations, as several case reports have noted elevated levels of CA19 to 9 and/or CEA in lymphoepithelial cysts.[82–84]

Gross examination shows a medium-size (mean size = 5 cm), encapsulated cystic lesion.

Depending on the degree of keratin formation, cyst content may vary from serous to cheesy/caseous-appearing. Microscopically, there is a dense band of mature lymphoid tissue with prominent, well-formed germinal centers subtending a cyst lining of mature stratified squamous epithelium occasionally containing keratinaceous debris (**Fig. 9**). The adjacent pancreas may have granulomas, collections of foamy histiocytes and fat necrosis[77,78] (**Fig. 10**).

*Fig.* 8. Proliferation of generally bland spindle mesenchymal cells arranged in irregular fascicles into a stroma with lymphocytes, plasma cells, and histiocytes is characteristic in inflammatory myofibroblastic tumor (H&E, ×200).

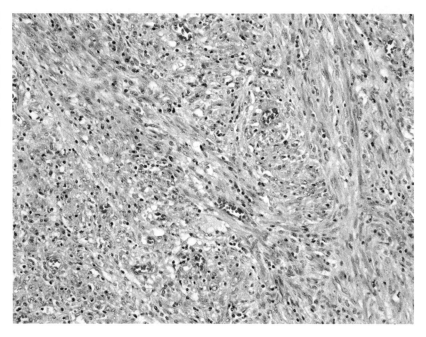

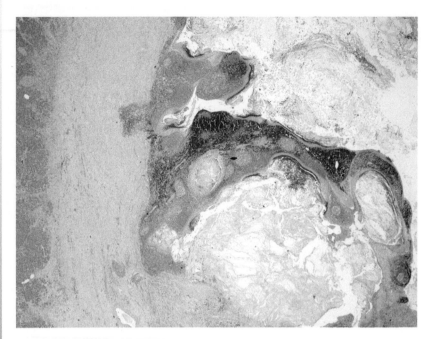

*Fig. 9.* A lymphoepithelial cyst lined by mature, stratified squamous epithelium with keratinization. Note the lymphoid tissue with germinal center formation immediately beneath the epithelium (H&E, ×20).

Although lymphoepithelial cysts might contain sebaceous glands, they are distinct from dermoid cysts (cystic monodermal teratomas) or teratomas because of the large amount of organized lymphoid tissue present and the lack of hair, cartilage, and occasionally neural tissue.[77,85]

Pancreatic lymphoepithelial cyst can be cured by conservative resection but if it is asymptomatic and diagnosed before surgery, no treatment is necessary. Neither malignant transformation nor recurrence after resection has been reported.[86]

---

### Key Features
#### LYMPHOEPITHELIAL CYST

*Clinical*
- Mostly in male patients
- Medium-size, peripancreatic cyst

*Microscopic*
- Has variable lining ranging from attenuated to transitional to stratified squamous epithelium with keratinization
- Goblet cells or scanty sebaceous elements may be seen
- Distinct band of lymphoid tissue, sometimes with prominent, well-formed germinal centers, composed of mature T lymphocytes surrounds the epithelium

---

## EPIDERMOID CYST IN INTRAPANCREATIC ACCESSORY SPLEEN

These are very rare lesions seen in younger adults (second to third decades). They occur almost exclusively in the tail of the pancreas where accessory spleens are not uncommon. Of note, accessory spleens are most frequently found at the perihilar region of the spleen (80% of cases) followed by the pancreatic tail.[87]

Similar to lymphoepithelial cyst, epidermoid cyst in intrapancreatic accessory spleen can also be misdiagnosed preoperatively as a cystic pancreatic neoplasm, such as intraductal papillary mucinous neoplasm or mucinous cystic neoplasm, especially in the setting of elevated serum CA19 to 9 levels.[88,89]

Grossly, a well-circumscribed dark red mass with a unilocular or multilocular cyst in the pancreatic tail is characteristic.[88] The cyst contains serous fluid or keratinaceous debris and is lined by benign multilayered epithelium, which is reminiscent of squamous epithelium or urothelium, surrounded by unremarkable splenic tissue.[78,88,90] The lining epithelium shows stratified cuboidal or columnar cell morphology in some areas, whereas it is flattened and attenuated in other areas (**Fig. 11**).[91]

---

## SQUAMOID CYST OF PANCREATIC DUCTS

Squamoid cysts of pancreatic ducts are relatively small cysts, with a median size of 1.5 cm, and

*Fig. 10.* Epithelioid granulomas and cholesterol clefts may also be present beneath the lining epithelium of lymphoepithelial cysts (H&E, ×200).

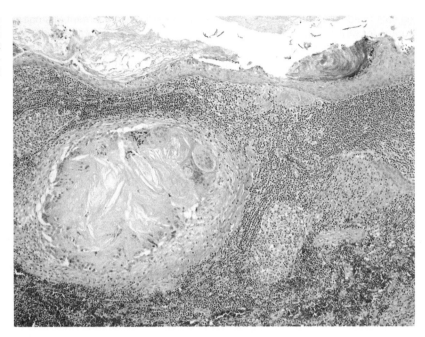

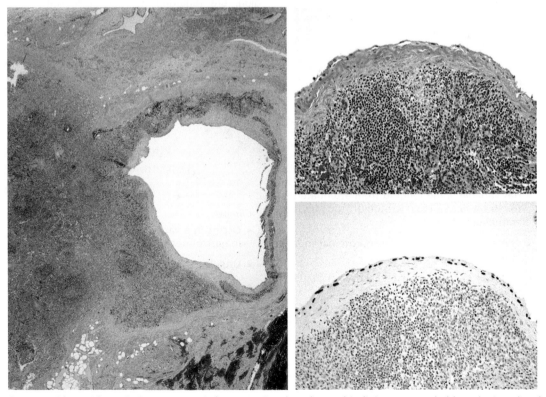

*Fig. 11.* Epidermoid cyst in intrapancreatic heterotopic spleen has a thin lining surrounded by splenic red and white pulp (*left*, H&E, ×20). Recognition of the splenic elements allows a correct diagnosis even if the squamous nature of the attenuated lining epithelium (*top right*, H&E, ×200) may not be appreciated without immunohistochemical staining (*bottom right*, p63 immunohistochemical stain, ×200).

the vast majority of the cases are detected during workup for other conditions.[92,93] These cysts typically result from unilocular cystic dilatation of the ducts and have variable lining ranging from attenuated, flat, nonstratified squamous, to transitional, to mucosal-type stratified squamous epithelium (Fig. 12) as well as mucoproteinaceous acidophilic secretions within the lumen. The wall of the cyst is composed of a thin band of fibrous tissue, focally showing tributary ducts. Neither acute nor chronic inflammation is a feature of this lesion.

Immunohistochemically, nuclear p63 expression is present in all cases, a finding that is not seen in any normal component of pancreas or in nonsquamous cystic lesions of this organ.[94]

It is important to distinguish squamoid cysts of pancreatic ducts from other cystic lesions, in particular, from mucinous tumors, as the latter often have malignant potential, whereas squamoid cysts of pancreatic ducts are innocuous lesions.[95] Preoperative differential diagnosis of these may be difficult, especially in the setting of elevated fluid CEA levels and acellular cytology.[96,97] However, their distinction at the microscopic level is fairly straightforward.[92]

---

### Key Features
#### SQUAMOID CYST OF PANCREATIC DUCTS

*Clinical*

- Usually small, unilocular cyst

- Some might undergo resection with the clinical impression of being an intraductal papillary mucinous neoplasm

*Microscopic*

- Has variable lining ranging from attenuated to transitional to stratified squamous epithelium

- Contains distinctive mucoproteinaceous acidophilic secretions

- The wall is composed of thin fibrous tissue devoid of any lymphoid tissue

- Nuclear p63 expression confirms the nature of the lining

---

## HETEROTOPIC PANCREAS

Heterotopic (ectopic) pancreatic tissue, independent from the vascular supply or anatomic connection to the pancreas, may occur from displacement of small amounts of pancreas during embryologic development.[98–100] It is located most frequently in the stomach and proximal small intestine (Fig. 13), but can be identified in other organs, such as esophagus, gallbladder, hepatic or common bile ducts, spleen, and Meckel diverticulum.[101–103]

Depending on the size, location, and the pathologic changes similar to those observed in case of the normal pancreas, patients may present with symptoms such as epigastric pain, nausea, vomiting, ulcer, obstruction, and weight loss. However, it is often an incidental finding. Radiographically or endoscopically, it may be a challenge to differentiate it from a neoplasm.[104,105]

If it is large enough to be seen on gross inspection, it appears as a firm, pale, nodular mass. Microscopically, it has been classified into 3 types according to the histologic components (Heinrich classification). Type I is composed of complete structures consisting of ducts, acini, and islets of Langerhans cells (see Fig. 13). Type II is composed of ducts and acini. Type III is composed of ducts alone.[106] Histologic type is not related to the clinical symptoms.[107] Of note, small collections of acinar cells in other organs, such as gastroesophageal region, are regarded as metaplasia rather than heterotopia.[108]

In symptomatic cases, surgical excision relieves symptoms. However, rarely, a more extensive treatment may be necessary due to secondary pancreatic neoplasms, including adenocarcinomas arising within ectopic pancreatic tissue.[103,109–114]

---

### Key Features
#### HETEROTOPIC PANCREAS

*Clinical*

- Occurs in a variety of organs; most common in gastrointestinal tract

- Usually an incidental finding

- May rarely cause symptoms due to local complications or secondary pancreatic pathology

*Microscopic*

- Components of the pancreas (acini, ducts, or islets) in different combinations

---

## PANCREATIC HAMARTOMA

The term hamartoma refers to a focal overgrowth of cells and tissues native to the organ in which it

*Fig. 12.* Squamoid cyst of pancreatic duct showing unilocular and well-circumscribed cyst filled with dense mucoproteinaceous material, characteristic of enzymatic concretions (H&E, ×40).

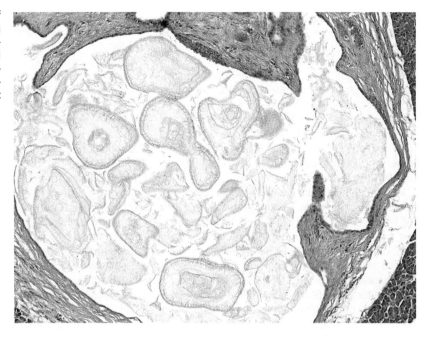

occurs. Thus, hamartoma is regarded as a malformation rather than a true neoplasm.[98,115]

Pancreatic hamartoma is rare, accounting for fewer than 1% of occurrences of tumorlike lesions.[116] Usually presents as a well-demarcated, solid, or solid and cystic mass. It is often located in the head of the pancreas.[117–121] Cases with multiple lesions have been reported.[117,118]

Microscopically, it is characterized by small to medium-sized ductal structures, lined by

*Fig. 13.* Heterotopic pancreas, containing all of the normal pancreatic elements, in the duodenal submucosa (H&E, ×40).

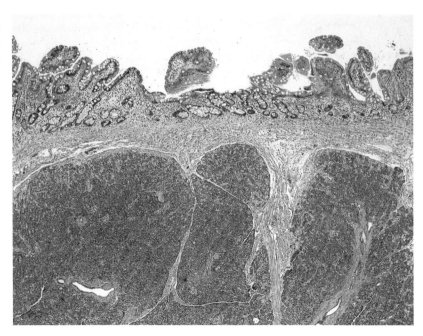

columnar epithelium without atypia, surrounded by disarranged acini and reveals various amounts of fibrous stroma (Fig. 14). Well-formed islets of Langerhans are not common. In fact, Pauser and colleagues[120,122] and Yamaguchi and colleagues[123] defined the criteria for the diagnosis of pancreatic hamartoma as (1) forming a well-demarcated mass, (2) being composed of mature acini and ducts with distorted architecture, and (3) lacking discrete islets of Langerhans. Adjacent pancreatic parenchyma is usually unremarkable.

Immunohistochemically, both acinar cells and ductal cells are positive for epithelial markers (AE1/AE3, CAM5.2, and EMA), and the acinar cells are positive for exocrine markers (eg, trypsin, chymotrypsin), similar to what is observed in a normal pancreas. The stromal spindle cells reportedly express CD34 and CD117 but are usually negative for S100, SMA, desmin, and bcl-2.[118–123]

Although pancreatic hamartoma is usually not aggressive, it typically requires surgical resection because of the difficulty in prospective clinical imaging diagnosis.[124–126]

## NESIDIOBLASTOSIS

Nesidioblastosis is a descriptor of the morphologic changes seen in functional disorders of the endocrine pancreas, characterized by persistent hyperinsulinemic hypoglycemia, due to defective non-neoplastic β-cells.[2] It is usually seen in newborns[30,31] (also known as congenital hyperinsulinism[127,128]); however, rare cases of adult nesidioblastosis do occur.[98,129–133]

Nesidioblastosis can be diagnosed biochemically, usually within the first few weeks of life, through a series of highly specialized tests of glucose, insulin, C-peptide levels, ketones, and glucagon response coupled with arterial calcium stimulation or percutaneous transhepatic pancreatic venous sampling.[134] However, heterogeneous clinical manifestation causes risk of late diagnosis or even misdiagnosis, which can lead to serious and permanent damage to the central nervous system and, eventually, mental retardation.[135]

Currently, there are 3 histologic forms of nesidioblastosis: focal, diffuse, and atypical. Focal nesidioblastosis occurs when the abnormal islets are localized to a specific location in the pancreas. Diffuse form occurs when all the islets in the pancreas are abnormal. If a case is difficult to histologically categorize, it is regarded as atypical form.[128,136]

Alterations vary from patient to patient and may include the following:

- Relatively large collections of islet cells displacing acinar tissue,
- Neoproliferation of islet cells from ducts (ductuloinsular complexes),

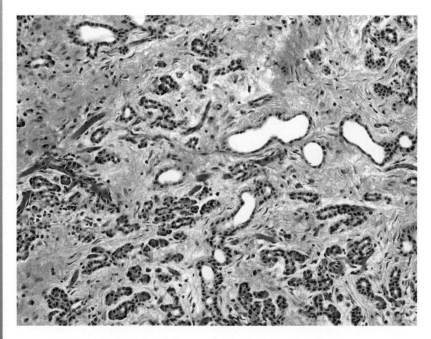

Fig. 14. Pancreatic hamartoma with cystic ductal structures and disorganized acini embedded in a fibroblastic stroma. Note that islets are not present (H&E, ×100).

- Islet cell "dysplasia" or nesidiodysplasia (loss of the usual centrilobular concentration of larger islets, increased numbers of small aggregates of islet cells distributed irregularly in the lobules, irregularity of the contour of the islets), or
- Scattered islet cells (mostly β-cells cells) with enlarged and hypertrophic nuclei.[132,137–140]

However, none of these changes are specific for nesidioblastosis and would be confirmatory only in the right clinical context. Also, it should be kept in mind that in adults, hyperinsulinemic hypoglycemia is usually the result of a neuroendocrine neoplasm releasing insulin. Therefore, before nesidioblastosis diagnosis can be rendered, a diligent search for a neuroendocrine tumor is essential. In fact, the patient ought to be considered to have a neuroendocrine tumor unless definitively proven otherwise by systemic examination of the resected pancreas.

At a molecular level, genetic abnormalities in 9 different genes (ATP-binding cassette subfamily C member 8 [ABCC8], potassium channel, inwardly rectifying subfamily J, member 11 [KCNJ11], glutamate dehydrogenase 1 [GLUD1], glucokinase [GCK], hepatocyte nuclear factor 4 homeobox A [HNF4A], HNF1A, SLC16A1 [also known as a monocarboxylate transporter, MCT1], uncoupling protein 2 [UCP2] and hydroxyacyl-CoA dehydrogenase [HADH]) have been identified in approximately half of the cases, indicating that there are as yet unidentified mechanisms involved in the regulation of insulin secretion.[135]

Genetic abnormalities are classified into 2 categories: "channelopathies" and "metabolopathies."[141] The former is attributed to the ATP-sensitive potassium channels ($K_{ATP}$) channel genes (ABCC8 and KCNJ11) and latter to genes regulating different metabolic pathways (GLUD1, GCK, HNF4A, HNF1A, SLC16A1, UCP2, and HADH). The most common disorders are those affecting the $K_{ATP}$ channel genes and these are predominantly autosomal recessive. The other 7 are less common but are autosomal dominant.[135,142,143] In most cases, diffuse form is inherited in an autosomal recessive manner, whereas focal form is sporadic.[144,145] Patients with a homozygous recessive or a compound heterozygote mutation in their ABCC8 or KCNJ11 genes are usually medically unresponsive.[142]

Partial to near-total pancreatectomy is the treatment of choice in cases refractory to aggressive medical management, although enucleation may be of value in controlling

the symptoms in cases with focal nesidioblastosis. Diabetes mellitus and pancreatic insufficiency (malabsorption) may develop after pancreatectomy.[129,146–148]

## Key Features
### NESIDIOBLASTOSIS

*Clinical*
- Functional disorder of the β-cells
- Associated with persistent hyperinsulinemic hypoglycemia

*Microscopic*
- Can be focal or diffuse
- Pathologic findings vary greatly patient to patient
- Enlarged islets, abnormally shaped islets, ductuloinsular complexes, and enlarged (a threefold increase relative to the nuclei of adjacent islet cells) and hyperchromatic β-cell nuclei are common
- However, none of these changes are specific and would be confirmatory only in the right clinical context
- An insulinoma must be excluded by pathologic examination before nesidioblastosis diagnosis can be rendered

*Molecular*
- Genetic abnormalities in 9 different genes (ABCC8, KCNJ11, GLUD1, GCK, HNF4A, HNF1A, SLC16A1, UCP2, and HADH) have been identified in approximately half of the cases

## LIPOMATOUS PSEUDOHYPERTROPHY

Focal replacement of the exocrine pancreas with mature adipose tissue is common in the pancreas and usually correlates directly with body mass index.[149–151] In contrast, lipomatous pseudohypertrophy is a distinct entity characterized by pseudotumor formation by adipose tissue, replacing almost an entire segment of exocrine parenchyma.[152]

Most common symptom at presentation is abdominal pain.[152] In some cases, lipomatous pseudohypertrophy seems to be associated with specific syndromes such as Shwachman-Diamond or Johanson-Blizzard[153,154] syndromes. Because it forms a mass, it is often mistaken for a malignancy.[155] On the other hand, if proper radiological evaluation is performed, it can be recognized that the lesion is actually composed of fat. Fine-needle aspiration biopsy showing mature fat cells, without any atypia, might be helpful in such cases.[156]

Approximately in 70% of the cases, there is a diffuse involvement of the pancreas; in 30%, the tumor is located in the head, body, or tail only.[152] Macroscopically, the appearance and consistency are those of adipose tissue. Histologic examination shows massive replacement of pancreatic parenchyma by mature adipose tissue. Although it does not appear to have a well-formed capsule, it has well-defined borders (Fig. 15). The islets of Langerhans are relatively preserved, and typically there are scattered, small but well-preserved acinar elements. There is no significant inflammation. Adjacent pancreatic or soft tissue may show signs of compression.

At the microscopic level, the main differential diagnosis is with a well-differentiated liposarcoma, which is reported in the literature as individual case reports.[66,157] The findings that speak against this possibility are the perfect maturation of lipocytes, sharp demarcation of the lesion, lack of lipoblasts, and admixture of normal pancreatic parenchyma within the lesion.[152]

### Key Features
#### LIPOMATOUS PSEUDOHYPERTROPHY

*Clinical*
- May be mistaken for a malignancy

*Microscopic*
- Can be focal or diffuse

- Characterized by mature adipose tissue replacing the pancreatic parenchyma, leaving only scattered clusters of pancreatic elements

- Lipocytes are entirely normal, no lipoblast present

## PARADUODENAL (GROOVE) PANCREATITIS

Paraduodenal pancreatitis (also known as groove pancreatitis or cystic dystrophy of heterotopic pancreas) is a distinctive form of pancreatitis that occurs in the tissue between the duodenal wall and the pancreatic head. It often surrounds the minor ampulla and accessory duct.[158–160]

The vast majority of patients are young men with a history of alcohol abuse. The most common symptom is severe waxing and waning upper abdominal pain. Frequent clinical findings include stenosis of duodenum, disordered gastric emptying, and

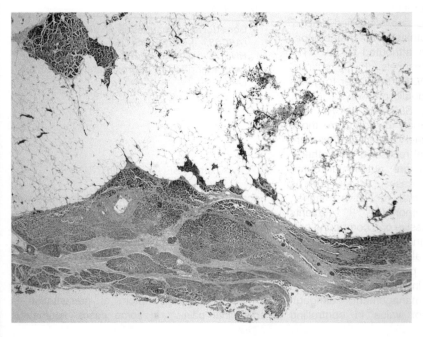

Fig. 15. Well-circumscribed lipomatous pseudohypertrophy, composed of mature adipose tissue, pushing into the adjacent pancreas is illustrated. Scattered acini within the adipose tissue are also visible (H&E, ×200).

postprandial vomiting. Weight loss is also a common finding and can be severe in some cases, complicating the differential diagnosis with pancreas cancer.[91,161,162] local thickening and abnormal enhancement of the second portion of the duodenum and "tubulocystic" change in the vicinity of the accessory duct are specific features of this entity.[90,163,164] Those who have predominantly solid lesions, often related to the sclerotic changes in the periampullary region, are commonly diagnosed as "pancreas cancer" or "ampullary/periampullary neoplasm."[90,160]

The reasons for this process to develop are not known; however, the macroscopic and microscopic findings are quite distinctive: the process leads to narrowing of the duodenal lumen and the duodenal mucosa often acquires a nodular or cobblestone appearance.[165] On sectioning, the duodenal wall shows a trabeculated appearance, often accompanied by cystic change, especially in the vicinity of the minor ampulla. In some cases, cyst formation may be prominent, measuring up to several centimeters in size, mimicking intestinal duplication.

Microscopically, the duodenal mucosa often reveals Brunner gland hyperplasia and there is an exuberant myofibroblastic proliferation, often arranged in fascicles (**Fig. 16**) accompanied by small, well-circumscribed lobules of pancreatic tissue ("myoadenomatosis" pattern) or variably sized ducts ("cystic dystrophy of heterotopic pancreas"). These ducts may contain inspissated acinar enzymes. The cyst contents may extravasate and lead to the development of a foreign-body giant cell reaction and stromal eosinophilia. Some cysts are devoid of epithelium (**Fig. 17**). Instead, they are lined by more cellular fibroblastic tissue.[160,164] Prominence of nerve bundles mimicking traumatic neuroma is also common.

It should be kept in mind that, as in any case of pancreatic pathology, before the diagnosis of paraduodenal pancreatitis is rendered, the possibility of adenocarcinoma ought to be carefully excluded, because it can mimic any form of pancreatitis, and be associated with any of the changes characteristic of this lesion.

---

### *Key Features*
#### PARADUODENAL PANCREATITIS

*Clinical*

- Predominantly in men 40 to 50 years old

- History of alcohol abuse is common

- Patients present with waxing and waning severe upper abdominal pain and postprandial vomiting

- Predominantly solid ones radiographically mimic pancreatic or ampullary/periampullary tumors

*Macroscopic*

- Often centered in the region of minor papilla

- Trabeculation of duodenal musculature with occasional cysts is common

- Paraduodenal wall cyst (measuring up to 10 cm) mimicking intestinal duplication may occur

*Microscopic*

- Dense myoid stromal proliferation with intervening rounded lobules of pancreatic tissue ("myoadenomatosis")

- Brunner gland hyperplasia

- Extravasated (stromal) mucoprotein plugs surrounded by eosinophiles or multinucleated giant cells

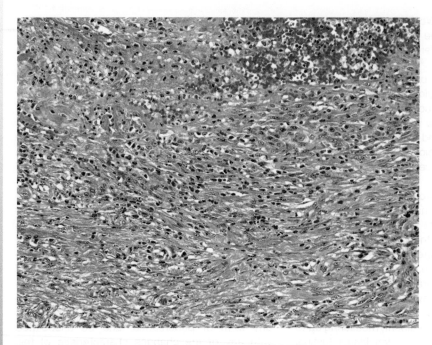

*Fig. 16.* In paraduodenal (groove) pancreatitis, there is a striking reactive spindle cell proliferation, including, smooth muscle cells and myofibroblasts, associated with inflammatory cells (H&E, ×200).

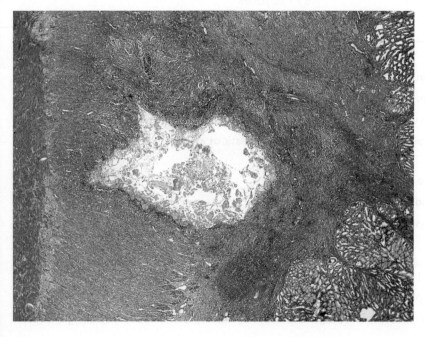

*Fig. 17.* Characteristically, the cysts of paraduodenal (groove) pancreatitis contain eosinophilic, amorphous inspissated enzymatic secretions and are surrounded by markedly inflamed fibrous tissue. Note the abundant Brunner glands on the right (H&E, ×40).

## SUMMARY

Benign neoplasms and tumorlike (pseudotumoral) lesions of the pancreas can be challenging, mostly due to lack of familiarity because of the lower number of cases, compared with malignant neoplasms, pathologists encounter on a daily basis.

Well-demarcated and spongelike appearance with innumerable small cysts of *microcystic* serous cystadenomas is so characteristic and usually does not create any diagnostic problems. In contrast, macrocytic serous cystadenomas can be difficult to diagnose, as the lining epithelium might be extremely attenuated. Inflammatory myofibroblastic tumors may have overlapping morphologic features with IgG4-related autoimmune pancreatitis (discussed separately in this issue). However, it is different from autoimmune pancreatitis in terms of the ALK expression, low level of IgG4+ cell infiltration, and lack of obstructive phlebitis.

A variety of non-neoplastic conditions may also form a cystic or solid mass mimicking a malignant neoplasm in the pancreas. Up to 5% of pancreatectomies performed with the preoperative clinical diagnosis of malignant neoplasm will prove to be non-neoplastic by pathologic examination, although this figure is decreasing with improved diagnostic modalities. Lymphoepithelial cyst, epidermoid cyst in intrapancreatic accessory spleen, and squamoid cyst of pancreatic ducts are all cystic lesions lined by usually squamous epithelium and recognition of the accompanying elements (eg, lymphoid tissue with or without germinal centers, splenic tissue) is necessary for a correct diagnosis. Heterotopic pancreas may form a well-defined nodule within the duodenum and is typically mistaken for neuroendocrine neoplasm. Hamartomas are very rare if the entity is defined strictly. They are characterized by irregularly arranged mature pancreatic elements admixed with stromal tissue. None of the pathologic findings of nesidioblastosis, such as enlarged islets, abnormally shaped islets, ductuloinsular complexes, and enlarged/hyperchromatic β-cell nuclei are specific and would be confirmatory only in the right clinical context. Lipomatous hypertrophy is the replacement of pancreatic tissue with mature adipose tissue that occasionally leads to moderate to marked enlargement of the pancreas. Chronic inflammatory lesions are the leading cause of "pseudotumoral pancreatitis," and among these, autoimmune and paraduodenal pancreatitides are most important.

In conclusion, it is important to recognize all these benign neoplasms and types of conditions that form pseudotumors in the pancreas so that they can be distinguished from malignant neoplasms, especially ductal adenocarcinomas.

## REFERENCES

1. Reid MD, Choi HJ, Memis B, et al. Serous neoplasms of the pancreas: a clinicopathologic analysis of 193 cases and literature review with new insights on macrocystic and solid variants and critical reappraisal of so-called "serous cystadenocarcinoma". Am J Surg Pathol 2015;39: 1597–610.
2. Hruban R, Pitman MB, Klimstra DS. Tumors of the pancreas. AFIP atlas of tumor pathology. Washington, DC: American Registry of Pathology; 2007.
3. Kobayashi N, Sato T, Kato S, et al. Imaging findings of pancreatic cystic lesions in von Hippel-Lindau disease. Intern Med 2012;51:1301–7.
4. Kanno A, Satoh K, Hamada S, et al. Serous cystic neoplasms of the whole pancreas in a patient with von Hippel-Lindau disease. Intern Med 2011;50: 1293–8.
5. Matsubayashi H, Uesaka K, Kanemoto H, et al. Multiple endocrine neoplasms and serous cysts of the pancreas in a patient with von Hippel-Lindau disease. J Gastrointest Cancer 2010;41:197–202.
6. Moore PS, Zamboni G, Brighenti A, et al. Molecular characterization of pancreatic serous microcystic adenomas: evidence for a tumor suppressor gene on chromosome 10q. Am J Pathol 2001;158: 317–21.
7. Mohr VH, Vortmeyer AO, Zhuang Z, et al. Histopathology and molecular genetics of multiple cysts and microcystic (serous) adenomas of the pancreas in von Hippel-Lindau patients. Am J Pathol 2000;157:1615–21.
8. Vortmeyer AO, Lubensky IA, Fogt F, et al. Allelic deletion and mutation of the von Hippel-Lindau (VHL) tumor suppressor gene in pancreatic microcystic adenomas. Am J Pathol 1997;151:951–6.
9. Jais B, Rebours V, Malleo G, et al. Serous cystic neoplasm of the pancreas: a multinational study of 2622 patients under the auspices of the International Association of Pancreatology and European Pancreatic Club (European Study Group on Cystic Tumors of the Pancreas). Gut 2016;65:305–12.
10. Reid MD, Choi H, Balci S, et al. Serous cystic neoplasms of the pancreas: clinicopathologic and molecular characteristics. Semin Diagn Pathol 2014;31:475–83.
11. Fukasawa M, Maguchi H, Takahashi K, et al. Clinical features and natural history of serous cystic neoplasm of the pancreas. Pancreatology 2010;10: 695–701.
12. Colonna J, Plaza JA, Frankel WL, et al. Serous cystadenoma of the pancreas: clinical and

pathological features in 33 patients. Pancreatology 2008;8:135–41.

13. Kosmahl M, Pauser U, Peters K, et al. Cystic neoplasms of the pancreas and tumor-like lesions with cystic features: a review of 418 cases and a classification proposal. Virchows Arch 2004;445:168–78.

14. Bassi C, Salvia R, Molinari E, et al. Management of 100 consecutive cases of pancreatic serous cystadenoma: wait for symptoms and see at imaging or vice versa? World J Surg 2003;27:319–23.

15. Yasuhara Y, Sakaida N, Uemura Y, et al. Serous microcystic adenoma (glycogen-rich cystadenoma) of the pancreas: study of 11 cases showing clinicopathological and immunohistochemical correlations. Pathol Int 2002;52:307–12.

16. Procacci C, Carbognin G, Biasiutti C, et al. Serous cystadenoma of the pancreas: imaging findings. Radiol Med 2001;102:23–31.

17. Capella C, Solcia E, Kloppel G, et al. Serous cystic neoplasms of the pancreas. Tumors of the exocrine pancreas. In: Hamilton SR, Aaltonen LA, editors. Pathology and genetics of tumours of the digestive system. Lyon (France): IARCPress; 2000. p. 231–3.

18. Compton CC. Serous cystic tumors of the pancreas. Semin Diagn Pathol 2000;17:43–55.

19. Sperti C, Pasquali C, Perasole A, et al. Macrocystic serous cystadenoma of the pancreas: clinicopathologic features in seven cases. Int J Pancreatol 2000;28:1–7.

20. Alpert LC, Truong LD, Bossart MI, et al. Microcystic adenoma (serous cystadenoma) of the pancreas. A study of 14 cases with immunohistochemical and electron-microscopic correlation. Am J Surg Pathol 1988;12:251–63.

21. Compagno J, Oertel JE. Microcystic adenomas of the pancreas (glycogen-rich cystadenomas): a clinicopathologic study of 34 cases. Am J Clin Pathol 1978;69:289–98.

22. Kimura W, Moriya T, Hirai I, et al. Multicenter study of serous cystic neoplasm of the Japan Pancreas Society. Pancreas 2012;41:380–7.

23. Galanis C, Zamani A, Cameron JL, et al. Resected serous cystic neoplasms of the pancreas: a review of 158 patients with recommendations for treatment. J Gastrointest Surg 2007;11:820–6.

24. Charlesworth M, Verbeke CS, Falk GA, et al. Pancreatic lesions in von Hippel-Lindau disease? A systematic review and meta-synthesis of the literature. J Gastrointest Surg 2012;16:1422–8.

25. Khashab MA, Shin EJ, Amateau S, et al. Tumor size and location correlate with behavior of pancreatic serous cystic neoplasms. Am J Gastroenterol 2011;106:1521–6.

26. Mukhopadhyay B, Sahdev A, Monson JP, et al. Pancreatic lesions in von Hippel-Lindau disease. Clin Endocrinol (Oxf) 2002;57:603–8.

27. Girelli R, Bassi C, Falconi M, et al. Pancreatic cystic manifestations in von Hippel-Lindau disease. Int J Pancreatol 1997;22:101–9.

28. Berman L, Mitchell KA, Israel G, et al. Serous cystadenoma in communication with the pancreatic duct: an unusual radiologic and pathologic entity. J Clin Gastroenterol 2010;44:e133–5.

29. Garcea G, Ong SL, Rajesh A, et al. Cystic lesions of the pancreas. A diagnostic and management dilemma. Pancreatology 2008;8:236–51.

30. Kim SY, Lee JM, Kim SH, et al. Macrocystic neoplasms of the pancreas: CT differentiation of serous oligocystic adenoma from mucinous cystadenoma and intraductal papillary mucinous tumor. AJR Am J Roentgenol 2006;187:1192–8.

31. Lal A, Bourtsos EP, DeFrias DV, et al. Microcystic adenoma of the pancreas: clinical, radiologic, and cytologic features. Cancer 2004;102:288–94.

32. Chatelain D, Hammel P, O'Toole D, et al. Macrocystic form of serous pancreatic cystadenoma. Am J Gastroenterol 2002;97:2566–71.

33. Kobayashi T, Shimura T, Araki K, et al. Macrocystic serous cystadenoma mimicking branch duct intraductal papillary mucinous neoplasm. Int Surg 2009;94:176–81.

34. Lee SE, Kwon Y, Jang JY, et al. The morphological classification of a serous cystic tumor (SCT) of the pancreas and evaluation of the preoperative diagnostic accuracy of computed tomography. Ann Surg Oncol 2008;15:2089–95.

35. Yamaguchi H, Ishigami K, Inoue T, et al. Three cases of serous oligocystic adenomas of the pancreas; evaluation of cyst wall thickness for preoperative differentiation from mucinous cystic neoplasms. J Gastrointest Cancer 2007;38:52–8.

36. Collins BT. Serous cystadenoma of the pancreas with endoscopic ultrasound fine needle aspiration biopsy and surgical correlation. Acta Cytol 2013;57:241–51.

37. Salomao M, Remotti H, Allendorf JD, et al. Fine-needle aspirations of pancreatic serous cystadenomas: improving diagnostic yield with cell blocks and alpha-inhibin immunohistochemistry. Cancer Cytopathol 2014;122(1):33–9.

38. Belsley NA, Pitman MB, Lauwers GY, et al. Serous cystadenoma of the pancreas: limitations and pitfalls of endoscopic ultrasound-guided fine-needle aspiration biopsy. Cancer 2008;114:102–10.

39. Huang P, Staerkel G, Sneige N, et al. Fine-needle aspiration of pancreatic serous cystadenoma: cytologic features and diagnostic pitfalls. Cancer 2006;108:239–49.

40. Lewandrowski K, Lee J, Southern J, et al. Cyst fluid analysis in the differential diagnosis of pancreatic cysts: a new approach to the preoperative assessment of pancreatic cystic lesions. AJR Am J Roentgenol 1995;164:815–9.

41. Wu J, Matthaei H, Maitra A, et al. Recurrent GNAS mutations define an unexpected pathway for pancreatic cyst development. Sci Transl Med 2011;3:92ra66.

42. Yip-Schneider MT, Wu H, Dumas RP, et al. Vascular endothelial growth factor, a novel and highly accurate pancreatic fluid biomarker for serous pancreatic cysts. J Am Coll Surg 2014;218:608–17.

43. Panarelli NC, Park KJ, Hruban RH, et al. Microcystic serous cystadenoma of the pancreas with subtotal cystic degeneration: another neoplastic mimic of pancreatic pseudocyst. Am J Surg Pathol 2012;36:726–31.

44. Tseng JF, Warshaw AL, Sahani DV, et al. Serous cystadenoma of the pancreas: tumor growth rates and recommendations for treatment. Ann Surg 2005;242:413–9.

45. Thirabanjasak D, Basturk O, Altinel D, et al. Is serous cystadenoma of the pancreas a model of clear-cell-associated angiogenesis and tumorigenesis? Pancreatology 2009;9:182–8.

46. Yamazaki K, Eyden B. An immunohistochemical and ultrastructural study of pancreatic microcystic serous cyst adenoma with special reference to tumor-associated microvasculature and vascular endothelial growth factor in tumor cells. Ultrastruct Pathol 2006;30:119–28.

47. Basturk O, Singh R, Kaygusuz E, et al. GLUT-1 expression in pancreatic neoplasia: implications in pathogenesis, diagnosis, and prognosis. Pancreas 2011;40:187–92.

48. Ji Y, Wang XN, Lou WH, et al. Serous cystic neoplasms of the pancreas: a clinicopathologic and immunohistochemical analysis. Chin J Dig Dis 2006;7:39–44.

49. Kosmahl M, Wagner J, Peters K, et al. Serous cystic neoplasms of the pancreas: an immunohistochemical analysis revealing alpha-inhibin, neuron-specific enolase, and MUC6 as new markers. Am J Surg Pathol 2004;28:339–46.

50. Wu J, Jiao Y, Dal Molin M, et al. Whole-exome sequencing of neoplastic cysts of the pancreas reveals recurrent mutations in components of ubiquitin-dependent pathways. Proc Natl Acad Sci U S A 2011;108:21188–93.

51. Malleo G, Bassi C, Rossini R, et al. Growth pattern of serous cystic neoplasms of the pancreas: observational study with long-term magnetic resonance surveillance and recommendations for treatment. Gut 2012;61:746–51.

52. El-Hayek KM, Brown N, O'Rourke C, et al. Rate of growth of pancreatic serous cystadenoma as an indication for resection. Surgery 2013;154: 794–800, [discussion: 800–20].

53. Valsangkar NP, Morales-Oyarvide V, Thayer SP, et al. 851 resected cystic tumors of the pancreas: a 33-year experience at the Massachusetts General Hospital. Surgery 2012;152:S4–12.

54. Zanini N, Fantini L, Casadei R, et al. Serous cystic tumors of the pancreas: when to observe and when to operate: a single-center experience. Dig Surg 2008;25:233–9, [discussion: 240].

55. Wargo JA, Fernandez-del-Castillo C, Warshaw AL. Management of pancreatic serous cystadenomas. Adv Surg 2009;43:23–34.

56. Oh HC, Seo DW. Endoscopic ultrasonography-guided pancreatic cyst ablation (with video). J Hepatobiliary Pancreat Sci 2015;22:16–9.

57. DiMaio CJ, DeWitt JM, Brugge WR. Ablation of pancreatic cystic lesions: the use of multiple endoscopic ultrasound-guided ethanol lavage sessions. Pancreas 2011;40:664–8.

58. Terris B, Fukushima N, Hruban RH. Serous neoplasms of the pancreas. In: Bosman FT, Carneiro F, Hruban RH, et al, editors. WHO classification of tumours of the digestive system. Lyon (France): IARC Press; 2010. p. 296–9.

59. Zhu H, Qin L, Zhong M, et al. Carcinoma ex microcystic adenoma of the pancreas: a report of a novel form of malignancy in serous neoplasms. Am J Surg Pathol 2012;36:305–10.

60. Lee SD, Han SS, Hong EK. Solid serous cystic neoplasm of the pancreas with invasive growth. J Hepatobiliary Pancreat Sci 2013;20:454–6.

61. Yasuda A, Sawai H, Ochi N, et al. Solid variant of serous cystadenoma of the pancreas. Arch Med Sci 2011;7:353–5.

62. Casadei R, D'Ambra M, Pezzilli R, et al. Solid serous microcystic tumor of the pancreas. JOP 2008;9:538–40.

63. Stern JR, Frankel WL, Ellison EC, et al. Solid serous microcystic adenoma of the pancreas. World J Surg Oncol 2007;5:26.

64. Reese SA, Traverso LW, Jacobs TW, et al. Solid serous adenoma of the pancreas: a rare variant within the family of pancreatic serous cystic neoplasms. Pancreas 2006;33:96–9.

65. Hoang MP, Hruban RH, Albores-Saavedra J. Clear cell endocrine pancreatic tumor mimicking renal cell carcinoma: a distinctive neoplasm of von Hippel-Lindau disease. Am J Surg Pathol 2001;25:602–9.

66. Kim JY, Song JS, Park H, et al. Primary mesenchymal tumors of the pancreas: single-center experience over 16 years. Pancreas 2014;43: 959–68.

67. Mizukami H, Yajima N, Wada R, et al. Pancreatic malignant fibrous histiocytoma, inflammatory myofibroblastic tumor, and inflammatory pseudotumor related to autoimmune pancreatitis: characterization and differential diagnosis. Virchows Arch 2006;448:552–60.

68. Yamamoto H, Watanabe K, Nagata M, et al. Inflammatory myofibroblastic tumor (IMT) of the pancreas. J Hepatobiliary Pancreat Surg 2002;9: 116–9.

69. Yamamoto H, Yamaguchi H, Aishima S, et al. Inflammatory myofibroblastic tumor versus IgG4-related sclerosing disease and inflammatory pseudotumor: a comparative clinicopathologic study. Am J Surg Pathol 2009;33:1330–40.

70. Casadei R, Piccoli L, Valeri B, et al. Inflammatory pseudotumor of the pancreas resembling pancreatic cancer: clinical, diagnostic and therapeutic considerations. Chir Ital 2004;56:849–58.

71. Wreesmann V, van Eijck CH, Naus DC, et al. Inflammatory pseudotumour (inflammatory myofibroblastic tumour) of the pancreas: a report of six cases associated with obliterative phlebitis. Histopathology 2001;38:105–10.

72. Tothova Z, Wagner AJ. Anaplastic lymphoma kinase-directed therapy in inflammatory myofibroblastic tumors. Curr Opin Oncol 2012;24:409–13.

73. Griffin CA, Hawkins AL, Dvorak C, et al. Recurrent involvement of 2p23 in inflammatory myofibroblastic tumors. Cancer Res 1999;59:2776–80.

74. Bridge JA, Kanamori M, Ma Z, et al. Fusion of the ALK gene to the clathrin heavy chain gene, CLTC, in inflammatory myofibroblastic tumor. Am J Pathol 2001;159:411–5.

75. Ma Z, Hill DA, Collins MH, et al. Fusion of ALK to the Ran-binding protein 2 (RANBP2) gene in inflammatory myofibroblastic tumor. Genes Chromosomes Cancer 2003;37:98–105.

76. Ohara H, Nakazawa T, Sano H, et al. Histopathologic similarities of inflammatory pseudotumor to autoimmune pancreatitis: a morphologic and immunohistochemical study of 4 cases. Pancreas 2006;32:115–7.

77. Adsay NV, Hasteh F, Cheng JD, et al. Lymphoepithelial cysts of the pancreas: a report of 12 cases and a review of the literature. Mod Pathol 2002; 15:492–501.

78. Adsay NV, Hasteh F, Cheng JD, et al. Squamous-lined cysts of the pancreas: lymphoepithelial cysts, dermoid cysts (teratomas), and accessory-splenic epidermoid cysts. Semin Diagn Pathol 2000;17:56–65.

79. Bedat B, Genevay M, Dumonceau JM, et al. Association between lymphoepithelial cysts of the pancreas and HIV infection. Pancreatology 2012; 12:61–4.

80. Kim WH, Lee JY, Park HS, et al. Lymphoepithelial cyst of the pancreas: comparison of CT findings with other pancreatic cystic lesions. Abdom Imaging 2013;38:324–30.

81. Vandenbussche CJ, Maleki Z. Fine-needle aspiration of squamous-lined cysts of the pancreas. Diagn Cytopathol 2014;42(7):592–9.

82. Tewari N, Rollins K, Wu J, et al. Lymphoepithelial cyst of the pancreas and elevated cyst fluid carcinoembryonic antigen: a diagnostic challenge. JOP 2014;15:504–7.

83. Raval JS, Zeh HJ, Moser AJ, et al. Pancreatic lymphoepithelial cysts express CEA and can contain mucous cells: potential pitfalls in the preoperative diagnosis. Mod Pathol 2010;23:1467–76.

84. Yamaguchi T, Takahashi H, Kagawa R, et al. Lymphoepithelial cyst of the pancreas associated with elevated CA 19-9 levels. J Hepatobiliary Pancreat Surg 2008;15:652–4.

85. Nakamura T, Osaka Y, Ishikawa S, et al. Uncommon lymphoepithelial cyst with sebaceous glands of the pancreas. JOP 2013;14:632–5.

86. Mege D, Gregoire E, Barbier L, et al. Lymphoepithelial cyst of the pancreas: an analysis of 117 patients. Pancreas 2014;43:987–95.

87. Halpert B, Gyorkey F. Accessory spleen in the tail of the pancreas. AMA Arch Pathol 1957;64:266–9.

88. Hwang HS, Lee SS, Kim SC, et al. Intrapancreatic accessory spleen: clinicopathologic analysis of 12 cases. Pancreas 2011;40:956–65.

89. Motosugi U, Yamaguchi H, Ichikawa T, et al. Epidermoid cyst in intrapancreatic accessory spleen: radiological findings including superparamagnetic iron oxide-enhanced magnetic resonance imaging. J Comput Assist Tomogr 2010;34:217–22.

90. Kalb B, Martin DR, Sarmiento JM, et al. Paraduodenal pancreatitis: clinical performance of MR imaging in distinguishing from carcinoma. Radiology 2013;269:475–81.

91. Kloppel G, Adsay NV. Chronic pancreatitis and the differential diagnosis versus pancreatic cancer. Arch Pathol Lab Med 2009;133:382–7.

92. Othman M, Basturk O, Groisman G, et al. Squamoid cyst of pancreatic ducts: a distinct type of cystic lesion in the pancreas. Am J Surg Pathol 2007;31:291–7.

93. Adsay NV. Cystic lesions of the pancreas. Mod Pathol 2007;20(Suppl 1):S71–93.

94. Basturk O, Khanani F, Sarkar F, et al. DeltaNp63 expression in pancreas and pancreatic neoplasia. Mod Pathol 2005;18:1193–8.

95. Basturk O, Coban I, Adsay NV. Pancreatic cysts: pathologic classification, differential diagnosis, and clinical implications. Arch Pathol Lab Med 2009;133:423–38.

96. Hanson JA, Salem RR, Mitchell KA. Squamoid cyst of pancreatic ducts: a case series describing novel immunohistochemistry, cytology, and quantitative cyst fluid chemistry. Arch Pathol Lab Med 2014; 138:270–3.

97. Milanetto AC, Iaria L, Alaggio R, et al. Squamoid cyst of pancreatic ducts: a challenging differential diagnosis among benign pancreatic cysts. JOP 2013;14:657–60.

98. Thompson LDR, Basturk O, Adsay V. Pancreas. In: Mills S, editor. Sternberg's diagnostic surgical pathology. (China): Wolters Kluwer Health; 2015. p. 1577–662.

99. Ormarsson OT, Gudmundsdottir I, Marvik R. Diagnosis and treatment of gastric heterotopic pancreas. World J Surg 2006;30:1682–9.

100. Eisenberger CF, Gocht A, Knoefel WT, et al. Heterotopic pancreas–clinical presentation and pathology with review of the literature. Hepatogastroenterology 2004;51:854–8.

101. Lawrence AJ, Thiessen A, Morse A, et al. Heterotopic pancreas within the proximal hepatic duct, containing intraductal papillary mucinous neoplasm. Case Rep Surg 2015;2015:816960.

102. Sumiyoshi T, Shima Y, Okabayashi T, et al. Heterotopic pancreas in the common bile duct, with a review of the literature. Intern Med 2014;53:2679–82.

103. Cates JM, Williams TL, Suriawinata AA. Intraductal papillary mucinous adenoma that arises from pancreatic heterotopia within a Meckel diverticulum. Arch Pathol Lab Med 2005;129:e67–9.

104. Lin M, Fu Y, Yu H, et al. Gastric heterotopic pancreas masquerading as a stromal tumor: a case report. Oncol Lett 2015;10:2355–8.

105. Zinczuk J, Bandurski R, Pryczynicz A, et al. Ectopic pancreas imitating gastrointestinal stromal tumor (GIST) in the stomach. Pol Przegl Chir 2015;87:268–71.

106. von Heinrich H. Ein Beitrag zur Histologie des sogen akzessorischen Pankreas. Virchows Archiv Pathol 1909;198:392–401.

107. Lai EC, Tompkins RK. Heterotopic pancreas. Review of a 26 year experience. Am J Surg 1986;151:697–700.

108. Schneider NI, Plieschnegger W, Geppert M, et al. Pancreatic acinar cells—a normal finding at the gastroesophageal junction? Data from a prospective Central European multicenter study. Virchows Arch 2013;463:643–50.

109. Fukino N, Oida T, Mimatsu K, et al. Adenocarcinoma arising from heterotopic pancreas at the third portion of the duodenum. World J Gastroenterol 2015;21:4082–8.

110. Lee SH, Kim WY, Hwang DY, et al. Intraductal papillary mucinous neoplasm of the ileal heterotopic pancreas in a patient with hereditary nonpolyposis colorectal cancer: a case report. World J Gastroenterol 2015;21:7916–20.

111. Abraham J, Agrawal V, Behari A. Mucinous cystic neoplasm in heterotopic pancreas presenting as colonic polyp. JOP 2013;14:671–3.

112. Ginori A, Vassallo L, Butorano MA, et al. Pancreatic adenocarcinoma in duodenal ectopic pancreas: a case report and review of the literature. Pathologica 2013;105:56–8.

113. Yan ML, Wang YD, Tian YF, et al. Adenocarcinoma arising from intrahepatic heterotopic pancreas: a case report and literature review. World J Gastroenterol 2012;18:2881–4.

114. Chetty R, Weinreb I. Gastric neuroendocrine carcinoma arising from heterotopic pancreatic tissue. J Clin Pathol 2004;57:314–7.

115. Basturk O, Adsay NV. Pancreas. In: Cheng L, Bostwick DG, editors. Essentials of anatomic pathology. 4th Edition. London: Springer; 2016. p. 1945–68.

116. Kim HH, Cho CK, Hur YH, et al. Pancreatic hamartoma diagnosed after surgical resection. J Korean Surg Soc 2012;83:330–4.

117. Matsushita D, Kurahara H, Mataki Y, et al. Pancreatic hamartoma: a case report and literature review. BMC Gastroenterol 2016;16:3.

118. Kawakami F, Shimizu M, Yamaguchi H, et al. Multiple solid pancreatic hamartomas: a case report and review of the literature. World J Gastrointest Oncol 2012;4:202–6.

119. Nagata S, Yamaguchi K, Inoue T, et al. Solid pancreatic hamartoma. Pathol Int 2007;57:276–80.

120. Pauser U, Kosmahl M, Kruslin B, et al. Pancreatic solid and cystic hamartoma in adults: characterization of a new tumorous lesion. Am J Surg Pathol 2005;29:797–800.

121. Flaherty MJ, Benjamin DR. Multicystic pancreatic hamartoma: a distinctive lesion with immunohistochemical and ultrastructural study. Hum Pathol 1992;23:1309–12.

122. Pauser U, da Silva MT, Placke J, et al. Cellular hamartoma resembling gastrointestinal stromal tumor: a solid tumor of the pancreas expressing c-kit (CD117). Mod Pathol 2005;18:1211–6.

123. Yamaguchi H, Aishima S, Oda Y, et al. Distinctive histopathologic findings of pancreatic hamartomas suggesting their "hamartomatous" nature: a study of 9 cases. Am J Surg Pathol 2013;37:1006–13.

124. Al-Hawary MM, Kaza RK, Azar SF, et al. Mimics of pancreatic ductal adenocarcinoma. Cancer Imaging 2013;13:342–9.

125. Kersting S, Janot MS, Munding J, et al. Rare solid tumors of the pancreas as differential diagnosis of pancreatic adenocarcinoma. JOP 2012;13:268–77.

126. Raman SP, Hruban RH, Cameron JL, et al. Pancreatic imaging mimics: part 2, pancreatic neuroendocrine tumors and their mimics. AJR Am J Roentgenol 2012;199:309–18.

127. Fournet JC, Junien C. Genetics of congenital hyperinsulinism. Endocr Pathol 2004;15:233–40.

128. Sempoux C, Guiot Y, Jaubert F, et al. Focal and diffuse forms of congenital hyperinsulinism: the keys for differential diagnosis. Endocr Pathol 2004;15:241–6.

129. Kloppel G, Anlauf M, Raffel A, et al. Adult diffuse nesidioblastosis: genetically or environmentally induced? Hum Pathol 2008;39:3–8.

130. Rumilla KM, Erickson LA, Service FJ, et al. Hyperinsulinemic hypoglycemia with nesidioblastosis: histologic features and growth factor expression. Mod Pathol 2009;22:239–45.

131. Raffel A, Krausch MM, Anlauf M, et al. Diffuse nesidioblastosis as a cause of hyperinsulinemic hypoglycemia in adults: a diagnostic and therapeutic challenge. Surgery 2007;141:179–84.

132. Anlauf M, Wieben D, Perren A, et al. Persistent hyperinsulinemic hypoglycemia in 15 adults with diffuse nesidioblastosis: diagnostic criteria, incidence, and characterization of beta-cell changes. Am J Surg Pathol 2005;29:524–33.

133. Service FJ, Natt N, Thompson GB, et al. Noninsulinoma pancreatogenous hypoglycemia: a novel syndrome of hyperinsulinemia hypoglycemia in adults independent of mutations in Kir6.2 and SUR1 genes. J Clin Endocrinol Metab 1998;84:1582–9.

134. Thompson SM, Vella A, Thompson GB, et al. Selective arterial calcium stimulation with hepatic venous sampling differentiates insulinoma from nesidioblastosis. J Clin Endocrinol Metab 2015;100: 4189–97.

135. Gilis-Januszewska A, Piatkowski J, Skalniak A, et al. Noninsulinoma pancreatogenous hypoglycaemia in adults–a spotlight on its genetics. Endokrynol Pol 2015;66:344–54.

136. Goossens A, Gepts W, Saudubray JM, et al. Diffuse and focal nesidioblastosis. A clinicopathological study of 24 patients with persistent neonatal hyperinsulinemic hypoglycemia. Am J Surg Pathol 1989; 13:766–75.

137. Suchi M, MacMullen C, Thornton PS, et al. Histopathology of congenital hyperinsulinism: retrospective study with genotype correlations. Pediatr Dev Pathol 2003;6:322–33.

138. Delonlay P, Simon A, Galmiche-Rolland L, et al. Neonatal hyperinsulinism: clinicopathologic correlation. Hum Pathol 2007;38:387–99.

139. Ismail D, Werther G. Persistent hyperinsulinaemic hypoglycaemia of infancy: 15 years' experience at the Royal Children's Hospital (RCH), Melbourne. J Pediatr Endocrinol Metab 2005;18:1103–9.

140. Fournet JC, Mayaud C, de LP, et al. Unbalanced expression of 11p15 imprinted genes in focal forms of congenital hyperinsulinism: association with a reduction to homozygosity of a mutation in ABCC8 or KCNJ11. Am J Pathol 2001;158: 2177–84.

141. Dunne MJ, Cosgrove KE, Shepherd RM, et al. Hyperinsulinism in infancy: from basic science to clinical disease. Physiol Rev 2004;84:239–75.

142. Rahman SA, Nessa A, Hussain K. Molecular mechanisms of congenital hyperinsulinism. J Mol Endocrinol 2015;54:R119–29.

143. Senniappan S, Arya VB, Hussain K. The molecular mechanisms, diagnosis and management of congenital hyperinsulinism. Indian J Endocrinol Metab 2013;17:19–30.

144. Henquin JC, Nenquin M, Sempoux C, et al. In vitro insulin secretion by pancreatic tissue from infants with diazoxide-resistant congenital hyperinsulinism deviates from model predictions. J Clin Invest 2011;121:3932–42.

145. Huopio H, Reimann F, Ashfield R, et al. Dominantly inherited hyperinsulinism caused by a mutation in the sulfonylurea receptor type 1. J Clin Invest 2000;106:897–906.

146. Suchi M, MacMullen CM, Thornton PS, et al. Molecular and immunohistochemical analyses of the focal form of congenital hyperinsulinism. Mod Pathol 2006;19:122–9.

147. Meissner T, Wendel U, Burgard P, et al. Long-term follow-up of 114 patients with congenital hyperinsulinism. Eur J Endocrinol 2003;149:43–51.

148. Adzick NS, Thornton PS, Stanley CA, et al. A multidisciplinary approach to the focal form of congenital hyperinsulinism leads to successful treatment by partial pancreatectomy. J Pediatr Surg 2004;39:270–5.

149. Pezzilli R, Calculli L. Pancreatic steatosis: is it related to either obesity or diabetes mellitus? World J Diabetes 2014;5:415–9.

150. Stamm BH. Incidence and diagnostic significance of minor pathologic changes in the adult pancreas at autopsy: a systematic study of 112 autopsies in patients without known pancreatic disease. Hum Pathol 1984;15:677–83.

151. Olsen TS. Lipomatosis of the pancreas in autopsy material and its relation to age and overweight. Acta Pathol Microbiol Scand A 1978; 86A:367–73.

152. Altinel D, Basturk O, Sarmiento JM, et al. Lipomatous pseudohypertrophy of the pancreas: a clinicopathologically distinct entity. Pancreas 2010;39: 392–7.

153. Maunoury V, Nieuwarts S, Ferri J, et al. Pancreatic lipomatosis revealing Johanson-Blizzard syndrome. Gastroenterol Clin Biol 1999;23:1099–101, [in French].

154. MacMaster SA, Cummings TM. Computed tomography and ultrasonography findings for an adult with Shwachman syndrome and pancreatic lipomatosis. Can Assoc Radiol J 1993;44:301–3.

155. Okun SD, Lewin DN. Non-neoplastic pancreatic lesions that may mimic malignancy. Semin Diagn Pathol 2016;33:31–42.

156. Masuda A, Tanaka H, Ikegawa T, et al. A case of lipomatous pseudohypertrophy of the pancreas diagnosed by EUS-FNA. Clin J Gastroenterol 2012;5:282–6.

157. Dodo IM, Adamthwaite JA, Jain P, et al. Successful outcome following resection of a pancreatic liposarcoma with solitary metastasis. World J Gastroenterol 2005;11:7684–5.

158. Zamboni G, Capelli P, Scarpa A, et al. Nonneoplastic mimickers of pancreatic neoplasms. Arch Pathol Lab Med 2009;133:439–53.

159. Chatelain D, Vibert E, Yzet T, et al. Groove pancreatitis and pancreatic heterotopia in the minor duodenal papilla. Pancreas 2005;30:e92–5.

160. Adsay NV, Zamboni G. Paraduodenal pancreatitis: a clinico-pathologically distinct entity unifying "cystic dystrophy of heterotopic pancreas", "paraduodenal wall cyst", and "groove pancreatitis. Semin Diagn Pathol 2004;21:247–54.

161. Klöppel G. Chronic pancreatitis, pseudotumors and other tumor-like lesions. Mod Pathol 2007; 20(Suppl 1):S113–31.

162. Adsay NV, Bandyopadhyay S, Basturk O, et al. Chronic pancreatitis or pancreatic ductal adenocarcinoma? Semin Diagn Pathol 2004;21:268–76.

163. Manzelli A, Petrou A, Lazzaro A, et al. Groove pancreatitis. A mini-series report and review of the literature. JOP 2011;12:230–3.

164. Castell-Monsalve FJ, Sousa-Martin JM, Carranza-Carranza A. Groove pancreatitis: MRI and pathologic findings. Abdom Imaging 2008;33: 342–8.

165. Casetti L, Bassi C, Salvia R, et al. Paraduodenal" pancreatitis: results of surgery on 58 consecutives patients from a single institution. World J Surg 2009;33:2664–9.

# Chronic Pancreatitis

Michelle Stram, MD, Shu Liu, PhD, Aatur D. Singhi, MD, PhD*

**KEYWORDS**

- Pancreas • Etiology • Pathology • Alcohol • Obstruction • Paraduodenal • Autoimmune
- Hereditary

---

**Key points**

- Chronic pancreatitis is a progressive, fibroinflammatory disease characterized by irreversible damage to the pancreas.
- The underlying cause of chronic pancreatitis is multifactorial and involves a complex interaction of environmental, genetic, and/or other risk factors.
- The pathology of chronic pancreatitis is highly variable and dependent on the pathogenesis of the disease.
- The main differential diagnosis of chronic pancreatitis is pancreatic ductal adenocarcinoma and differentiating between these 2 entities remains a significant clinical and diagnostic challenge.

---

## ABSTRACT

Chronic pancreatitis is a debilitating condition often associated with severe abdominal pain and exocrine and endocrine dysfunction. The underlying cause is multifactorial and involves complex interaction of environmental, genetic, and/or other risk factors. The pathology is dependent on the underlying pathogenesis of the disease. This review describes the clinical, gross, and microscopic findings of the main subtypes of chronic pancreatitis: alcoholic chronic pancreatitis, obstructive chronic pancreatitis, paraduodenal ("groove") pancreatitis, pancreatic divisum, autoimmune pancreatitis, and genetic factors associated with chronic pancreatitis. As pancreatic ductal adenocarcinoma may be confused with chronic pancreatitis, the main distinguishing features between these 2 diseases are discussed.

## OVERVIEW

Chronic pancreatitis was first reported in the medical literature by Sir Thomas Cawley in 1788.[1] He described a "free living young man" who died of diabetes and on autopsy was found to have a pancreas filled with calculi. Since this landmark publication, there have been major advances in our understanding of the pathogenesis and pathophysiology of chronic pancreatitis that include etiologic risk factors, natural history, and associated genetic changes. Based on numerous studies, chronic pancreatitis is considered to be a progressive, fibroinflammatory disease characterized by irreversible damage to the pancreas.[2] In the United States, the overall incidence of chronic pancreatitis ranges from 4.4 to 11.9 cases per 100,000 per year, and the prevalence ranges from 36.9 to 41.8 cases per 100,000.[3–5] Patients often present with severe abdominal pain and both exocrine and endocrine dysfunction. Treatment for chronic pancreatitis is mostly supportive and, thus, patients repeatedly seek medical attention, which strains medical resources and represents a huge financial burden. In fact, despite the low prevalence of chronic pancreatitis within the United States, it ranks seventh for hospital admissions, and eighth for overall costs among digestive diseases.[6] Moreover, patients with long-standing chronic pancreatitis are at increased risk for developing pancreatic ductal adenocarcinoma.[7] The underlying cause of chronic pancreatitis is multifactorial and involves a complex interaction of environmental, genetic, and/or other risk factors.[2,8] The

---

Funding Support: None.

Disclosure/Conflict of Interest: The authors have no conflicts of interest to declare.

Department of Pathology, University of Pittsburgh Medical Center, Pittsburgh, PA, USA

\* Corresponding author. UPMC Presbyterian Hospital, 200 Lothrop Street, Room A616.2, Pittsburgh, PA 15213.

*E-mail address:* singhiad@upmc.edu

pathology of chronic pancreatitis is equally intricate and can vary significantly based on the pathogenesis of the disease. Herein, we review the key clinical and pathologic features of the major subtypes of chronic pancreatitis. Further, as chronic pancreatitis may closely mimic pancreatic ductal adenocarcinoma, we discuss their distinguishing features.

## ALCOHOLIC CHRONIC PANCREATITIS

### BACKGROUND

In western countries, heavy and prolonged alcohol use is a major cause of chronic pancreatitis. Patients are typically young-to-middle aged (30–50 years) men, who develop chronic pancreatitis after repeated attacks of acute pancreatitis as they continue to drink.[9] Interestingly, fewer than 5% of alcoholic individuals develop chronic pancreatitis. This observation implies the involvement of additional insults or factors. In fact, smoking, a high-fat diet, obesity, genetics, and infectious agents have been suggested to contribute to pancreatic disease in alcoholic individuals.[9–11] Similar to other etiologies of chronic pancreatitis, alcoholic chronic pancreatitis is clinically characterized by frequent episodes of epigastric/abdominal pain in the early stages of the disease. Over time, the pain attacks decrease in frequency and intensity, which parallel the progressive destruction of the gland and eventual endocrine and exocrine insufficiency. Patients with this disease have an elevated risk of pancreatic ductal adenocarcinoma, but comparable to other forms of chronic pancreatitis.

---

### Key Points

- In western countries, heavy and prolonged alcohol use is a major cause of chronic pancreatitis.

- Patients are typically young-to-middle aged (30–50 years) men.

- Fewer than 5% of alcoholic individuals develop chronic pancreatitis which implies the involvement of additional cofactors.

- Gross and microscopic findings consist of progressive perilobular and interlobular fibrosis with ductal dilatation, distortion and squamous metaplasia.

- Advanced cases include intralobular fibrosis, pseudocyst formation, and intraductal calculi.

---

## GROSS FEATURES

The gross findings of alcoholic chronic pancreatitis can differ in the early and late stages of this disease.[12] Early alcoholic chronic pancreatitis commonly shows an uneven distribution of perilobular and interlobular parenchymal fibrosis. On cut surface, these findings impart an indurated appearance to the gland with variation in size and accentuation of individual pancreatic lobules. The pancreatic ducts in affected areas, which are often embedded in fibrosis, display dilatation and/or distortion. Pseudocysts may be encountered, but are small and located within the periphery of the pancreatic body and tail.

In the latter stages of alcoholic chronic pancreatitis, the pancreas appears opaque, shrunken, and reduced in size due to parenchymal atrophy and continuing fibrosis. There is extensive loss of normal pancreatic lobular architecture with replacement by diffuse fibrosis.[13] Pancreatic ductal changes are also more prominent and range from obstruction to overt dilatation and/or distortion (Fig. 1A). Calculi, which are composed of calcium carbonate, are frequently present within the main pancreatic duct and branch ducts, and vary in size from 0.1 cm to larger than 1.0 cm in diameter. Pseudocysts are present in 25% to 50% of cases and can exceed 10 cm in greatest dimension (Fig. 1B).[14] They are filled with turbid, necrotic debris, which is rich in exocrine enzymes. In some cases, pseudocysts may connect to the ductal system, erode through major vessels, or rupture within the retroperitoneum.

## MICROSCOPIC FEATURES

Analogous to the gross findings, microscopic examination of early alcoholic chronic pancreatitis reveals perilobular and interlobular fibrosis, which is composed of scattered, spindled fibroblasts and thin wavy collagen (Fig. 2A, B).[12,13] A patchy distribution of T-cell lymphocytes, plasma cells, and macrophages are frequently associated with these areas of fibrosis. The intralobular ducts are focally dilated and/or distorted, and contain intraluminal proteinaceous plugs. In addition, the ductal epithelium may be hyperplastic or undergo squamous metaplasia. Foci of resolving fat necrosis characterized by partially necrotic adipose tissue with foamy macrophages, multinucleated giant cells, and chronic inflammation also may be present.

In advanced cases, there is extensive loss of pancreatic acinar, ductal, and islet cell parenchyma with replacement by not only perilobular and interlobular fibrosis, but also intralobular

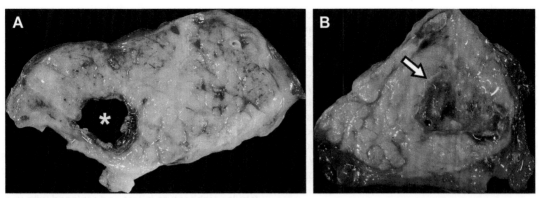

Fig. 1. Alcoholic chronic pancreatitis. (A) Grossly, alcoholic chronic pancreatitis is characterized by prominent periloboular and interlobular parenchymal fibrosis with loss of normal pancreatic lobular architecture. Pancreatic ductal dilatation (asterisk) and/or distortion are also common findings. (B) Pseudocysts, filled with turbid, necrotic debris, (white arrow) may also be identified in advanced stages.

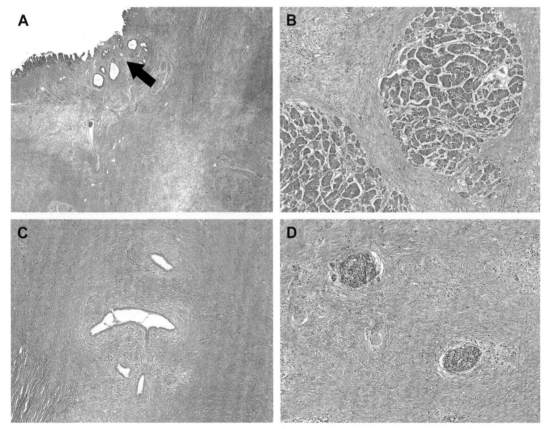

Fig. 2. Alcoholic chronic pancreatitis. (A) Consistent with the gross findings, the microscopic findings include main pancreatic duct dilatation (black arrow) with associated loss of pancreatic parenchyma and replacement by both perilobular and interlobular fibrosis (hematoxylin-eosin [H&E], original magnification ×40). (B) Embedded within the interlobular fibrosis are islands of remnant acinar epithelium (H&E, original magnification ×200). (C) In advanced cases, there is extensive loss of pancreatic parenchyma with little to no residual acinar parenchyma. The pancreatic ducts are often dilated and/or distorted (H&E, original magnification ×100). (D) Scant areas with residual islets of Langerhans may be identified, and are often encircled by thick bundles of collagenous fibrosis (H&E, original magnification ×200).

fibrosis (**Fig.** 2C). Within the intralobular fibrosis may be remnant acinar epithelium, dilated and/or distorted ducts, and islet cell aggregates (**Fig.** 2D).[15] The ductal epithelium can be atrophic and flattened with intraluminal proteinaceous plugs and calculi. Pseudocysts, which may also be seen within the early phases of chronic pancreatitis, are composed of thick, fibrous walls that lack an epithelial lining, and are filled with necrotic debris, fibrin, blood, and macrophages. In addition to the pancreatic parenchyma, the fibrofatty peripancreatic soft tissue is often replaced by prominent fibrosis.

## OBSTRUCTIVE CHRONIC PANCREATITIS

### BACKGROUND

Obstruction of the main pancreatic duct or its branches by tumors, scars, strictures, ductal stones, paraduodenal wall cysts, congenital anomalies, and stenosis of the ampulla of Vater or minor papilla can result in chronic pancreatitis.[16] However, in contrast to alcoholic chronic pancreatitis, chronic pancreatitis due to an obstruction affects the gland distal to the site of obstruction and tends to be uneven in distribution.[17] Based on the etiology of the obstruction, obstructive chronic pancreatitis can present in men and women equally, and occur over a wide age range. As expected, treatment for obstructive chronic pancreatitis involves removing the offending agent or underlying cause. Thus, treatment can range from endoscopic therapy to surgical resection.[16]

---

### Key Points

- Due to obstruction of the main pancreatic duct or its branches by tumors, scars, strictures, ductal stones, paraduodenal wall cysts, congenital anomalies, and stenosis of the ampulla of Vater or minor papilla.

- While dependent on etiology, this entity presents in men and women equally and over a wide age range.

- Gross parenchymal changes are restricted to the portion of pancreas distal to the obstruction; however, uneven in distribution.

- Results in distal duct dilatation and obstruction with concomitant and progressive fibrosis.

- Long-standing cases develop diffuse parenchymal fibrosis and retention cysts.

---

## GROSS FEATURES

Although the gross findings for obstructive chronic pancreatitis will vary depending on the underlying etiology, the pancreatic parenchymal changes are restricted to the portion of the pancreas distal to the obstruction (**Fig.** 3). However, these changes are uneven in distribution. The affected area of the pancreas is typically reduced in size with irregular contours due to parenchymal atrophy. Obstruction of the main pancreatic duct or its branches results in distal ductal dilatation and distortion.[18] On cut section, the normal pancreatic lobular architecture is lost and replaced with variable perilobular and interlobular fibrosis. Long-standing cases of obstructive chronic pancreatitis are characterized by diffuse parenchymal fibrosis and retention cysts. Although uncommon, pseudocysts also may be present, but are often not as large as those found in the setting of alcoholic chronic pancreatitis.

## MICROSCOPIC FEATURES

Similar to the gross features, the histologic findings of obstructive chronic pancreatitis are confined to the pancreatic parenchyma distal to the obstruction. Pancreatic acinar, ductal, and islet cell parenchyma are replaced by variable amounts of perilobular and interlobular fibrosis (see **Fig.** 3B). Due to the obstruction, the ductal epithelium may undergo hyperplasia and squamous metaplasia. Intraluminal proteinaceous plugs may also be seen; however, calculi are rarely ever present, unless they are the cause of the obstruction (see **Fig.** 3C). Advanced cases of obstructive chronic pancreatitis show extensive loss of pancreatic parenchyma and prominent fibrosis (see **Fig.** 3D). Retention cysts are frequently observed and represent dilated ducts that are lined by reactive cuboidal-to-columnar epithelium with intraluminal proteinaceous plugs and serous fluid. Small pseudocysts also may be seen and, similar to alcoholic chronic pancreatitis, composed of a thick fibrous wall that lack a true epithelial lining and filled with necrotic debris and macrophages.

## PARADUODENAL ("GROOVE") PANCREATITIS

### BACKGROUND

A rare form of obstructive chronic pancreatitis that deserves special mention is paraduodenal or groove pancreatitis. Paraduodenal pancreatitis affects the anatomic region between the superior aspect of the pancreatic head, duodenum, and common bile duct, which is referred to as the

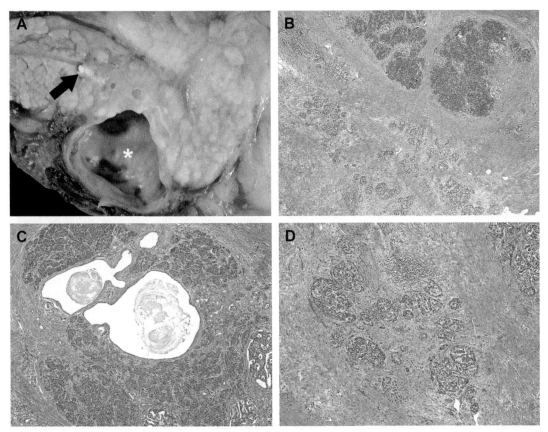

*Fig. 3.* Obstructive chronic pancreatitis. (*A*) Although dependent on the etiology (calculus, *black arrow*), the gross changes in obstructive chronic pancreatitis are confined to the pancreatic parenchyma distal to the obstruction. In addition, long-standing cases may develop retention cysts (*asterisk*). (*B*) Microscopically, pancreatic acinar, ductal and islet cell parenchyma are replaced by variable amounts of perilobular and interlobular fibrosis (H&E, original magnification ×40). (*C*) Due to the obstruction, normal concretions from the pancreatic ducts cannot exit the pancreas and result in ductal dilatation with intraluminal proteinaceous plugs (H&E, original magnification ×200). (*D*) As chronic pancreatitis continues, further fibrosis and parenchymal loss is identified with islets of Langerhans often found in aggregates (H&E, original magnification ×200).

groove area.[19–23] Most patients with paraduodenal pancreatitis are men between the ages of 40 and 50 years with a history of alcohol abuse and smoking.[24] The clinical symptoms are severe upper abdominal pain, postprandial vomiting, and weight loss due to duodenal stenosis. Although the pathogenesis of paraduodenal pancreatitis remains unclear, it is postulated to be attributed to obstruction of the minor papilla. Imaging reveals thickening of the duodenum with associated cyst formation within the duodenal wall or groove area that radiographically may resemble a pseudocyst or cystic pancreatic neoplasm. Cases without cystic change may mimic a pancreatic or periampullary malignancy.[25] Treatment options for paraduodenal pancreatitis can vary, but pancreaticoduodenectomy is currently the treatment of choice when symptoms do not improve or if the condition is difficult to distinguish from a carcinoma.

### Key Points

- A rare form of obstructive chronic pancreatitis occurring within the pancreatoduodenal groove area.

- Most patients are men between the ages of 40 and 50 years with a history of alcohol and smoking abuse.

- Between the major and minor papillae, the duodenal wall and underlying pancreatic parenchyma are thickened and fibrotic.

- The minor papilla may be absent or partially to completely obstructed by calcified, proteinaceous material.

- Within zones of fibrosis are often multiple cysts that are lined by eroded, ductal epithelium and an associated myofibroblastic reaction.

## GROSS FEATURES

On gross examination, the duodenal wall and underlying pancreatic parenchyma are thickened and fibrotic between the major and minor papillae. The duodenal mucosa often acquires a nodular or cobblestone appearance (Fig. 4A).[26] The minor papilla may be absent or partially to completely obstructed by calcified, proteinaceous material.[19] On cut section, the epicenter of this disease process is within the space between the duodenum and pancreas, which can be relatively gelatinous to solid, or contain cysts (Fig. 4B). The cysts can range in size from subcentimeter to 10 cm and generally have a smooth, opaque cyst wall. The cysts are filled with proteinaceous debris, and, within larger cysts, may contain small calculi. Although the fibrosis is typically confined to the groove area, it may spill into the adjacent pancreatic tissue and lead to stenosis of the common bile duct and main pancreatic duct. However, diffuse pancreatic parenchymal fibrosis is not consistent with paraduodenal pancreatitis.

## MICROSCOPIC FEATURES

Microscopically, there is marked fibrosis of the duodenal wall around the minor papilla that extends into the adjacent pancreatic parenchyma and soft tissue within the groove area (Fig. 5A).[12] Admixed within the fibrosis are myoid cells that consist of either smooth muscle cells and/or myofibroblasts. Prominent Brunner gland hyperplasia is also present and contributes to the thickening of the duodenal mucosa and submucosa. Multiple cysts, lined by ductal epithelium, are often identified within the zones of fibrosis. However, the ductal epithelium is eroded with associated acute and chronic inflammation, and reactive myofibroblasts (Fig. 5B). The cysts contain small calculi that may extravasate and cause a foreign body giant cell reaction and stromal eosinophilia (Fig. 5C, D). Within the groove area, the underlying pancreatic parenchyma demonstrates atrophy, fat necrosis, and dense fibrosis.

## PANCREATIC DIVISUM

### BACKGROUND

Embryologically, the pancreas develops from 2 outgrowths of endoderm (the dorsal and ventral buds) at the junction of the foregut and midgut. The dorsal bud develops into the pancreatic tail and body, and the ventral bud gives rise to the pancreatic head and uncinate process. With growth and rotation of the duodenum, the ventral bud joins the dorsal bud. During the union of both buds, the duct of Wirsung within the ventral bud and the duct of Santorini within the dorsal bud fuse establishing pancreatic drainage through the duct of Wirsung and the major papilla.

In 5% to 10% of the general population, the ducts of Wirsung and Santorini fail to properly fuse, which is known as pancreatic divisum.[27,28] Although most individuals with this congenital anomaly are asymptomatic, a subset will present with chronic pancreatitis. Some studies suggest pancreatic divisum is a predisposing factor for ductal stenosis or obstruction. Moreover, patients with symptomatic pancreatic divisum are more likely to harbor germline mutations in genes associated with chronic pancreatitis, such as CFTR and SPINK1.[29,30]

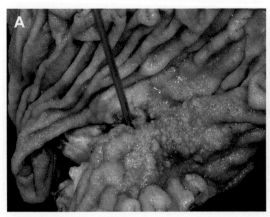
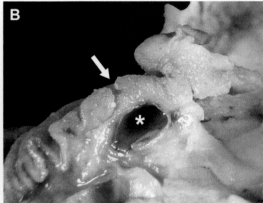

*Fig. 4.* Paraduodenal ("groove") pancreatitis. (A) In paraduodenal pancreatitis, the duodenal wall between the major (probe) and minor papillae is thickened and acquires a cobblestone appearance. (B) On cut section, the duodenal wall (*white arrow*) and underlying pancreas are characterized by fibrosis and smooth, opaque cysts (*asterisk*).

## Key Points

- Most common congenital anomaly of the pancreas.

- Unlikely a cause of chronic pancreatitis, but possibly a predisposing factor or associated with genetic risk factors of chronic pancreatitis.

- A diagnosis often made at the time of gross examination.

- Subdivided into 3 types: type 1 (classic pancreatic divisum) is defined by the lack of communication between the ducts of Wirsung and Santorini; type 2 (absent ventral duct) is characterized by the absence of the duct of Wirsung; and type 3 (incomplete or functional divisum) where there is a filamentous or inadequate connection between the ventral and dorsal ducts.

- There is often an associated stenosis or obstruction with distal parenchymal atrophy and fibrosis.

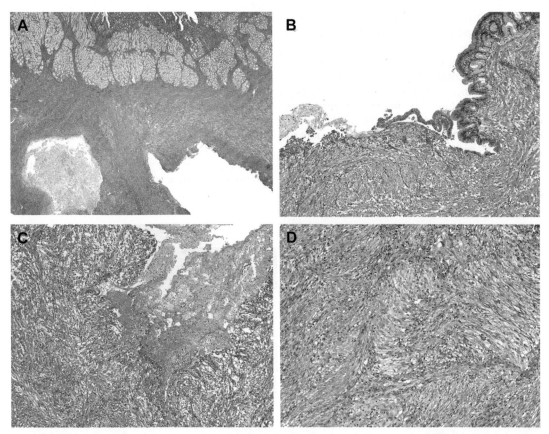

*Fig. 5.* Paraduodenal ("groove") pancreatitis. (*A*) At low magnification, there is marked fibrosis of the duodenal wall that extends into the adjacent pancreatic parenchyma. Multiple cysts are often identified within zones of fibrosis (H&E, original magnification ×20). (*B*) These cysts are lined by pancreatic ductal epithelium, but are typically eroded or ulcerated (H&E, original magnification ×100). (*C*) In some cases, the epithelium is completely lost and the cysts are characterized by intraluminal proteinaceous debris and associated acute and chronic inflammation (H&E, original magnification ×100). (*D*) Cyst rupture is associated with a storiform myofibroblastic proliferation, and both acute and chronic inflammation (H&E, original magnification ×200).

## GROSS AND MICROSCOPIC FEATURES

A diagnosis of pancreatic divisum is typically made at the time of gross examination. Pancreatic divisum is divided into 3 types.[31] Type 1 or classic pancreatic divisum is the most common form and is defined by the complete lack of communication between the ducts of Wirsung and Santorini, which occurs in 70% of cases (Fig. 6A). Type 2 or absent ventral duct occurs in 20% to 25% of cases and is characterized by the absence of duct of Wirsung. Due to the loss of the duct of Wirsung, the entire pancreas drains through the duct of Santorini and minor papilla, whereas the major papilla drains the bile duct. Type 3 or incomplete (functional) pancreatic divisum represents 5% of cases with a filamentous or inadequate connection between the ventral and dorsal ducts. In addition to pancreatic divisum, there is often an associated proximal area of stenosis or obstruction with distal parenchymal atrophy and fibrosis. Further, distal pancreatic ductal dilatation is a frequent occurrence. Over time, retention cysts may also develop in a background of further parenchymal loss and fibrotic replacement.

The microscopic assessment of chronic pancreatitis associated with pancreatic divisum shows overlapping features with obstructive chronic pancreatitis. The findings include loss of pancreatic acinar, ductal, and islet cell parenchyma with replacement by variable amounts of perilobular and interlobular fibrosis. Ductal changes consist of hyperplasia, squamous metaplasia, and intraluminal proteinaceous plugs. In advanced cases, retention cysts in a background of extensive intralobular fibrosis may be observed.

## AUTOIMMUNE PANCREATITIS

### BACKGROUND

Autoimmune pancreatitis is a rare form of chronic pancreatitis and is characterized by obstructive jaundice, prominent inflammatory infiltrate, and a therapeutic response to corticosteroids.[32] Recent studies have demonstrated that autoimmune pancreatitis represents a heterogeneous disease process and is composed of 2 subtypes (type 1 and type 2). Type 1 autoimmune pancreatitis is also called lymphoplasmacytic sclerosing pancreatitis.[33,34] It is within the spectrum of immunoglobulin (Ig)G4-related diseases that often affects multiple organs and shares similar clinical, serologic and pathologic features.[35] At clinical presentation, patients are generally men, older than 60 years, and seropositive for IgG4. Despite corticosteroid response, patients are prone to frequent relapse.

In contrast, type 2 autoimmune pancreatitis affects younger individuals within 40 to 50 years of age and is evenly distributed between genders.[36,37] Clinical presentation is limited to the pancreas, but approximately 15% of patients have concurrent inflammatory bowel disease.[37,38] Although most patients with type 2 autoimmune pancreatitis are reported to be IgG4 seronegative, a subset can have elevated serum IgG4.[39] As with type 1 autoimmune pancreatitis, type 2 autoimmune pancreatitis is a corticosteroid-responsive disorder; however, relapses are uncommon.

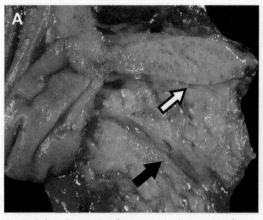 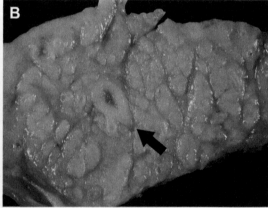

*Fig. 6.* (*A*) A diagnosis of pancreatic divisum is often made at the time of gross examination. The most common type, type 1 or classic pancreatic divisum, is characterized by the complete lack of communication between the ducts of Santorini (*black arrow*) and Wirsung (not shown). The common bile duct empties through the major papilla (*white arrow*). (*B*) Types 1 and 2 autoimmune pancreatitis show similar gross findings that include parenchymal enlargement, accentuation of the lobules and ducts (*black arrow*) with a white to yellow discoloration.

## Key Points

- Rare form of chronic pancreatitis that is characterized by obstructive jaundice, prominent inflammatory infiltrate, and a therapeutic response to corticosteroids.

- A heterogeneous disease composed of 2 subtypes (type 1 and type 2) with different clinicopathologic features.

- Type 1 autoimmune pancreatitis (lymphoplasmacytic sclerosing pancreatitis) generally affects men older than 60 years and seropositive for IgG4. The histologic features consist of a dense lymphoplasmacytic infiltrate, ductitis, and venulitis. There is often a predominance of IgG4-positive plasma cells (>10 per high-power field). Despite corticosteroid response, patients are prone to frequent relapse.

- Type 2 autoimmune pancreatitis affects both genders equally, between the ages of 40 and 50 years and typically IgG4 seronegative. Similar microscopic features of type 1 autoimmune pancreatitis; however, with pathognomonic granulocytic epithelial lesions. This entity is also responsive to corticosteroids and relapses are uncommon.

## GROSS FEATURES

The gross findings of types 1 and 2 autoimmune pancreatitis are indistinguishable.[37] The affected pancreas may show a localized "pseudotumor," discrete nodules or diffuse parenchymal enlargement (Fig. 6B). There is effacement of the normal pancreatic lobular architecture with a white to yellow discoloration and indurated appearance.[37] These changes extend to involve the pancreatic and biliary ductal system resulting in obstruction. Pseudocysts and retention cyst are typically not observed. In addition, calculi are usually absent.

## MICROSCOPIC FEATURES

The histologic features of type 1 autoimmune pancreatitis are a dense lymphoplasmacytic infiltrate, periductal fibrosis and venulitis.[40–42] The inflammation is composed of predominantly T-cell lymphocytes and plasma cells that are centered around and within medium-to-large interlobular ducts. This results in ductal epithelial infolding and, consequently, narrowing of the ductal lumen (Fig. 7A). In addition, the inflammatory infiltrate extends into the surrounding acinar parenchyma with secondary atrophy and fibrosis.

Inflammation is also present around and within the venule and venous walls (Fig. 7B). Over time, the inflammatory infiltration of the vessel wall may become deeper and lead to destruction (obliterative phlebitis) and fibrosis (Fig. 7C). Perineural inflammation is also a frequent finding. Although not diagnostic, IgG4 immunolabeling highlights prominent IgG4-positive plasma cells (>10 IgG4-positive plasma cells per high-power field) (Fig. 7D).[43] In the later stages of this disease process, the fibrotic changes become more extensive. Myofibroblastlike cells with intermixed dense chronic inflammation extend from the ducts and veins into the surrounding pancreatic parenchyma within a whorled or storiform pattern.

Similar to type 1 autoimmune pancreatitis, type 2 autoimmune pancreatitis demonstrates periductal lymphoplasmacytic inflammation with associated acinar atrophy and periductal fibrosis.[44] However, these histologic findings are less pronounced in type 2 autoimmune pancreatitis. A distinguishing and diagnostic feature of type 2 autoimmune pancreatitis is the presence of granulocytic epithelial lesions (Fig. 8).[37] These lesions are characterized by periductal acute inflammation composed of neutrophils that cluster underneath the ductal epithelium and within the lumen. The acute inflammatory infiltrate leads to ductal epithelial detachment, destruction and obliteration. Another less specific finding for type 2 autoimmune pancreatitis is scant-to-absent immunolabeling for IgG4-positive plasma cells.[23]

## GENETIC FACTORS IN CHRONIC PANCREATITIS

### BACKGROUND

Genetic factors play a critical role in both the susceptibility and predisposition of developing chronic pancreatitis.[8] The genetic patterns of chronic pancreatitis can be broadly grouped into 3 categories: autosomal dominant, autosomal recessive, and modifier gene mutations that confer varying levels of risk for chronic pancreatitis. The first breakthrough in the genetics of chronic pancreatitis came with the discovery that gain-of-function mutations in the gene that encodes cationic trypsinogen (PRSS1) cause hereditary pancreatitis, which comprises 2% to 3% of patients with chronic pancreatitis.[45,46] Most affected individuals develop symptoms before the age of 20 years, and often before the age of 5. Of particular importance, patients with PRSS1-related hereditary pancreatitis have a lifetime risk for pancreatic ductal adenocarcinoma of 40% at 70 years of age.[47]

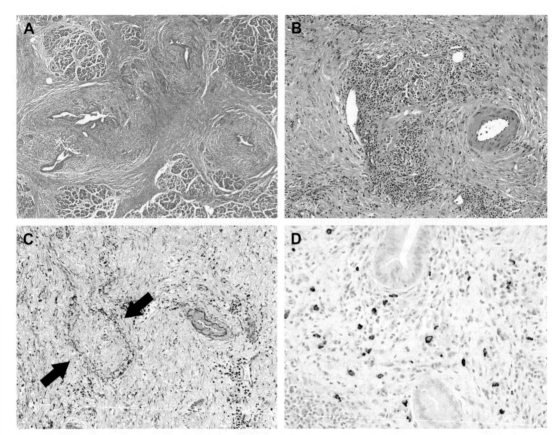

*Fig. 7.* Type 1 autoimmune pancreatitis. (*A*) The histologic features of type 1 autoimmune pancreatitis are a peri-ductal and perivenular, dense lymphoplasmacytic infiltrate and fibrosis. The chronic inflammatory infiltrate ex-tends into the ductal epithelium, resulting in epithelial infolding and narrowing of the ductal lumen (H&E, original magnification ×100). (*B*) Inflammation around and within the venules and veins is a hallmark finding and typically present within the periphery of this lesion (H&E, original magnification ×200). (*C*) Overtime, the in-flammatory infiltration of the vessel wall may become deep and lead to destruction (*black arrows*) or obliterative phlebitis (Verhoeff-Van Gieson stain, original magnification ×200). (*D*) Although not diagnostic, IgG4 immuno-labeling highlights prominent IgG4-positive plasma cells of more than 10 per high-power field (IgG4, original magnification ×400).

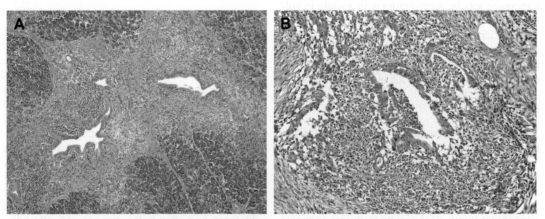

*Fig. 8.* Type 2 autoimmune pancreatitis. (*A*) A prominent periductal acute and chronic inflammatory infiltrate with associated fibrosis that extends to the surrounding acinar parenchyma is characteristic of type 2 autoim-mune pancreatitis (H&E, original magnification ×100). (*B*) The ductal epithelium is disrupted and destroyed by neutrophilic granulocytes, collectively termed as granulocytic epithelial lesion (H&E, original magnification ×200).

The most common etiology of chronic pancreatitis in children is cystic fibrosis, an autosomal recessive disorder caused by *CFTR* mutations.[48] Cystic fibrosis is a multiorgan syndrome associated with impaired transport of chloride ions and movement of water in and out of cells. As a result, cells that line the passageways of the lungs, pancreas, and other organs produce mucous that is abnormally thick that obstructs airways and glands. In the vast majority of patients, exocrine pancreatic insufficiency occurs in utero or soon after birth. However, minor *CFTR* mutations have been identified in children and young adults with idiopathic chronic pancreatitis, in the absence of other organ manifestations of this disease.[49]

In addition to *PRSS1* and *CFTR*, mutations in *SPINK1* have also been shown to be associated with hereditary and idiopathic chronic pancreatitis.[50] *SPINK1* is a potent protease inhibitor and a specific inactivation factor of intrapancreatic trypsin activity. Mutated *SPINK1* genes seem to behave as disease modifiers that either lower the threshold of initiating pancreatitis or worsen the severity of pancreatitis caused by other genetic or environmental factors. A high prevalence of *SPINK1* mutations is associated with tropical chronic pancreatitis, a distinctive disorder affecting young adults in developing countries.[8]

## Key Points

- The 3 most common germline alterations associated with chronic pancreatitis involve the genes *PRSS1*, *CFTR*, and *SPINK1*.

- Germline gain-of-function mutations in *PRSS1* are responsible for hereditary pancreatitis, with most afflicted individuals developing chronic pancreatitis before the age of 20 years.

- The most common etiology of chronic pancreatitis in children is cystic fibrosis, which is associated with autosomal recessive alterations in *CFTR*. Although *CFTR* mutations frequently affect multiple organs, minor recessive *CFTR* mutations have been identified and associated with chronic pancreatitis alone.

- *SPINK1* mutations are considered to be disease modifiers, which either lower the threshold of initiating pancreatitis or worsen its severity due to other risk factors.

- The pathology of *PRSS1* and *CFTR*-related chronic pancreatitis is progressive lipomatous atrophy. In contrast, *SPINK1* mutations are associated with progressive fibrosis.

## GROSS FEATURES

Although most etiologies of chronic pancreatitis are associated with fibrosis, *PRSS1*-related hereditary pancreatitis demonstrates progressive atrophy and diffuse fatty replacement of the pancreas (lipomatous atrophy).[51] Lipomatous atrophy of the pancreas is a frequent occurrence and seen with increasing age. In fact, it is the most common degenerative lesion of the pancreas and regarded as a normal finding in the obese and elderly.[52,53] However, it typically presents focally and is not as extensive as seen in patients with *PRSS1*. Considering the increased risk of pancreatic ductal adenocarcinoma in patients with *PRSS1*, it is not surprising that lipomatous atrophy may mimic a pancreatic mass lesion. Pancreatic ductal dilatation and intraductal calculi are also common findings in patients with *PRSS1*.

As mentioned previously, patients with cystic fibrosis develop intraductal mucinous plugs with secondary obstruction and ductal dilatation. Interestingly, the pancreas in cystic fibrosis shows prominent lipomatous atrophy. Considering the presence of intraductal calculi in patients with *PRSS1*, obstruction may be responsible for the pathologic similarities between these genetically related disorders. Limited information has been reported on pathologic findings associated with *SPINK1* mutations, but anecdotal evidence suggests features analogous to alcoholic chronic pancreatitis.

## MICROSCOPIC FEATURES

The microscopic features of *PRSS1*-related hereditary pancreatitis are dependent on patient age.[51] In pediatric cases, there is central parenchymal loss with accompaniment by mild chronic inflammation and loosely packed perilobular and interlobular fibrosis (Fig. 9A). More significantly, the periphery of the pancreas exhibits patchy parenchymal replacement with mature adipose tissue. These changes are more developed with increasing patient age. The fatty replacement of the pancreatic parenchyma extends from the periphery to the central portions of the pancreas (Fig. 9B). Although fibrosis may be present; it is often thin and loosely packed as compared with alcoholic or obstructive chronic pancreatitis. With advanced age, pancreata from patients with *PRSS1* show marked atrophy and extensive replacement by mature adipose tissue with scattered islets of Langerhans and rare islands of acinar epithelium concentrated near the main pancreatic duct (Fig. 10). The ductal epithelium

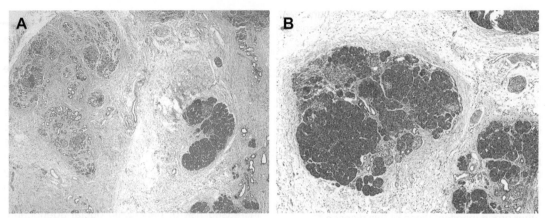

*Fig. 9.* The histopathology of *PRSS1*-related hereditary pancreatitis is progressive lipomatous atrophy. (*A*) In pediatric cases, there is central parenchymal loss and loosely packed perilobular and interlobular fibrosis (H&E, original magnification ×40). (*B*) With increasing patient age, these changes become more developed with fatty replacement of the pancreatic parenchyma that extends from the periphery to the central portions of the pancreas (H&E, original magnification ×100).

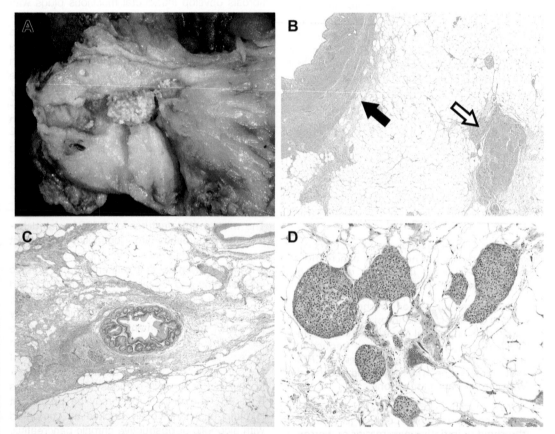

*Fig. 10.* (*A*) In advanced cases, *PRSS1*-related hereditary pancreatitis is characterized by marked pancreatic atrophy, fatty replacement, and large, intraductal calculi. (*B*) At low magnification, there is periductal fibrosis (main pancreatic duct, *black arrow*; interlobular duct, *white arrow*) and extensive parenchymal replacement by mature adipose tissue (H&E, original magnification ×40). (*C*) Within the adipose tissue are residual ducts that may show low-grade pancreatic intraepithelial neoplasia (PanIN) (H&E, original magnification ×100). (*D*) In addition, scattered, aggregates of islets of Langerhans are also often present within the fatty tissue (H&E, original magnification ×200).

may undergo neoplastic changes that are consistent with low-grade and intermediate-grade pancreatic intraepithelial neoplasia (PanIN), which are more noticeable in older patients.[54]

Less is known about the progression of histologic findings in patients with *CFTR* and *SPINK1*. However, *CFTR* mutations are associated with prominent intraductal mucinous plugs, dilated ducts, and periductal fibrosis (Fig. 11A, B). There is marked fatty replacement of the pancreatic parenchyma and patchy aggregates of residual islets of Langerhans. In contrast, *SPINK1* mutations are characterized by loss of pancreatic acinar, ductal and islet cell parenchyma with concomitant perilobular and interlobular fibrosis (Fig. 11C, D). The ductal epithelium can be atrophic with intraluminal proteinaceous plugs and calculi. Pseudocysts with thick fibrous walls and intracystic debris and retention cysts can be found in a subset of patients.

## DIFFERENTIAL DIAGNOSIS OF CHRONIC PANCREATITIS

Although with improvements in radiographic imaging and serologic studies, the diagnosis of chronic pancreatitis remains challenging, especially when the changes of chronic pancreatitis suggest a mass lesion. The main differential diagnosis includes pancreatic ductal adenocarcinoma.[55,56] The diagnostic difficulty is understandable when considering pancreatic ductal adenocarcinoma often comes to clinical presentation as the tumor causes ductal obstruction and, consequently, obstructive chronic pancreatitis. Moreover, chronic pancreatitis is a significant risk factor for the development of pancreatic ductal adenocarcinoma.

Despite many of the similarities between chronic pancreatitis and pancreatic ductal adenocarcinoma, patients with pancreatic ductal adenocarcinoma

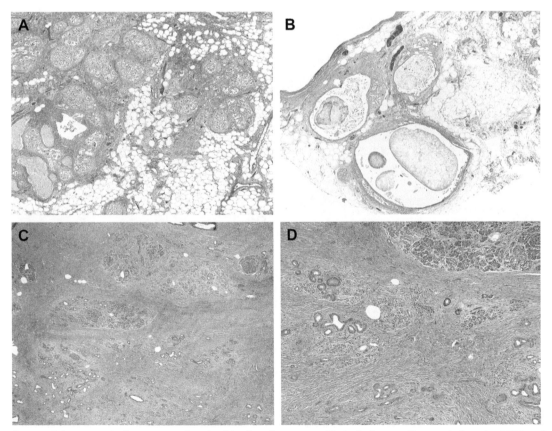

*Fig. 11.* Other genetic factors associated with chronic pancreatitis include germline mutations in *CFTR* and *SPINK1*. (*A, B*) Mutations in *CFTR* are associated with prominent intraductal mucinous/proteinaceous plugs, dilated ducts, periductal fibrosis and progressive lipomatous atrophy (H&E, original magnification ×100). (*C, D*) In contrast to *PRSS1* and *CFTR*, *SPINK1* mutations are characterized by loss of pancreatic acinar, ductal and islet cell parenchyma with concomitant perilobular and interlobular fibrosis (H&E, original magnification ×100 and ×200, respectively).

are typically older, have no history of pancreatitis, and present with painless jaundice of relatively short duration.[55] Microscopically, pancreatic ductal adenocarcinoma is composed of neoplastic glands in a haphazard growth pattern (**Fig. 12**A).[57] The glands are embedded within variable amounts of cellular and fibrotic stroma that may mimic the fibrosis seen in chronic pancreatitis. The neoplastic glands are attracted to muscular vessels and nerves, which also include vascular and perineural invasion (**Fig. 12**B). It is worth noting that when neoplastic glands infiltrate into vessels, they have a tendency to grow along the intimal surface of the vessel. In these instances, the malignant glands lining the vascular intima can be mistaken for low-grade PanIN (**Fig. 12**C).[58] The neoplastic cells form incomplete glands, cribriform structures, and/or papillae without fibrovascular cores (**Fig. 12**D). Intraglandular necrosis and debris is a frequent finding, but should not be misinterpreted as benign, such as in the setting of

chronic pancreatitis. Significant nuclear anisonucleosis can be appreciated with nuclei in a single gland varying in size by a ratio of greater than 4 to 1. Mitoses, including abnormal mitotic figures, as well as a prominent nucleolus, also may be present. Although many of these features can be identified within resection specimens, they may be inconspicuous in needle biopsies. Under these circumstances, immunolabeling for abnormal p53 expression that is characterized by strong nuclear labeling in more than 80% of tumor nuclei or complete absence of staining, may be of diagnostic value. van Heek and colleagues[59] reported p53 immunohistochemistry had a 48% sensitivity and 97% specificity for malignancy. However, in combination with cytologic assessment and additional molecular markers, the investigators achieved a sensitivity and specificity of 86% and 94%, respectively. Similarly, Smad4 immunohistochemistry can aid in the diagnosis of malignancy on biopsies and

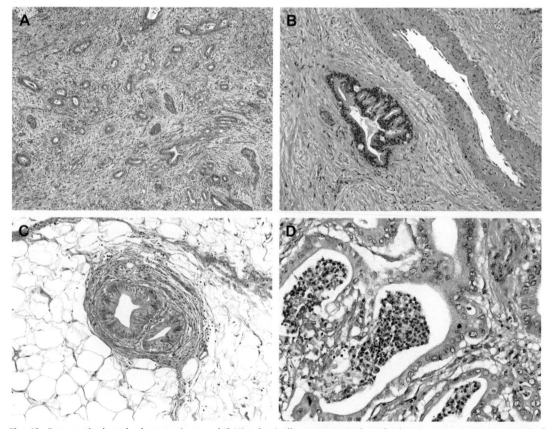

*Fig. 12.* Pancreatic ductal adenocarcinoma. (*A*) Histologically, pancreatic ductal adenocarcinoma is composed of neoplastic glands in a haphazard growth pattern within variable amounts of cellular and fibrotic stroma (H&E, original magnification ×100). (*B*) The neoplastic glands often grow next to nerves and muscular vessels (H&E, original magnification ×200). (*C*) Infiltrative glands have a tendency to grow along the intimal surface of vessels, mimicking low-grade PanIN (H&E, original magnification ×200). (*D*) The neoplastic cells form incomplete glands and/or cribriform structures with intraglandular debris and significant anisonucleosis (H&E, original magnification ×400).

cytologic specimens. Complete loss of staining is seen in 55% of pancreatic ductal adenocarcinomas, but preserved in chronic pancreatitis.[57]

## FUTURE TRENDS

Although we have described chronic pancreatitis as relatively distinct subtypes, it is very much an individualized disease process. With few exceptions, the exact etiology or etiologies of chronic pancreatitis are only partially known. For example, heavy and prolonged alcohol use alone does not cause chronic pancreatitis. Thus, other genetic or environmental factors must be present before alcoholic chronic pancreatitis can ensue. Likewise, several of the genetic mutations associated with chronic pancreatitis, such as mutations in *SPINK1*, cannot be disease causing, because only a small fraction of individuals who inherit these mutations will develop chronic pancreatitis. Therefore, determination of the etiology or etiologies of chronic pancreatitis continues to grow in importance. In the future, as our understanding of the pathogenesis of chronic pancreatitis evolves, many of the subtypes outlined herein may be replaced or alternatively described by risk factors that are associated with a spectrum of clinical and pathologic features.

---

### Pitfalls

*Pancreatic Ductal Adenocarcinoma*

! The key differential diagnosis of chronic pancreatitis and a significant clinicopathologic challenge.

! In contrast to chronic pancreatitis, patients with pancreatic ductal adenocarcinoma are often older, have no history of pancreatitis, and present with painless jaundice of relatively short duration.

! Microscopic features that support a diagnosis of pancreatic ductal adenocarcinoma include a haphazard growth pattern of ducts; growth of ducts near muscular vessels and nerves; perineural and lymphovascular invasion; glandular necrotic debris; incomplete lumen formation; variation in nuclear size by more than 4:1 in a single gland; prominent, irregular nucleoli; and mitoses, especially abnormal mitotic figures.

! Immunohistochemistry for p53 and Smad4 can be helpful in certain cases.

---

## REFERENCES

1. Cawley T. A singular case of diabetes, consisting entirely in the quantity of urine: with an inquirey into the different theories of the disease. London Medical Journal 1788;9:286–308.
2. Etemad B, Whitcomb DC. Chronic pancreatitis: diagnosis, classification, and new genetic developments. Gastroenterology 2001;120:682–707.
3. Lankisch PG, Assmus C, Maisonneuve P, et al. Epidemiology of pancreatic diseases in Luneburg County. A study in a defined German population. Pancreatology 2002;2:469–77.
4. Dite P, Stary K, Novotny I, et al. Incidence of chronic pancreatitis in the Czech Republic. Eur J Gastroenterol Hepatol 2001;13:749–50.
5. Yadav D, Timmons L, Benson JT, et al. Incidence, prevalence, and survival of chronic pancreatitis: a population-based study. Am J Gastroenterol 2011; 106:2192–9.
6. Everhart JE, Ruhl CE. Burden of digestive diseases in the United States Part III: liver, biliary tract, and pancreas. Gastroenterology 2009;136:1134–44.
7. Lowenfels AB, Maisonneuve P, Cavallini G, et al. Pancreatitis and the risk of pancreatic cancer. International Pancreatitis Study Group. N Engl J Med 1993;328:1433–7.
8. Whitcomb DC. Genetic risk factors for pancreatic disorders. Gastroenterology 2013;144:1292–302.
9. Yadav D, Whitcomb DC. The role of alcohol and smoking in pancreatitis. Nat Rev Gastroenterol Hepatol 2010;7:131–45.
10. Muniraj T, Aslanian HR, Farrell J, et al. Chronic pancreatitis, a comprehensive review and update. Part I: epidemiology, etiology, risk factors, genetics, pathophysiology, and clinical features. Dis Mon 2014;60:530–50.
11. Apte MV, Wilson JS, Korsten MA. Alcohol-related pancreatic damage: mechanisms and treatment. Alcohol Health Res World 1997;21:13–20.
12. Kloppel G. Chronic pancreatitis, pseudotumors and other tumor-like lesions. Mod Pathol 2007;20(Suppl 1):S113–31.
13. Ammann RW, Heitz PU, Kloppel G. Course of alcoholic chronic pancreatitis: a prospective clinicomorphological long-term study. Gastroenterology 1996; 111:224–31.
14. Kloppel G. Pseudocysts and other non-neoplastic cysts of the pancreas. Semin Diagn Pathol 2000; 17:7–15.
15. Detlefsen S, Sipos B, Feyerabend B, et al. Fibrogenesis in alcoholic chronic pancreatitis: the role of tissue necrosis, macrophages, myofibroblasts and cytokines. Mod Pathol 2006;19:1019–26.
16. Forsmark CE. Chronic pancreatitis. In: Feldman M, Friedman LS, Brandt LJ, editors. Sleisenger and

Fordtran's gastrointestinal and liver disease. Philadelphia: Elsevier Saunders; 2016. p. 994–1026.

17. Kloppel G, Maillet B. Pathology of acute and chronic pancreatitis. Pancreas 1993;8:659–70.

18. Sarles H. Etiopathogenesis and definition of chronic pancreatitis. Dig Dis Sci 1986;31:91S–107S.

19. Adsay NV, Zamboni G. Paraduodenal pancreatitis: a clinico-pathologically distinct entity unifying "cystic dystrophy of heterotopic pancreas", "para-duodenal wall cyst", and "groove pancreatitis". Semin Diagn Pathol 2004;21:247–54.

20. Flejou JF, Potet F, Molas G, et al. Cystic dystrophy of the gastric and duodenal wall developing in heterotopic pancreas: an unrecognised entity. Gut 1993; 34:343–7.

21. Balakrishnan V, Chatni S, Radhakrishnan L, et al. Groove pancreatitis: a case report and review of literature. JOP 2007;8:592–7.

22. Chatelain D, Vibert E, Yzet T, et al. Groove pancreatitis and pancreatic heterotopia in the minor duodenal papilla. Pancreas 2005;30:e92–5.

23. Bill K, Belber JP, Carson JW. Adenomyoma (pancreatic heterotopia) of the duodenum producing common bile duct obstruction. Gastrointest Endosc 1982;28:182–4.

24. Casetti L, Bassi C, Salvia R, et al. "Paraduodenal" pancreatitis: results of surgery on 58 consecutive patients from a single institution. World J Surg 2009;33:2664–9.

25. Adsay NV, Basturk O, Klimstra DS, et al. Pancreatic pseudotumors: non-neoplastic solid lesions of the pancreas that clinically mimic pancreas cancer. Semin Diagn Pathol 2004;21:260–7.

26. DeSouza K, Nodit L. Groove pancreatitis: a brief review of a diagnostic challenge. Arch Pathol Lab Med 2015;139:417–21.

27. DiMagno MJ, Wamsteker EJ. Pancreas divisum. Curr Gastroenterol Rep 2011;13:150–6.

28. Delhaye M, Engelholm L, Cremer M. Pancreas divisum: congenital anatomic variant or anomaly? Contribution of endoscopic retrograde dorsal pancreatography. Gastroenterology 1985;89: 951–8.

29. DiMagno MJ, Dimagno EP. Pancreas divisum does not cause pancreatitis, but associates with CFTR mutations. Am J Gastroenterol 2012;107:318–20.

30. Bertin C, Pelletier AL, Vullierme MP, et al. Pancreas divisum is not a cause of pancreatitis by itself but acts as a partner of genetic mutations. Am J Gastroenterol 2012;107:311–7.

31. Warshaw AL, Simeone JF, Schapiro RH, et al. Evaluation and treatment of the dominant dorsal duct syndrome (pancreas divisum redefined). Am J Surg 1990;159:59–64, [discussion: 64–6].

32. Hart PA, Zen Y, Chari ST. Recent advances in autoimmune pancreatitis. Gastroenterology 2015;149: 39–51.

33. Yoshida K, Toki F, Takeuchi T, et al. Chronic pancreatitis caused by an autoimmune abnormality. Proposal of the concept of autoimmune pancreatitis. Dig Dis Sci 1995;40:1561–8.

34. Hamano H, Kawa S, Horiuchi A, et al. High serum IgG4 concentrations in patients with sclerosing pancreatitis. N Engl J Med 2001;344: 732–8.

35. Kamisawa T, Funata N, Hayashi Y, et al. A new clinicopathological entity of IgG4-related autoimmune disease. J Gastroenterol 2003;38:982–4.

36. Ectors N, Maillet B, Aerts R, et al. Non-alcoholic duct destructive chronic pancreatitis. Gut 1997; 41:263–8.

37. Zamboni G, Luttges J, Capelli P, et al. Histopathological features of diagnostic and clinical relevance in autoimmune pancreatitis: a study on 53 resection specimens and 9 biopsy specimens. Virchows Arch 2004;445:552–63.

38. Kamisawa T, Chari ST, Giday SA, et al. Clinical profile of autoimmune pancreatitis and its histological subtypes: an international multicenter survey. Pancreas 2011;40:809–14.

39. Detlefsen S, Zamboni G, Frulloni L, et al. Clinical features and relapse rates after surgery in type 1 autoimmune pancreatitis differ from type 2: a study of 114 surgically treated European patients. Pancreatology 2012;12:276–83.

40. Zhang L, Chari S, Smyrk TC, et al. Autoimmune pancreatitis (AIP) type 1 and type 2: an international consensus study on histopathologic diagnostic criteria. Pancreas 2011;40:1172–9.

41. Notohara K, Burgart LJ, Yadav D, et al. Idiopathic chronic pancreatitis with periductal lymphoplasmacytic infiltration: clinicopathologic features of 35 cases. Am J Surg Pathol 2003;27:1119–27.

42. Kawaguchi K, Koike M, Tsuruta K, et al. Lymphoplasmacytic sclerosing pancreatitis with cholangitis: a variant of primary sclerosing cholangitis extensively involving pancreas. Hum Pathol 1991;22: 387–95.

43. Zhang L, Notohara K, Levy MJ, et al. IgG4-positive plasma cell infiltration in the diagnosis of autoimmune pancreatitis. Mod Pathol 2007;20:23–8.

44. Kloppel G, Detlefsen S, Chari ST, et al. Autoimmune pancreatitis: the clinicopathological characteristics of the subtype with granulocytic epithelial lesions. J Gastroenterol 2010;45:787–93.

45. Whitcomb DC, Gorry MC, Preston RA, et al. Hereditary pancreatitis is caused by a mutation in the cationic trypsinogen gene. Nat Genet 1996;14: 141–5.

46. Whitcomb DC, Preston RA, Aston CE, et al. A gene for hereditary pancreatitis maps to chromosome 7q35. Gastroenterology 1996;110:1975–80.

47. Lowenfels AB, Maisonneuve P, DiMagno EP, et al. Hereditary pancreatitis and the risk of pancreatic

cancer. International Hereditary Pancreatitis Study Group. J Natl Cancer Inst 1997;89:442–6.

48. Park RW, Grand RJ. Gastrointestinal manifestations of cystic fibrosis: a review. Gastroenterology 1981; 81:1143–61.

49. Atlas AB, Orenstein SR, Orenstein DM. Pancreatitis in young children with cystic fibrosis. J Pediatr 1992;120:756–9.

50. Witt H, Luck W, Hennies HC, et al. Mutations in the gene encoding the serine protease inhibitor, Kazal type 1 are associated with chronic pancreatitis. Nat Genet 2000;25:213–6.

51. Singhi AD, Pai RK, Kant JA, et al. The histopathology of PRSS1 hereditary pancreatitis. Am J Surg Pathol 2014;38:346–53.

52. Walters MN. Adipose atrophy of the exocrine pancreas. J Pathol Bacteriol 1966;92:547–57.

53. Altinel D, Basturk O, Sarmiento JM, et al. Lipomatous pseudohypertrophy of the pancreas: a clinicopathologically distinct entity. Pancreas 2010;39: 392–7.

54. Rebours V, Boutron-Ruault MC, Schnee M, et al. Risk of pancreatic adenocarcinoma in patients with hereditary pancreatitis: a national exhaustive series. Am J Gastroenterol 2008;103:111–9.

55. Adsay NV, Bandyopadhyay S, Basturk O, et al. Chronic pancreatitis or pancreatic ductal adenocarcinoma? Semin Diagn Pathol 2004;21: 268–76.

56. Kloppel G, Adsay NV. Chronic pancreatitis and the differential diagnosis versus pancreatic cancer. Arch Pathol Lab Med 2009;133:382–7.

57. Hruban RH, Fukushima N. Pancreatic adenocarcinoma: update on the surgical pathology of carcinomas of ductal origin and PanINs. Mod Pathol 2007;20(Suppl 1):S61–70.

58. Hong SM, Goggins M, Wolfgang CL, et al. Vascular invasion in infiltrating ductal adenocarcinoma of the pancreas can mimic pancreatic intraepithelial neoplasia: a histopathologic study of 209 cases. Am J Surg Pathol 2012;36:235–41.

59. van Heek T, Rader AE, Offerhaus GJ, et al. K-ras, p53, and DPC4 (MAD4) alterations in fine-needle aspirates of the pancreas: a molecular panel correlates with and supplements cytologic diagnosis. Am J Clin Pathol 2002;117:755–65.

# Pancreatic Cytopathology

Jennifer A. Collins, DO, MPH, Syed Z. Ali, MD, FRCPath, FIAC,
Christopher J. VandenBussche, MD, PhD*

## KEYWORDS

- Cytopathology • Fine-needle aspiration • Pancreatic cytopathology • Cytology • FNA • Pancreas

## Key points

- The sensitivity and specificity of endoscopic ultrasound-guided fine-needle aspiration (EUS-FNA) of pancreatic lesions both approach 95% with a low complication rate.
- Familiarity with benign elements, in particular contaminating gastrointestinal epithelium, is critical for arriving at an accurate diagnosis.
- EUS-FNA is the method of choice for the procurement of cytologic material for diagnosis in the setting of a cystic lesion; aspirates are often acellular and cytology alone is inferior compared to a combination of cytology with cyst fluid analysis.
- Well-established cytomorphological features of pancreatic adenocarcinoma include loss of organization, anisonucleosis, irregular nuclear membranes, nuclear crowding, nuclear overlap, high nuclear-to-cytoplasmic ratios, 3-dimensional architecture, and single cells.
- Recently, cyst fluid analysis has incorporated the detection of molecular markers through techniques such as gene sequencing, proteomic analysis, and detection of microRNA species to diagnosis premalignant and malignant cystic neoplasms, specifically in specimens with limited material.

## ABSTRACT

Pancreatic cytopathology, particularly through the use of endoscopic ultrasound-guided fine-needle aspiration (FNA), has excellent specificity and sensitivity for the diagnosis of pancreatic lesions. Such diagnoses can help guide preoperative management of patients, provide prognostic information, and confirm diagnoses in patients who are not surgical candidates. Furthermore, FNA can be used to obtain cyst fluid for ancillary tests that can improve the diagnosis of cystic lesions. In this article, we describe the cytomorphological features and differential diagnoses of the most commonly encountered pancreatic lesions on FNA.

## OVERVIEW TO PANCREATIC FINE-NEEDLE ASPIRATION

Current clinical management is dependent on the rapid and accurate diagnosis of pancreatic lesions. Although clinical and radiological findings can suggest malignancy, current management strategies rely on pathologic diagnosis, particularly in nonsurgical patients.[1-3] Pancreatic adenocarcinoma is the fourth leading cause of cancer-related death with a projected rise to the second leading by 2020.[4,5] Survival is poor with a 5-year survival of 7% and less than 20% of patients considered surgically resectable at diagnosis.[4-6] Although surgical and neoadjuvant management of the disease has advanced, overall mortality has continued to increase.[4] However, patients with early localized disease have shown an improved 5-year survival, up to 30%, following complete surgical resection.[7,8] Therefore, an early definitive diagnosis appears to be the most critical step in current management algorithms.[9]

Initial evaluation of pancreatic lesions is performed with imaging studies, preferably multidetector computer tomography (CT), MRI, or magnetic resonance cholangiopancreatography

Disclosure: The authors have nothing to disclose.
Department of Pathology, The Johns Hopkins Hospital, The Johns Hopkins University School of Medicine, 600 North Wolfe Street, Baltimore, MD 21287, USA
* Corresponding author.
E-mail address: cjvand@jhmi.edu

surgpath.theclinics.com

(MRCP), depending on the presence of a cystic component.[10–12] Although biopsy may not be required in the setting of highly suspicious clinical and radiologic findings, it is necessary in most cases in which neoadjuvant therapy is the initial management.[13] Modalities for image-guided pancreatic tissue sampling have evolved over time from transabdominal ultrasound-guided and CT to more recently endoscopic ultrasound (EUS). Endoscopic retrograde cholangiopancreatography (ERCP) is restricted to ductal sampling in the setting of biliary stricture with cytologic sampling restricted to exfoliative cells in bile and/or brush samples. These samples have been shown to have low sensitivity (6%–32%) and have been replaced over time by EUS in the diagnosis of solid neoplasms.[14–17] Although transabdominal ultrasound biopsy is the least invasive, it has an overall low sensitivity for detecting small lesions, particularly in the pancreatic head/uncinate, the most common site for adenocarcinoma.[18–20] CT-guided biopsy also appears inferior because of its expense, radiation exposure, and lack of real-time guidance.[18] The advent of EUS has changed pancreatic lesion evaluation significantly by allowing for simultaneous nonradiation imaging combined with the ability for cytologic sampling. EUS has been shown to have greater accuracy for small lesions (<3 cm) relative to both ultrasound or CT with less risk for peritoneal seeding when compared with percutaneous core needle biopsy.[21–24] Multiple systematic reviews have shown the pooled sensitivity and specificity of EUS approach 95% with a complication rate similar to percutaneous FNA, ranging from 0% to 5%.[25–28] EUS-FNA, introduced more than 20 years ago, has accumulated extensive support in the literature and is now the modality of choice in procuring specimen material for diagnosing pancreatic neoplasia, including nonadenocarcinoma.[26,29,30]

Cytology specimens, therefore, play a key role in the initial diagnosis and management of solid and cystic pancreatic lesions, including pancreatobiliary strictures.[31] This has led to a particularly important emphasis on the terminology and nomenclature in pancreatobiliary cytology reporting. Currently there is no standard or universal reporting format for pancreas cytology; however, the Papanicolaou Society of Cytopathology recently published a proposed standardized nomenclature, see Table 1.[32] The proposed 6-tier scheme has divided the conventional *Other* category into Atypical (Category III) and *Neoplastic: Benign* or *Neoplastic: Other* (Category IV), creating, functionally, 7 discrete categories. This modification allows for the discrimination of "atypical" findings, not including reactive, from benign and low-grade neoplasms. This is particularly relevant to diagnosing specimens with limited material, whereby secondary to low cellularity or preparation artifact, a definitive diagnosis of premalignant, suspicious, or benign cannot be made. Lesions classified within the *Neoplastic* category have more cellularity that show specific architectural and cytologic features that allow for a reproducible diagnosis of a benign entity (cystadenoma, neuroendocrine microadenoma, and lymphangioma) or low-grade neoplasms (premalignant mucin-producing cystic lesions, intraductal pancreatic mucinous neoplasm [IPMN] and mucinous cystic neoplasm [MCN], pancreatic neuroendocrine tumor [PanNET] and solid pseudopapillary neoplasm [SPN]) specified as *Other*.[32,33] The authors' intent for this latter category IV was to allow for ease of correlation to the 2010 World Health Organization (WHO) classification of pancreatic lesions and thus drive cytologic diagnoses into a reproducibly correlative format.[32,34] Another advantage of the new classification scheme is that a lack of epithelial cells no longer precludes a diagnostic specimen but rather allows for ancillary fluid chemistry testing to have diagnostic value. This is reflected by the use of *Neoplastic: Other* in the setting of an elevated carcinoembryonic antigen (CEA) without an epithelial component. The remaining diagnostic categories show features consistent with conventional diagnostic criteria. The WHO and the Papanicolaou Society for Cytopathology have suggested classification of *Malignant* (category V) to include adenocarcinoma (and its variants), acinar cell carcinoma, poorly differentiated neuroendocrine carcinoma (including large cell neuroendocrine carcinoma), pancreatoblastoma, lymphoma, and metastatic lesions.[32,34] Recently, Saieg and colleagues[35] showed that reclassification of 55 specimens using the proposed Papanicolaou categories has the greatest effect on the atypical and suspicious categories. They found that reclassification allowed for 94% of their atypical specimens to be diagnosed as *Neoplastic: Other*, including 33% nondiagnostic and 23% of negatives.[35] The latter of which is the result of an elevated CEA value considered sufficient for the diagnosis.[35] The positive predictive value for their diagnoses was 88.9%.[35] Thus, in the context of a multidisciplinary and multimodality approach to pancreatic lesion diagnosis and therapy, a standardized nomenclature would have the benefit of predictably guiding management algorithms while improving the correlation of future studies.

**Table 1**
**Papanicolaou Society of Cytopathology guidelines: standardized terminology and nomenclature for pancreatobiliary cytology**

| Numeric Category | Classification Terminology | Diagnostic Entities |
|---|---|---|
| I | Nondiagnostic | • Acellular<br>• Nonspecific cyst contents (volume inadequate for ancillary testing)<br>• Benign pancreatic parenchyma (with a mass present on imaging studies)<br>• Gastrointestinal contamination only |
| II | Negative (for malignancy) | • Benign pancreatic parenchyma (no discrete mass)<br>• Acute pancreatitis<br>• Chronic pancreatitis<br>• Autoimmune pancreatitis<br>• Pseudocyst<br>• Lymphoepithelial cyst<br>• Splenule (accessory spleen) |
| III | Atypical | Atypical features not consistent with normal or reactive changes and insufficient to classify as suspicious or neoplastic |
| IV | Neoplastic: benign or other | Benign:<br>• Serous cystadenoma<br>• Cystic teratoma<br>• Schwannoma<br>Other:<br>• Intraductal pancreatic mucinous neoplasm<br>• MCN (includes mucin in the absence of epithelium; epithelial dysplasia should be noted)<br>• Pancreatic neuroendocrine tumor<br>• Solid pseudopapillary neoplasm<br>• Gastrointestinal stromal tumor |
| V | Suspicious (for malignancy) | Cytologic features suggestive of malignancy with insufficient qualitative or quantitative material |
| VI | Positive/malignant | • Pancreatic ductal adenocarcinoma<br>• Colloid/mucinous carcinoma<br>• Medullary carcinoma<br>• Adenosquamous carcinoma<br>• Undifferentiated carcinoma with osteoclastlike giant cells<br>• Undifferentiated carcinoma<br>• Acinar cell carcinoma<br>• Poorly differentiated neuroendocrine, pancreatoblastoma<br>• Lymphoma<br>• Metastasis |

## NORMAL FINDINGS AND GASTROINTESTINAL CONTAMINATION

Aspiration of a pancreatic lesion requires familiarity with the structures the needle will traverse in addition to the benign native parenchyma that one will encounter. Depending on the location of the lesion, the gastrointestinal tract (stomach and/or duodenal epithelium) will be sampled.[36,37] Therefore, the identification of gastrointestinal (GI) epithelium within the specimen should be distinguished from that of lesional epithelium.

This can present as a challenge in the setting of cystic lesions. Nagle and colleagues[36] showed that duodenal mucosa is commonly found as a monolayer and composed of cells with nonvacuolated, dense cytoplasm, round to oval nuclei, often with a brush border and present in conjunction with goblet cells and intraepithelial lymphocytes, see **Fig.** 1A. Gastric mucosa, in contrast, can show some mucinous cytoplasm; however, it is limited to the upper one-third and forms a "cup shape."[36] The epithelial cells will show benign-appearing nuclear features and although rare,

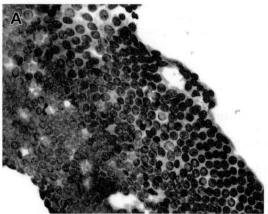
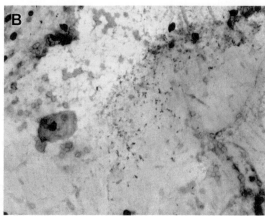

**Fig. 1.** Gastrointestinal contamination from the duodenum (*A*) is recognizable by its monolayer architecture, dense nonvacuolated cytoplasm, and the presence of goblet cells (Diff-Quick stain, ×200). An accompanying feature of esophageal and gastrointestinal contamination is "dirty mucin" (*B*), which contains bacterial organisms, stripped nuclei, and mature benign squamous cells (Diff-Quick stain, ×200).

goblet cells may be present in cases with intestinal metaplasia.[36] Gastric mucosa can represent side branch IPMN epithelium; however, the concern for a "false negative" is low because these are considered, clinically, to behave in a "benign" fashion.[38,39] Although goblet cells can be present in some cystic neoplasms, the presence of clean, thick colloid-type mucin, which should be distinguished from contaminating mucin (**Fig. 1**B), appears to be the most helpful distinguishing feature, see **Fig. 3**A.[36,40–42] For the most part, pancreatic parenchyma consists of acinar cells. Therefore, in sampling normal pancreas, the aspiration should consist predominantly of cohesive groups of acinar cells with only a minor component of ductal epithelium. Normal ductal epithelium will be both sparse and show monotonous honeycomb architecture. Islet cells make up less than 2% of the pancreatic tissue mass and are minimally sampled.[43] Mesothelial cells can also be present; however, they are often scant.

## CHRONIC PANCREATITIS

Chronic pancreatitis is largely diagnosed based on imaging and clinical findings; however, the associated reactive changes following injury can be challenging on FNA. Chronic pancreatitis is largely subclassified, radiologically, into 1 of 3 groups: chronic calcifying (alcohol related), chronic obstructive, and autoimmune.[44] Acknowledgement of acute and chronic pancreatitis, including autoimmune (immunoglobulin [Ig]G4 associated) in the differential diagnosis is often necessary so as to not overcall the reparative and reactive atypia present. Chronic pancreatitis shows a continuum of histologic changes from acute/recurrent to

chronic.[45] This spectrum of changes is characterized predominantly by an increase in fibrosis, inflammation, and loss of acini. Cytologic specimens typically will have decreased cellularity with a mixture of fibrotic stromal fragments and increased ductal epithelium in a background of mixed inflammation. Calcifications when abundant can be highly suggestive of pancreatitis in the correct clinical and radiologic context but for the most part are nonspecific.[46–48] Ductal atypia can be significant, often concurrent with pancreatic intraepithelial neoplasia (PanIN), which can create significant difficulty in distinguishing it from a well-differentiated adenocarcinoma.[49] Layfield and Jarboe[50] showed that a lack of nuclear atypia, characterized by hyperchromasia, membrane abnormalities, variability in size, and mitoses in a background of cohesive acinar cells, together, are critical in the discrimination of pancreatitis from malignancies.

Autoimmune pancreatitis (IgG4-related) can be particularly challenging because the patient demographics, clinical symptoms and even radiologic findings can be suspicious for adenocarcinoma.[51,52] In 2012, international consensus diagnostic criteria (ICDC) were created and used 5 features to subclassify autoimmune pancreatitis into 2 types: type 1IgG4–related or type 2 granulocytic epithelial lesion. The criteria included imaging, serology, multiorgan involvement, steroid responsiveness, and the gold standard, histology.[53,54] There have been several retrospective studies that reviewed cytologic features associated with a subsequent diagnosis of autoimmune pancreatitis and together conclude that the specimens are commonly hypocellular and composed of cellular stromal fragments with discohesive fibroblasts.[55,56] A background inflammatory component does not appear to be a consistent feature.[55,56] Although ICDC recognizes EUS Trucut biopsy or resection as "suitable" for pathologic diagnosis, many follow-up studies have shown EUS-FNA to provide adequate material for diagnosis and in some cases allowing for determination of subtype.[57,58] Last, IgG4 immunohistochemistry, although not currently supported in the literature, may be helpful on cell block material in which focal nonspecific ductal atypia is identified.

## CYSTIC LESIONS

Pancreatic cysts are not uncommon and have been identified in up to 19% of abdominal imaging studies.[59–61] Recent studies have shown an increase in the detection and diagnosis of smaller IPMNs.[62–64] Pancreatic cysts can be classified into non-neoplastic, neoplastic, and cystic necrosis within a solid tumor. Non-neoplastic cysts include pseudocysts and lymphoepithelial cysts, among others. Neoplastic cysts include MCN, IPMN, serous cystadenoma, SPN, and cystic neuroendocrine tumors. The malignant potential of these entities is variable, some with high potential, such as IPMN, and others with little to no malignant potential, such as serous cystadenoma. Therefore, an accurate diagnosis is critical to patient management. EUS-FNA is the method of choice for the procurement of fluid and cytologic material for diagnostic means in this setting. Aspirates are often acellular and cytology alone is inferior (<50% sensitivity) compared with a combination of cytology with cyst fluid analysis.[65–67] Management algorithms, therefore, typically rely on both cytologic diagnosis as well as cyst fluid analysis.

## NONMUCINOUS CYSTIC LESIONS

Pseudocyst is the most common cystic lesion in the pancreas, accounting for 80% of cystic lesions, is related to injury from alcohol or biliary complication, and predominantly identified in adult men.[68] These lesions contain pancreatic enzymatic secretions (amylase) and inflammatory cells encapsulated by fibrotic granulation tissue without an epithelial lining. The cytologic specimens consist of variable amounts of mixed inflammatory cells, histiocytes, fibroblasts, and granular debris, including bile pigment, in the absence of an epithelial component; see **Fig. 2**A.

Lymphoepithelial cysts are rare benign cysts that are more common in men without preference for a specific site. The cyst epithelium is squamous and fluid contains benign squamous cells, keratinaceous debris, cholesterol crystals, macrophages, and, rarely, lymphoid cells; see **Fig. 2**B.[69,70] However, the findings of the squamous component can be variable and, therefore, onsite evaluation maybe of great utility in this setting.[69]

Serous cystadenomas are rare, accounting for only 1% to 2% of pancreatic neoplasms, and commonly afflict middle-aged women (sixth to seventh decade).[71] The neoplasm arises from the centroacinar cells and, thus, the epithelium is composed of cuboidal, glycogen-rich cells that form cystic spaces filled with serous fluid. These lesions are predominantly benign, although can become bulky and rarely show dysplastic features that would classify them as cystadenocarcinoma.

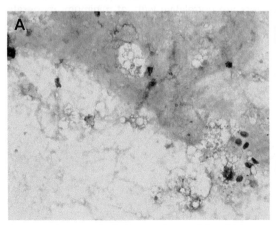 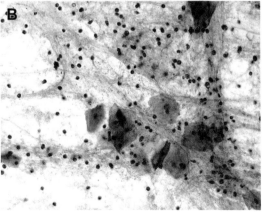

**Fig. 2.** Benign cysts include pseudocysts (*A*), which are recognizable by the presence of numerous macrophages, granular debris, including bile pigment, and lack of epithelial cells (Diff Quick stain, ×100). Lymphoepithelial cysts (*B*) can show variable numbers of lymphocytes with scattered mature squamous cells in a background of granular debris (Pap stain, ×100).

The yield of EUS-FNA cytology is poor, in part because of the amount of vascularity present.[72] Multiple studies have shown that the most common finding is hypocellularity, and when cells are present they are bland, cuboidal glandular cells with clear or granular cytoplasm often forming a monolayer.[72–74] The nucleus is round with smooth contours and finely distributed chromatin. The background typically lacks histiocytes or macrophages, a common finding in cystic lesions.[73] Although these findings are nonspecific, rendering a diagnosis of Neoplasm: benign, through recognition of its low cellularity and bland epithelium can have a significant impact on patient management.

## MUCINOUS CYSTIC LESIONS

Mucinous cysts are typically defined in concert with the new Papanicolaou Society of Cytopathology nomenclature to have one of the following: thick extracellular clean mucin (including mucin with evidence of cellular cyst debris, see Fig. 3A), mucinous epithelium (Fig. 3B) and/or elevated CEA (laboratory dependent but approximately >192 ng/mL).[32,65,75,76] Cutoffs lower than this have shown to be less sensitive and specific relative to EUS characteristics, cytology, and CEA levels combined.[77] Elevated CEA levels even in the absence of epithelium or mucin strongly support a neoplastic cystic lesion; however, they do not differentiate between benign and malignant.[65,75,78] Amylase levels in the thousands are supportive of a pseudocyst but when elevated in concert with CEA do not distinguish MCN from IPMN.[38,78,79] Amylase levels less than 250 U/L can rule out a pseudocyst with 98% specificity and is often seen in the context of a serous cystadenoma among others.[78] Once there is a diagnosis of a mucin-producing neoplasm, the second cytopathologic assessment is the identification of high-grade dysplasia. Criteria for distinguishing high-grade dysplasia include increased nuclear enlargement and coarse chromatin

identified in cells smaller than an enterocyte (12 μM) often with background necrosis.[80–84] This latter finding is particularly important in the management of low-risk IPMNs (side branch) in which frequency of malignancy is lower than that of the main duct and, as such, surveillance is commonly favored.[31,85–87]

Several studies have looked at the impact and criteria for grading dysplasia on EUS-FNA specimens of mucinous neoplasms and have identified common features that correlate with the grade of dysplasia on resection. Layfield and Cramer[88] showed that nuclear atypia defined by nuclear molding, prominent nucleoli, and membrane irregularity correlate with grade on resection; however, the study specimens were limited to only higher-grade IPMNs. Michaels and colleagues[89] looked at low-grade and high-grade IPMNs to show that the presence of necrosis, inflammation, epithelial clusters with high nuclear to cytoplasm ratio (cellular projections/papillary buds), parachromatin clearing, and nucleoli were all highly associated with higher-grade lesions, see Box 1 and Fig. 3C. Most recently, Pitman and colleagues[82] reconfirmed that the identification of background necrosis, increased nuclear to cytoplasm ratio, and an abnormal chromatin pattern (hypochromasia and hyperchromasia) are features of high-grade dysplasia in branch-duct IPMNs.[90] This discrimination is an important finding because it would directly change the course of treatment in this setting.[82,90] A particularly important criterion identified in the literature appears to be the identification of atypical epithelial cells (AECs) and their correlation with high-grade dysplasia or invasive adenocarcinoma on resection. Pitman and colleagues[91] showed that the presence of even limited numbers of these atypical epithelial clusters are correlative with, at minimum, moderate-grade dysplasia on resection, both retrospectively and prospectively.[83] Genevay and colleagues[84] showed that identification of AECs has greater sensitivity for high-grade dysplasia or an invasive

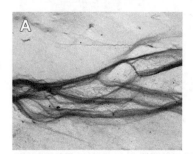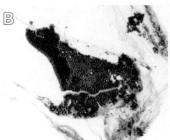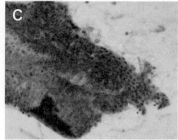

**Fig. 3.** Mucin-producing neoplasms commonly show "clean" thick mucin (A) (Diff Quick stain, ×100), often with fragments of columnar mucinous epithelium (B) (Diff Quick stain, ×40). Any feature suggestive of high-grade dysplasia (C) is a critical finding and includes increased nuclear-to-cytoplasmic ratio, nuclear overlap, presence of nucleoli, and parachromatin clearing (Pap stain, ×200).

> **Box 1**
> **High-grade features in an intraductal pancreatic mucinous neoplasm (IPMN)**
>
> *Features of High-Grade Dysplasia in IPMNs*
> - Architecture
>   - Atypical epithelial clusters (increased nuclear:cytoplasmic ratio)
>   - Presence of necrosis
> - Nuclear
>   - Prominent nucleoli
>   - Hyper and hypochromatic chromatin, including parachromatin clearing
>   - Nuclear molding
>   - Nuclear membrane irregularity
>   - Increased nuclear-to-cytoplasmic ratio

component than current radiologic features alone. The importance of this cytologic finding in cyst fluid is evident from the revisions in the 2012 Sendai guideline (international consensus guidelines for the management of patients with mucinous cysts), whereby this diagnosis was sufficient to define and treat these lesions as "high risk."[80,83,91–93]

## ADENOCARCINOMA

Pancreatic adenocarcinoma represents approximately 90% of the solid pancreatic lesions.[94,95] Definitive diagnosis of adenocarcinoma from nonadenocarcinoma malignancies is a critical distinction that has clear management implications. Several studies have identified discrete cytomorphologic features of adenocarcinoma and together have generated a general consensus on these findings. In early studies Lin and Staerkle[96] and separately Mitsuhashi and colleagues[97] showed that coarse hyperchromatic chromatin

with prominent nucleoli, irregular nuclear membranes, nuclear crowding and overlap with high nuclear-to-cytoplasmic ratios ($\geq 4$) and 3-dimensional architecture were highly correlative features, see **Fig. 4**A. Later Cohen and colleagues[98] determined anisonucleosis, macronuclei, and irregular nuclear membranes were highly correlated with adenocarcinoma. Others have shown the presence of cytoplasmic mucin as a reliable feature of adenocarcinoma.[99] Most recently, Huffmann and colleagues[100] set out to create a scoring system for the cytologic diagnosis of adenocarcinoma and identified 5 features that showed the strongest correlation with malignancy and include anisonucleosis, nuclear membrane irregularity, mitoses, dishesive atypical cells, and cribriform architecture. These cytologic criteria for the diagnostic category of *Malignancy: Adenocarcinoma* have been confirmed in the literature with several recent meta-analyses demonstrating a high sensitivity and specificity (both 90%) for its diagnosis, see **Box 2**.[25,101,102] It is important to keep in

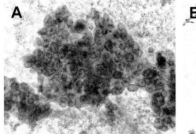 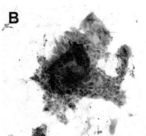 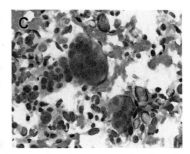

*Fig. 4.* Adenocarcinoma (*A*) can be distinguished by other entities from its increased nuclear-to-cytoplasmic ratio; coarse, hyperchromatic chromatin; prominent nucleoli; and necrotic background (Diff-Quick stain, ×400). The presence of atypical keratinizing squamous cells (*B*) can suggest a squamous component that has prognostic significance and should be noted (Pap Stain, ×200). Last, the identification of atypical osteoclastlike giant cells (*C*) is a discerning feature that would favor a variant of pancreatic carcinoma, undifferentiated carcinoma with osteoclastlike giant cells, which has a very poor prognosis (Diff-Quick stain, ×400).

---

**Box 2**
**Features of adenocarcinoma**

*Architecture*
- Three-dimensional clusters
- Disorganization ("drunken honeycomb")
- Discohesive cells

*Nuclear*
- Anisonucleosis
- Coarse hyperchromatic chromatin
- Macronuclei and macronucleoli
- Nuclear membrane irregularity
- Increased nuclear-to-cytoplasmic ratio

*Cytoplasmic*
- Mucin vacuoles

---

mind features of prognostically significant variants, including the presence of atypical or malignant squamous cells suggesting an adenosquamous or the characteristic osteoclastlike giant cells of an undifferentiated carcinoma, both of which can have important treatment implications; see **Fig. 4**B, C.[103]

## PANCREATIC NEUROENDOCRINE TUMORS

The diagnosis of PanNETs, although accounting for fewer than 5% of primary neoplasms, has increased in frequency over time.[104–106] Accurate diagnosis of PanNETs on EUS-FNA material is of particular importance because the prognostic and management implications differ significantly from that of adenocarcinoma.[107–109] Morphology of PanNET follows that of other neuroendocrine neoplasms on FNA. The first clue is typically the presence of numerous, monotonous, discohesive tumor cells that may at first blend into the background as lymphocytes or stripped epithelial cell nuclei, see **Fig. 5**A. The neoplasm also may be present as small or larger fragments that may maintain some identifiable microarchitecture, such as rosettes, sheets, or ribbons. Small fragments with rosettelike formations may mimic smeared fragments of pancreatic acini, or a well-differentiated adenocarcinoma. Individually, the neoplastic cells usually have round and eccentric nuclei with very regular nuclear borders.[110] The chromatin is typically speckled and nucleoli are not seen. Well-differentiated adenocarcinomas typically have higher nuclear to cytoplasmic ratios, with some nuclear border irregularities and nuclear pleomorphism; discohesive cells are not usually seen in adenocarcinoma in the absence of necrosis and/or marked pleomorphism.

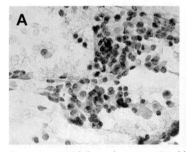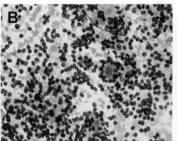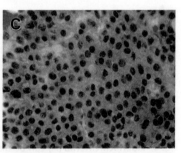

*Fig. 5.* PanNET (*A*) can be recognized by numerous discohesive, monotonous cells with eccentric nuclei that have fine chromatin, often with a background of stripped nuclei (Pap stain, ×200). SPN (*B*) shows small, monotonous cells with fine chromatin and oval nuclei, often forming rosettes and sometimes with the presence of hyaline globules (Diff-Quick stain, ×200). In contrast, ACC (*C*) will show monotonous cells often in sheets with prominent nucleoli and abundant granular cytoplasm with a vascular architecture (Diff-Quick stain, ×400).

Discerning a neoplastic process, especially in the context of a small number of neoplastic cells, can be challenging. Therefore, consideration of whether the FNA material represents a true neoplastic process is a critical one. Benign lesions, such as ectopic spleen and islet cell hyperplasia, have been misdiagnosed as PanNET on FNA. Cell block material is often crucial for confirming the diagnosis, as neuroendocrine markers can be ordered (CD56, synaptophysin, chromogranin).[110] The grading of PanNETs on FNA is controversial, because the limited tumor sampling may not be representative of higher-grade areas within the tumor.[111–114] Nevertheless, recent publications have explored the use of Ki-67 immunostaining for this intention but with variable results. Larghi and colleagues[111] recently have shown that a larger-gauge needle (19) in EUS-FNA tissue procurement had good correlation with histologic grade based on Ki67 immunostaining. Others have shown that Ki67 tends to underestimate the grade in cytology material and, therefore, the findings should be interpreted with caution.[114,115] High-grade tumors may have the morphology of small-cell carcinoma, which is described elsewhere.

The diagnosis of a cystic PanNET may be particularly difficult, as the number of neoplastic cells may be limited.[116,117] In such cases, there may be too few cells on a cell block for confirmatory staining. If the number of cells is limited but they possess neuroendocrine features, one may give the diagnosis "suspicious for a neoplasm with neuroendocrine features" or invoke the comment "if the cells present are representative of the entire lesion, it would be consistent with a pancreatic neuroendocrine tumor."

## SOLID PSEUDOPAPILLARY NEOPLASM

SPNs are rare neoplasms that occur in young women (third decade) in more than 90% of cases.[118] They classically appear as branching fragments with attached tumor cells in a background of dispersed single tumor cells.[119] The tumor cells are small and monotonous, with fine chromatin and oval nuclei, see Fig. 5B. If cell block material is available, cross sections of pseudopapillae demonstrate hyalinized fibrovascular cores. The presence of a dispersed cell population, especially when combined with areas showing rosette-like architecture, may be initially suggestive of a PanNET. The relative rarity of this lesion may also contribute to difficulty in diagnosis; thus, it must always be kept in mind, especially if the location and patient demographic are appropriate. As with other well-differentiated pancreatic neoplasms, immunostains performed on cell block material are often needed to confirm a diagnosis. Cytoplasmic and nuclear staining for beta-catenin, as well as immunoreactivity for CD99 and CD10 are commonly seen; it is important to note that SPN may express neuroendocrine markers, such as CD56 and synaptophysin.[120]

## ACINAR CELL CARCINOMA

Although acinar cell carcinoma (ACC) shares features of PanNET on FNA, their incidence is exceedingly rare.[121] The smears contain discohesive, monotonous individual cells that may also be present in fragments with an underlying acinar architecture.[122] The cells typically have abundant, granular cytoplasm and in contrast to PanNET, ACC cells often have prominent nucleoli; see Fig. 5C. The cells contain periodic acid-Schiff–positive, diastase-resistant granules. Immunostains for BCL10, trypsin, chymotrypsin, lipase, and amylase may be positive; however, trypsin and chymotrypsin positivity cannot definitively rule out an SPN.[121,123]

## PANCREATOBLASTOMA

Pancreatoblastoma is a rare pediatric tumor, with only 39 cases reported in adults since it was first described in 1957.[124,125] The cytomorphology varies by tumor, and depends on the area sampled by the FNA procedure. Cells may be epithelioid and have either acinar or undifferentiated morphology; immature spindlelike cells may be present (Fig. 6A).[126,127] On immunostains, neuroendocrine markers are at best focally positive; cells with acinar differentiation may be positive for pancreas enzyme markers, and if squamous morular cells are present, they may be positive for nuclear and cytoplasmic beta-catenin as well as alpha-fetoprotein. The presence of squamous morules on cell block material, as well as the patient's age, may be the first suggestion of this entity.

## LYMPHOMA

The diagnosis of primary pancreatic lymphoma (PPL) is rare and its identification on cytology is critical for its subsequent clinical management. Clinical criteria for its diagnosis appear widely accepted and include specific findings (pancreatic mass, absence of lymphadenopathy, hepatic or splenic involvement, and normal white blood cell count).[128] Several studies have shown 2 distinct radiological features in PPL and include location in the head and no dilatation of the main duct.[128,129] Multiple studies have shown the

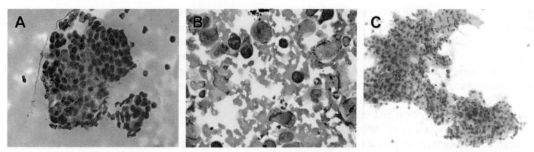

*Fig. 6.* Pancreatoblastoma (*A*), an extremely rare entity will show fragments of epithelioid cells with spindle or squamoid features (Diff-Quick, ×200). Lymphoma (*B*) shows abundant monotonous hematopoietic cells often with karyorrhexis and lymphoglandular bodies in the background and a notable absence of either ductal epithelium or acinar cells (Diff-Quick, ×400). Metastatic RCC (*C*), the most common metastasis to the pancreas and shows fragments of epithelioid cells that have a low nuclear-to-cytoplasmic ratio with dense cytoplasm, prominent nucleoli, and a prominent vascular architecture (Pap stain, ×200).

cytologic evaluation to reveal abundant discohesive lymphocytes (with or without atypia) in a background of karyorrhexis and lymphoglandular bodies in the absence of atypical epithelium or abundant acinar cells (**Fig. 6**B).[128,130–132] Rapid onsite evaluation for adequacy has been shown to be important for diagnostic accuracy by the addition of flow cytometric analysis.[132] The most common diagnosis among these series was non-Hodgkin large B-cell lymphoma.[128,130–132]

## METASTASES

Pancreatic masses rarely represent metastatic lesions with a prevalence reported from 2% to 8%.[39,133–135] Often there are clinical or radiological findings suggestive of metastases; however, none are definitive and with many overlapping features a metastasis should always be considered. The most common metastatic carcinoma identified throughout multiple studies and institutions is renal cell carcinoma (RCC) followed by lung, colon, melanoma, and breast (**Fig. 6**C).[133–145] The management of metastases depends on the primary and for some entities, namely RCC, surgical resection may not only be the treatment of choice but have a better prognosis than pancreatic adenocarcinoma.[146,147]

## FUTURE DIRECTIONS

Cytopathology, as with many areas of medicine, is moving in the direction of having to provide more accurate, and prognostically relevant diagnoses with less material. Medicine is continuously working toward minimally invasive procedures to diagnose and manage disease and molecular diagnostics are providing this niche. This situation is particularly important to neoplastic entities that are a challenge cytologically, such as in mucinous

neoplasms, whereby aspirates are commonly acellular but not benign. Recently, some molecular markers, specifically, *K-ras* in combination with loss of heterozygosity have been shown to be highly specific for malignancy in mucinous cyst fluid.[148] Al-Haddad and colleagues[149] have shown among diagnostically challenging mucinous cysts (those without "high-risk" features), accuracy increased with the addition of molecular studies (*K-ras*), particularly when CEA levels were indeterminate. *GNAS* is a second marker that has been targeted in several studies and its presence appears to strongly correlate with the diagnosis of an IPMN, particularly when found in combination with *K-ras* mutations.[150–152] Proteomic studies have shown that mucin proteomic profiling of cyst fluid can be highly accurate for the diagnosis of premalignant and malignant mucinous cysts, which is particularly useful in specimens with limited material.[153,154] Lastly, Brand and colleagues[155] recently showed that the detection of specific microRNAs, among FNA specimens that did not meet cytologic criteria for definitive diagnosis of adenocarcinoma (false negatives), increases the diagnostic probability of detecting adenocarcinoma preoperatively. Although no current studies, to date, have defined a clear use for the diagnostic utility of molecular studies; this area is still emerging and the populations that maybe impacted most are only now beginning to be identified. Molecular analysis of pancreatic cyst fluid is discussed in more depth in the article by Ngamruengphong S, Lennon AM: Analysis of Pancreatic Cyst Fluid, in this issue.

## REFERENCES

1. Erickson RA, Garza AA. Impact of endoscopic ultrasound on the management and outcome of

pancreatic carcinoma. Am J Gastroenterol 2000; 95(9):2248–50.

2. Fisher L, Segarajasingam DS, Stewart C, et al. Endoscopic ultrasound guided fine needle aspiration of solid pancreatic lesions: performance and outcomes. J Gastroenterol Hepatol 2009;24(1): 90–6.

3. Touchefeu Y, Le Rhun M, Coron E, et al. Endoscopic ultrasound-guided fine-needle aspiration for the diagnosis of solid pancreatic masses: the impact on patient management strategy. Aliment Pharmacol Ther 2009;30(10):1070–7.

4. Siegel R, Miller KD, Jemal A. Cancer statistics, 2015. CA Cancer J Clin 2015;65:5–29.

5. Rahib L, Smith BD, Aizenberg R, et al. Projecting cancer incidence and deaths to 2030: the unexpected burden of thyroid, liver, and pancreas cancers in the United States. Cancer Res 2014;74(11): 2913–21.

6. Al-Hawary MM, Kaza RK, Wasnik AP, et al. Staging of pancreatic cancer: role of imaging. Semin Roentgenol 2013;48(3):245–52.

7. Winter JM, Cameron JL, Campbell KA, et al. 1423 pancreaticoduodenectomies for pancreatic cancer: a single-institution experience. J Gastrointest Surg 2006;10(9):1199–210.

8. Sohn TA, Yeo CJ, Cameron JL, et al. Resected adenocarcinoma of the pancreas—616 patients: results, outcomes, and prognostic indicators. J Gastrointest Surg 2000;4(6):567–79.

9. Toomey P, Childs C, Luberice K, et al. Nontherapeutic celiotomy incidence is not affected by volume of pancreaticoduodenectomy for pancreatic adenocarcinoma. Am Surg 2013;79(8):781–5.

10. Edge SB, Compton CC. The American Joint Committee on Cancer: the 7th edition of the AJCC cancer staging manual and the future of TNM. Ann Surg Oncol 2010;17(6):1471–4.

11. Coley SC, Strickland NH, Walker JD, et al. Spiral CT and the preoperative assessment of pancreatic adenocarcinoma. Clin Radiol 1997;52(1):24–30.

12. Vedantham S, Lu DS, Reber HA, et al. Small peripancreatic veins: improved assessment in pancreatic cancer patients using thin-section pancreatic phase helical CT. AJR Am J Roentgenol 1998; 170(2):377–83.

13. Berland LL. The American College of Radiology strategy for managing incidental findings on abdominal computed tomography. Radiol Clin North Am 2011;49(2):237–43.

14. McIntyre CA, Winter JM. Diagnostic evaluation and staging of pancreatic ductal adenocarcinoma. Semin Oncol 2015;42(1):19–27.

15. Kurzawinski TR, Deery A, Dooley JS, et al. A prospective study of biliary cytology in 100 patients with bile duct strictures. Hepatology 1993; 18(6):1399–403.

16. Fogel EL, Sherman S. How to improve accuracy of diagnosis of malignant biliary strictures. Endoscopy 1999;31(9):758–60.

17. Malek M, Masuda D, Ogura T, et al. Yield of endoscopic ultrasound-guided fine needle aspiration and endoscopic retrograde cholangiopancreatography for solid pancreatic neoplasms. Scand J Gastroenterol 2016;5(3):360–7.

18. D'Onofrio M, DeRobertis R, Barbi E, et al. Ultrasound-guided percutaneous fine-needle aspiration of solid pancreatic neoplasms: 10-year experience with more than 2,000 cases and a review of the literature. Eur Radiol 2016;26(6):1801–7.

19. Adler D, Schmidt CM, Al-Haddad M. Clinical evaluation, imaging studies, indications for cytologic study and preprocedural requirements for duct brushing studies and pancreatic fine-needle aspiration: The Papanicolaou Society of Cytopathology guidelines. Cytojournal 2014;11(Suppl 1):1.

20. Yang RY, Ng D, Jaskolka JD, et al. Evaluation of percutaneous ultrasound-guided biopsies of solid mass lesions of the pancreas: a center's 10-year experience. Clin Imaging 2015;39(1):62–5.

21. Volmar KE, Vollmer RT, Jowell PS, et al. Pancreatic FNA in 1000 cases: a comparison of imaging modalities. Gastrointest Endosc 2005;61(7):854–61.

22. Micames C, Jowell PS, White R, et al. Lower frequency of peritoneal carcinomatosis in patients with pancreatic cancer diagnosed by EUS-guided FNA vs. percutaneous FNA. Gastrointest Endosc 2003;58(5):690–5.

23. Chong A, Venugopal K, Segarajasingam D, et al. Tumor seeding after EUS-guided FNA of pancreatic tail neoplasia. Gastrointest Endosc 2011; 74(4):933–45.

24. Ikezawa K, Uehara H, Sakai A, et al. Risk of peritoneal carcinomatosis by endoscopic ultrasound-guided fine needle aspiration for pancreatic cancer. J Gastroenterol 2013;48(8):966–72.

25. Puli SR, Bechtold ML, Buxbaum JL, et al. How good is endoscopic ultrasound-guided fine-needle aspiration in diagnosing the correct etiology for a solid pancreatic mass? A meta-analysis and systematic review. Pancreas 2013;42(1):20–6.

26. Chen J, Yang R, Lu Y, et al. Diagnostic accuracy of endoscopic ultrasound-guided fine-needle aspiration for solid pancreatic lesion: a systemic review. J Cancer Res Clin Oncol 2012;138(9): 1433–41.

27. Horwhat JD, Paulson EK, McGrath K, et al. A randomized comparison of EUS-guided FNA versus CT or US guided FNA for the evaluation of pancreatic mass lesions. Gastrointest Endosc 2006;63(7):966–75.

28. Affolter KE, Schmidt RL, Matynia AP, et al. Needle size has only a limited effect on outcomes in EUS-guided fine needle aspiration: a systematic

review and meta-analysis. Dig Dis Sci 2013;58(4): 1026–34.

29. Vilmann P, Jacobsen GK, Henriksen FW, et al. Endoscopic ultrasonography with guided fine needle aspiration biopsy on pancreatic disease. Gastrointest Endosc 1992;38(2):172–3.

30. Turner BG, Cizginer S, Agarwal D, et al. Diagnosis of pancreatic neoplasia with EUS and FNA: a report of accuracy. Gastrointest Endosc 2010; 71(1):91–8.

31. Tanaka M, Fernandez-del Castillo C, Adsay V, et al. International consensus guidelines 2012 for the management of IPMN and MCN of the pancreas. Pancreatology 2012;12(3):183–97.

32. Pitman MB, Centeno BA, Ali SZ, et al. Standardized terminology and nomenclature for pancreatobiliary cytology: The Papanicolaou Society of Cytopathology Guidelines. Cytojournal 2013;11(Suppl 1):3.

33. Yoon WJ, Bishop Pitman M. Cytology specimen management, triage and standardized reporting of fine needle aspiration biopsies of the pancreas. J Pathol Transl Med 2015;49(5):364–72.

34. Bosman FT, Carneiro F, Hruban RH, et al. WHO classification of tumours of the digestive system. Lyon (France): IARC Press; 2010.

35. Saieg MA, Munson V, Colletti S, et al. The impact of the new proposed Papanicolaou Society of Cytopathology Terminology for pancreaticobiliary cytology in endoscopic US-FNA: A single institutional experience. Cancer Cytopathol 2015;123(8):488–94.

36. Nagle JA, Wilbur DC, Pitman MB. Cytomorphology of gastric and duodenal epithelium and reactivity to B72.3: a baseline for comparison to pancreatic lesions aspirated by EUS-FNAB. Diagn Cytopathol 2005;33(6):381–6.

37. Brugge W, DeWitt J, Klapman JB, et al. Techniques for cytologic sampling of pancreatic and bile duct lesions. Diagn Cytopathol 2014;42(4):333–7.

38. Mino-Kenudson M, Fernandez-del Castillo C, Baba Y, et al. Prognosis of invasive intraductal mucinous neoplasm depends on histological and precursor epithelial subtypes. Gut 2011;60(12): 1712–20.

39. Adsay NV, Andrea A, Basturk O, et al. Secondary tumours of the pancreas: an analysis of a surgical and autopsy database and review of the literature. Virchows Arch 2004;444(6):527–35.

40. Stelow EB, Stanley MW, Bardales RH, et al. Intraductal papillary-mucinous neoplasm of the pancreas. The findings and limitations of cytologic samples obtained by endoscopic ultrasound-guided fine-needle aspiration. Am J Clin Pathol 2003;120(3):398–404.

41. Emerson RE, Randolph ML, Cramer HM. Endoscopic ultrasound-guided fine-needle aspiration cytology diagnosis of intraductal papillary mucinous neoplasm of the pancreas is highly predictive of pancreatic neoplasia. Diagn Cytopathol 2006;34(7):457–62.

42. Solé M, Iglesias C, Fernández-Esparrach G, et al. Fine-needle aspiration cytology of intraductal papillary mucinous tumors of the pancreas. Cancer 2005;105(5):298–303.

43. DeMay RM. Practical principles of cytopathology. Chicago: ASCP; 2007. p. 324.

44. Catalano MF, Sahai A, Levy M, et al. EUS-based criteria for the diagnosis of chronic pancreatitis: The Rosemont classification. Gastrointest Endosc 2009;69(7):1251–61.

45. Braganza JM, Lee SH, McCloy RF, et al. Chronic pancreatitis. Lancet 2011;377(9772):1184–97.

46. Furukawa H, Takayasu K, Mukai K, et al. Ductal adenocarcinoma of the pancreas and associated with intratumoral calcification. Int J Pancreatol 1995;17(3):291–6.

47. Kim T, Murakami T, Takahashi S, et al. Ductal adenocarcinoma of the pancreas with intratumoral calcification. Abdom Imaging 1999;24(6): 610–3.

48. Samad A, Attam R, Pambuccian SE. Calcifications in and endoscopic ultrasound-guided fine needle aspirate of chronic pancreatitis. Diagn Cytopathol 2013;41(12):1081–5.

49. Jarboe EA, Layfield LJ. Cytologic features of pancreatic intraepithelial neoplasia and pancreatitis: potential pitfalls in the diagnosis of pancreatic ductal carcinoma. Diagn Cytopathol 2011;39(8): 575–81.

50. Layfield LJ, Jarboe EA. Cytopathology of the pancreas: neoplastic and nonneoplastic entities. Ann Diagn Pathol 2010;14(2):140–51.

51. Abraham SC, Wilentz RE, Yeo CJ, et al. Pancreaticoduodenectomy (Whipple resections) in patients without malignancy: are they all 'chronic pancreatitis'? Am J Surg Pathol 2003;27(1):110–20.

52. Zamboni G, Lüttges J, Capelli P. Histopathological features of diagnostic and clinical relevance in autoimmune pancreatitis: a study on 53 resection specimens and 9 biopsy specimens. Virchows Arch 2004;445(6):552–63.

53. Shimosegawa T, Chari ST, Frulloni L, et al. International consensus diagnostic criteria for autoimmune pancreatitis: Guidelines of the International Association of Pancreatology. Pancreas 2011; 40(3):352–8.

54. Ohara H, Okazaki K, Tsubouchi H. Clinical diagnostic criteria of IgG4-related sclerosing cholangitis 2012. J Hepatobiliary Pancreat Sci 2012;19(5): 536–42.

55. Holmes BJ, Hruban RH, Wolfgang CL. Fine needle aspirate of autoimmune pancreatitis (lymphoplasmacytic sclerosing pancreatitis): cytomorphologic characteristics and clinical correlates. Acta Cytol 2012;56(3):228–32.

56. Deshpande V, Mino-Kenudson M, Brugge W, et al. More than just a pancreatic disease? A contemporary review of its pathology. Arch Pathol Lab Med 2005;129(9):1148–54.

57. Kanno A, Ishida K, Hamada S, et al. Diagnosis of autoimmune pancreatitis by EUS-FNA by using a 22-gauge needle based on the International Consensus Diagnostic Criteria. Gastrointest Endosc 2012;76(3):594–602.

58. Ishikawa T, Itoh A, Kawashima H, et al. Endoscopic ultrasound guided fine needle aspiration in the differentiation of type 1 and type 2 autoimmune pancreatitis. World J Gastroenterol 2012;18(29):3883–8.

59. Yoon WJ, Brugge WE. Pancreatic cystic neoplasms: diagnosis and management. Gastroenterol Clin North Am 2012;41(1):103–8.

60. Lees KS, Sekhar A, Rofsky NM, et al. Prevalence of incidental pancreatic cysts in the adult population on MR imaging. Am J Gastroenterol 2010;105(9):2079–84.

61. Laffan TA, Horton KM, Klein AP, et al. Prevalence of unsuspected pancreatic cysts on MDCT. AJR Am J Roentgenol 2008;191(3):802–7.

62. Chung JW, Chung MJ, Fockens P. Clinicopathologic features and outcomes of pancreatic cysts during a 12 year period. Pancreas 2013;42(2):230–8.

63. Klibansky DA, Reid-Lombardo KM, Gordon SR, et al. The clinical relevance of increasing incidence of intraductal papillary mucinous neoplasm. Clin Gastroenterol Hepatol 2012;10(5):555–8.

64. Morris-Stiff G, Falk GA, Chalikonda S, et al. Natural history of asymptomatic pancreatic cystic neoplasms. HPB (Oxford) 2013;15(3):175–81.

65. Brugge WR, Lewandrowski K, Lee-Lewandrowski E. Diagnosis of pancreatic cystic neoplasm: a report of the cooperative pancreatic cystic neoplasms: A report of the cooperative pancreatic study. Gastroenterology 2004;126(5):1330–6.

66. Maker AV, Lee LS, Raut CP, et al. Cytology from pancreatic cysts has marginal utility in surgical decision-making. Ann Surg Oncol 2008;15(11):3187–92.

67. Attasaranya S, Pais S, LeBlanc J, et al. Endoscopic ultrasound-guided fine needle aspiration and cyst fluid analysis for pancreatic cysts. JOP 2007;8(5):553–63.

68. Habashi S, Draganov PV. Pancreatic pseudocyst. World J Gastroenterol 2009;15(1):38–47.

69. VandenBussche CJ, Maleki Z. Fine needle aspiration of squamous-lined cysts of the pancreas. Diagn Cytopathol 2014;42(7):592–9.

70. Karim Z, Walker B, Lam E. Lymphoepithelial cysts of the pancreas: the use of endoscopic ultrasound-guided fine-needle aspiration in diagnosis. Can J Gastroenterol 2010;24(6):348–50.

71. Kosmahl M, Pauser U, Peters K, et al. Cystic neoplasms of the pancreas and tumor-like lesions with cystic features: a review of 418 cases and classification proposal. Virchows Arch 2004;445(2):168–78.

72. Belsley NA, Pitman MB, Lauwers GY, et al. Serous cystadenoma of the pancreas: limitations and pitfalls of endoscopic ultrasound-guided fine-needle aspiration biopsy. Cancer 2008;114(2):102–10.

73. Collins BT. Serous cystadenoma of the pancreas with endoscopic ultrasound fine needle aspiration biopsy and surgical correlation. Acta Cytol 2013;57(3):241–51.

74. Huang P, Staerkel G, Sneige N, et al. Fine needle aspiration of pancreatic serous cystadenoma: cytologic features and diagnostic pitfalls. Cancer 2006;108(4):239–49.

75. Cizginer S, Turner BG, Bilge AR, et al. Cyst fluid carcinoembryonic antigen is an accurate diagnostic marker of pancreatic mucinous cysts. Pancreas 2011;40(7):1024–8.

76. Lau SK, Lewandrowski KB, Brugge WR, et al. Diagnostic significance of mucin in fine needle aspiration samples of pancreatic cysts. Mod Pathol 2000;13(3):48A.

77. Oppong KW, Dawwas MF, Charnley RM, et al. EUS and EUS-FNA diagnosis of suspected cystic neoplasms: Is the sum of the parts greater than CEA? Pancreatology 2015;15(5):531–7.

78. Van der Waaij LA, van Dullemen HM, Porte RJ. Cyst fluid analysis in the differential diagnosis of pancreatic cystic lesions: a pooled analysis. Gastrointest Endosc 2005;62(3):383–9.

79. Adsay NV, Pierson C, Sarker F, et al. Colloid (mucinous noncystic) carcinoma of the pancreas. Am J Surg Pathol 2001;25(1):26–42.

80. Tanaka M, Chari S, Adsay V, et al. International consensus guidelines for management of intraductal papillary mucinous neoplasms and mucinous cystic neoplasms of the pancreas. Pancreatology 2006;6(1–2):17–32.

81. Pitman MB, Centeno BA, Genevay M, et al. Grading epithelial atypia in endoscopic ultrasound-guided fine needle aspiration of intraductal papillary mucinous neoplasms. Cancer Cytopathol 2013;121(12):729–36.

82. Pitman MB, Centeno BA, Daglilar ES. Cytological criteria of high-grade epithelial atypia in the cyst fluid of pancreatic intraductal papillary mucinous neoplasms. Cancer Cytopathol 2014;122(1):40–7.

83. Pitman MB, Yaeger KA, Brugge WR, et al. Prospective analysis of atypical epithelial cells as a high-risk cytologic feature for malignancy in pancreatic cysts. Cancer Cytopathol 2013;121(1):29–36.

84. Genevay M, Mino-Kenudson M, Yaeger K, et al. Cytology adds value to imaging studies for risk

assessment of malignancy in pancreatic mucinous cysts. Ann Surg 2011;254(6):977–83.

85. Buscaglia JM, Giday SA, Kantsevoy SV, et al. Patient and cyst-related factors for improved prediction of malignancy within cystic lesions of the pancreas. Pancreatology 2009;9(5):631–8.

86. Ferrone CR, Correa-Gallego C, Warshaw AL, et al. Current trends in pancreatic cysts. Arch Surg 2009; 144(5):448–54.

87. Lahav M, Maor Y, Avidan B, et al. Nonsurgical management of asymptomatic incidental pancreatic cysts. Clin Gastroenterol Hepatol 2007;5(7): 813–7.

88. Layfield LJ, Cramer H. Fine-needle aspiration cytology of intraductal papillary-mucinous tumors: a retrospective analysis. Diagn Cytopathol 2005; 32(1):16–20.

89. Michaels PJ, Brachtel EF, Bounds BC, et al. Intraductal papillary mucinous neoplasm of the pancreas. Cytologic features predict histologic grade. Cancer Cytopathol 2006;108(3):163–73.

90. Ono J, Yaeger KA, Genevay M, et al. Cytological analysis of small branch-duct intraductal papillary mucinous neoplasms provides a more accurate risk assessment of malignancy than symptoms. Cytojournal 2011;8:21.

91. Pitman MB, Genevay M, Yaeger K, et al. High-grade atypical epithelial cells in pancreatic mucinous cysts are a more accurate predictor of malignancy than "positive" cytology. Cancer Cytopathol 2010;118(6):434–40.

92. Schmidt CM, White PB, Waters JA, et al. Intraductal papillary mucinous neoplasms: predictors of malignant and invasive pathology. Ann Surg 2007; 246(4):644–51.

93. Wiesenauer CA, Schmidt CM, Cummings OW. Preoperative predictors of malignancy in pancreatic intraductal papillary mucinous neoplasms. Arch Surg 2003;138(6):610–7.

94. Krishna SG, Lee JH. Endosonography in solid and cystic pancreatic tumors. J Interv Gastroenterol 2011;1(4):193–201.

95. Gagovic V, Spier BJ, DeLee RJ, et al. Endoscopic ultrasound fine-needle aspiration characteristics of primary adenocarcinoma versus other malignant neoplasms of the pancreas. Can J Gastroenterol 2012;26(10):691–6.

96. Lin F, Staerkel G. Cytologic criteria for well differentiated adenocarcinoma of the pancreas in fine-needle aspiration biopsy specimens. Cancer 2003;99(1):44–50.

97. Mitsuhashi T, Ghafari S, Chang CY, et al. Endoscopic ultrasound- guided fine needle aspiration of the pancreas: cytomorphological evaluation with emphasis on adequacy assessment, diagnostic criteria and contamination from the gastrointestinal tract. Cytopathology 2006;17(1):34–41.

98. Cohen MB, Egerter DP, Holly EA, et al. Pancreatic adenocarcinoma: regression analysis to identify improved cytologic criteria. Diagn Cytopathol 1991;7(4):341–5.

99. Pitmen MB. The pancreas. In: Sidawy M, Ali S, editors. Fine needle aspiration cytology. Foundations in diagnostic pathology. Philadelphia: Churchill Livingstone; Elsevier; 2007. p. 80.

100. Huffman BM, Esebua M, Layfield LJ, et al. Risk stratification using cytomorphologic features in endoscopic ultrasonographic-guided fine-needle aspiration diagnosis of pancreatic ductal adenocarcinoma. Diagn Cytopathol 2015;43(8): 613–21.

101. Chen G, Liu S, Zhao Y, et al. Diagnostic accuracy of endoscopic ultrasound-guided fine-needle aspiration for pancreatic cancer: a meta-analysis. Pancreàtology 2013;13(3):298–304.

102. Hewitt MJ, McPhail MJ, Possamari L, et al. EUS-guided FNA for diagnosis of solid pancreatic neoplasms: a meta-analysis. Gastrointest Endosc 2012;75(2):319–31.

103. Olson MT, Siddiqui MT, Ali SZ. The differential diagnosis of squamous cells in pancreatic aspirates: from contamination to adenosquamous carcinoma. Acta Cytol 2013;57(2):139–46.

104. O'Grady HL, Conlon KC. Pancreatic neuroendocrine tumours. Eur J Surg Oncol 2008;34(3): 324–32.

105. Oberg K. Pancreatic endocrine tumors. Semin Oncol 2010;37(6):594–618.

106. Batcher E, Madaj P, Gianoukakis AG. Pancreatic neuroendocrine tumors. Endocr Res 2011;36(1): 35–43.

107. Artale S, Giannetta L, Cerea G, et al. Treatment of metastatic neuroendocrine carcinomas based on WHO classification. Anticancer Res 2005;25(6C): 4463–9.

108. Bajetta E, Catena L, Procopio G, et al. Is the new WHO classification of neuroendocrine tumours useful for selecting an appropriate treatment? Ann Oncol 2005;16(8):1374–80.

109. Plöckinger U, Rindi G, Arnold R, et al. Guidelines for the diagnosis and treatment of neuroendocrine gastrointestinal tumours. A consensus statement on behalf of the European Neuroendocrine Tumour Society (ENETS). Neuroendocrinology 2004;80(6): 394–424.

110. al-Kaisi N, Weaver MG, Abdul-Karim FW, et al. Fine needle aspiration cytology of neuroendocrine tumors of the pancreas. A cytologic, immunocytochemical and electron microscopic study. Acta Cytol 1992;36(5):655–60.

111. Larghi A, Capruso G, Carnuccio A, et al. Ki-67 grading of non-functioning pancreatic neuroendocrine tumours on histologic samples obtained by EUS-guided fine-needle tissue acquisition: a

prospective study. Gastrointest Endosc 2012; 76(3):570–7.

112. Piani C, Franchi GM, Cappelletti C, et al. Cytological Ki-67 in pancreatic endocrine tumours: an opportunity for pre-operative grading. Endocr Relat Cancer 2008;15(1):175–81.

113. Hasegawa T, Yamao K, Hijioka S, et al. Evaluation of Ki-67 index in EUS-FNA specimens for the assessment of malignancy risk in pancreatic neuroendocrine tumors. Endoscopy 2014;46(1):32–8.

114. Weynand B, Borbath I, Bernard V, et al. Pancreatic neuroendocrine tumour grading on endoscopic ultrasound-guided fine needle aspiration: high reproducibility and inter-observer agreement of the Ki-67 labelling index. Cytopathology 2014; 25(6):389–95.

115. Figueiredo FA, Giovannini M, Monges G, et al. EUS-FNA predicts 5-year survival in pancreatic endocrine tumours. Gastrointest Endosc 2009; 70(5):907–14.

116. Baker MS, Knuth JL, DeWitt J, et al. Pancreatic cystic neuroendocrine tumors: preoperative diagnosis with endoscopic ultrasound and fine-needle immunocytology. J Gastrointest Surg 2008;12(3): 450–6.

117. Morales-Oyarvide V, Yoon WJ, Ingkakul T, et al. Cystic pancreatic neuroendocrine tumors: the value of cytology in preoperative diagnosis. Cancer Cytopathol 2014;122(6):435–44.

118. Law JK, Ahmed A, Singh VK, et al. A systematic review of solid-pseudopapillary neoplasms: are these rare lesions? Pancreas 2014;43(3):331–7.

119. Pettinato G, Di Vizio D, Manivel JC, et al. Solid-pseudopapillary tumor of the pancreas: a neoplasm with distinct and highly characteristic cytological features. Diagn Cytopathol 2002;27(6): 325–34.

120. Notohara K, Hamazaki S, Tsukayama C, et al. Solid-pseudopapillary tumor of the pancreas: immunohistochemical localization of neuroendocrine markers and CD10. Am J Surg Pathol 2000; 24(10):1361–71.

121. Labate AM, Klimstra DL, Zakowski MF. Comparative cytologic features of pancreatic acinar cell carcinoma and islet cell tumor. Diagn Cytopathol 1997;16(2):112–6.

122. Stelow EB, Bardales RH, Shami VM, et al. Cytology of pancreatic acinar cell carcinoma. Diagn Cytopathol 2006;34(5):367–72.

123. La Rosa S, Franzi F, Marchet S, et al. The monoclonal anti-BCL10 antibody (clone 331.1) is a sensitive and specific marker of pancreatic acinar cell carcinoma and pancreatic metaplasia. Virchows Arch 2009;454(2):133–42.

124. Becker WF. Pancreatoduodenectomy for carcinoma of the pancreas in an infant; report of a case. Ann Surg 1957;145(6):864–70.

125. Argon A, Celik A, Oniz H, et al. Pancreatoblastoma, a rare childhood tumor. A case report. Turk Patoloji Derg 2014;11:1–5.

126. Silverman J, Holbrook C, Pories W, et al. Fine needle aspiration cytology of pancreatoblastoma with immunocytochemical and ultrastructural studies. Acta Cytol 1989;34(5):632–40.

127. Henke AC, Kelley CM, Jensen CS, et al. Fine-needle aspiration cytology of pancreatoblastoma. Diagn Cytopathol 2001;25(2):118–21.

128. Ramesh J, Herbert-Magee S, Kim H, et al. Frequency of occurrence and characteristics of primary pancreatic lymphoma during endoscopic ultrasound guided fine needle aspiration: a retrospective study. Dig Liver Dis 2014;46(5):470–3.

129. Khashab M, Mokadem M, DeWitt J. Endoscopic ultrasound-guided fine-needle aspiration with or without flow cytometry for the diagnosis of primary pancreatic lymphoma - a case series. Endoscopy 2010;42(3):228–31.

130. Nayer H, Weir EG, Sheth S, et al. Primary pancreatic lymphomas. Cancer 2004;102(5):315–21.

131. Ribeiro A, Pereira D, Escalón MP, et al. EUS-guided biopsy for the diagnosis and classification of lymphoma. Gastrointest Endosc 2010;71(4):851–5.

132. Al-Haddad M, Savabi MS, Sherman S, et al. Role of endoscopic ultrasound- guided fine-needle aspiration with flow cytometry to diagnose lymphoma: a single center experience. J Gastroenterol Hepatol 2009;24(12):1826–33.

133. Gilbert CM, Monaco SE, Cooper ST, et al. Endoscopic ultrasound-guided fine-needle aspiration of metastases to the pancreas: a study of 25 cases. Cytojournal 2011;8:7.

134. Layfield LJ, Hirschowitz SL, Adler DG. Metastatic disease to the pancreas documented by endoscopic ultrasound guided fine-needle aspiration: a seven-year experience. Diagn Cytopathol 2012; 40(3):228–33.

135. Olson MT, Wakely PE, Ali SZ. Metastases to the pancreas diagnosed by fine-needle aspiration. Acta Cytol 2013;57(5):473–80.

136. Smith AL, Odronic SI, Springer BS. Solid tumor metastases to the pancreas diagnosed by FNA: a single-institution experience and review of the literature. Cancer Cytopathol 2015;123(6):347–55.

137. Carson HJ, Green LK, Castelli MJ, et al. Utilization of fine-needle aspiration biopsy in the diagnosis of metastatic tumors to the pancreas. Diagn Cytopathol 1995;12(1):8–13.

138. Hijioka S, Matsuo K, Mizuno N, et al. Role of endoscopic ultrasound and endoscopic ultrasound-guided fine-needle aspiration in diagnosing metastasis to the pancreas: a tertiary center experience. Pancreatology 2011;11(4):390–8.

139. Arden JC, Lopes CV, Kemp R, et al. Accuracy of endoscopic ultrasound-guided fine-needle

aspiration in the suspicion of pancreatic metastases. BMC Gastroenterol 2013;11(13):63.

140. Eloubeidi MA, Tamhane AR, Buxbaum JL. Unusual,
metastatic, or neuroendocrine tumor of the
pancreas: a diagnosis with endoscopic ultrasound-
guided fine-needle aspiration and immunohistochemistry. Saudi J Gastroenterol 2012;18(2):
99–105.

141. DeWitt J, Jowell P, Leblanc J, et al. EUS-guided
FNA of pancreatic metastases: a multicenter experience. Gastrointest Endosc 2005;61(6):689–96.

142. Volmar KE, Jones CK, Xie HB. Metastases in the
pancreas from nonhematologic neoplasms: report
of 20 cases evaluated by fine-needle aspiration. Diagn Cytopathol 2004;31(4):216–20.

143. Mesa H, Stelow EB, Stanley MW, et al. Diagnosis of
nonprimary pancreatic neoplasms by endoscopic
ultrasound-guided fine-needle aspiration. Diagn
Cytopathol 2004;31(5):313–8.

144. El Hajj II, LeBlanc JK, Sherman S, et al. Endoscopic ultrasound-guided biopsy of pancreatic
metastases: a large single-center experience.
Pancreas 2013;42(3):524–30.

145. Atiq M, Bhutani MS, Ross WA, et al. Role of endoscopic ultrasonography in evaluation of metastatic
lesions to the pancreas: a tertiary cancer center
experience. Pancreas 2013;42(3):516–23.

146. Sellner F, Tykalsky N, DeSantes M, et al. Solitary
and multiple isolated metastasis of clear cell renal
cell carcinoma to the pancreas: an indication for
pancreatic surgery. Ann Surg Oncol 2006;13(1):
75–85.

147. Sweeney AD, Fisher WE, Wu MF, et al. Value of
pancreatic resection for cancer metastatic to the
pancreas. J Surg Res 2010;160(2):268–76.

148. Khalid A, Zahid M, Finkelstein SD, et al. Pancreatic
cyst fluid DNA analysis in evaluating pancreatic
cysts: a report of the PANDA study. Gastrointest
Endosc 2009;69(6):1095–102.

149. Al-Haddad M, DeWitt J, Sherman S. Performance
characteristics of molecular (DNA) analysis for
the diagnosis of mucinous pancreatic cysts. Gastrointest Endosc 2014;79(1):79–87.

150. Kanda M, Knight S, Topazian M, et al. Mutant
GNAS detected in duodenal collections of
secretin-stimulated pancreatic juice indicates the
presence or emergence of pancreatic cysts. Gut
2013;62(7):1024–33.

151. Amato E, Molin MD, Mafficini A, et al. Targeted
next-generation sequencing of cancer genes dissects the molecular profiles of intraductal papillary
neoplasms of the pancreas. J Pathol 2014;233(3):
217–27.

152. Singhi AD, Nikiforova MN, Fasanella KE, et al. Preoperative GNAS and KRAS testing in the diagnosis
of pancreatic mucinous cysts. Clin Cancer Res
2014;20(16):4381–9.

153. Jabbar KS, Verbeke C, Hyltander AG, et al. Proteomic mucin profiling for the identification of cystic
precursors of pancreatic cancer. J Natl Cancer
Inst 2014;106(2):djt439.

154. Cao Z, Maupin K, Curnutte B, et al. Specific glyco-
forms of MUC5AC and endorepellin accurately
distinguish mucinous from nonmucinous pancreatic cysts. Mol Cell Proteomics 2013;12(10):
2724–34.

155. Brand RE, Adai AT, Centeno BA, et al. A microRNA-
based test improves endoscopic ultrasound-
guided cytologic diagnosis of pancreatic cancer.
Clin Gastroenterol Hepatol 2014;12(10):1717–23.

# Analysis of Pancreatic Cyst Fluid

Saowanee Ngamruengphong, MD[a], Anne Marie Lennon, MD, PhD[b],*

## KEYWORDS

- Molecular markers • Pancreatic cyst • Cyst fluid • Intraductal papillary mucinous neoplasm
- Serous cystadenoma • Mucinous cysts

## Key points

- Pancreatic cysts are common, and are incidentally identified in between 2% and 13% of individuals undergoing cross-sectional imaging.

- Cyst fluid carcinoembryonic antigen is currently considered the most accurate marker for differentiating mucinous (intraductal papillary mucinous neoplasms [IPMNs] and mucinous cystic neoplasms [MCNs]) from nonmucinous cysts; however, recent studies suggest that its accuracy is approximately 65%.

- New molecular markers in cyst fluid have shown promise in differentiating serous cystadenomas, solid-pseudopapillary neoplasms, MCNs, and IPMNs, and identifying the presence of high-grade dysplasia or invasive adenocarcinoma.

## ABSTRACT

Pancreatic cysts are extremely common, and are identified in between 2% to 13% on abdominal imaging studies. Most pancreatic cysts are pseudocysts, serous cystic neoplasms, mucinous cystic neoplasms, or intraductal papillary mucinous neoplasms. The management of pancreatic cysts depends on whether a cyst is benign, has malignant potential, or harbors high-grade dysplasia or invasive carcinoma. The diagnosis of pancreatic cysts, and assessment of risk of malignant transformation, incorporates clinical history, computed tomography (CT), magnetic resonance imaging (MRI), endoscopic ultrasound, and fine-needle aspiration of cyst fluid. This article reviews the cyst fluid markers that are currently used, as well as promising markers under development.

## OVERVIEW

Advances in cross-sectional imaging have resulted in the frequent detection of pancreatic cysts that are incidentally identified in between 2% and 13% of cases.[1,2] There are a large number of different types of pancreatic cysts (Table 1), with the most common pancreatic cysts encountered in clinical practice being pseudocysts, serous cystadenomas (SCAs), mucinous cystic neoplasms (MCNs), and intraductal papillary mucinous neoplasm (IPMNs).[3] The management of pancreatic cysts is very much dependent on the type of pancreatic cyst (Fig. 1).[4] Those with no, or very low malignant potential, such as pseudocysts and SCAs, require minimal or no follow-up in the absence of symptoms related to the cyst.[5] Solid-pseudopapillary neoplasms

Disclosures: Dr S. Ngamruengphong has nothing to disclose. Dr A.M. Lennon is a consultant for Olympus and NovoNordisc.
Funded by: This work was supported by NIH grant P50 CA62924 and R01CA176828, the Lustgarten Foundation for Pancreatic Cancer Research, Susan Wojcicki and Dennis Troper, the Michael Rolfe Foundation, and the Benjamin Baker scholarship.
[a] Division of Gastroenterology and Hepatology, The Johns Hopkins Medical Institutions, 1800 Orleans Street, Sheikh Zayed Tower, Baltimore, MD 21287, USA; [b] Division of Gastroenterology and Hepatology, The Johns Hopkins Medical Institutions, 1800 Orleans Street, Sheikh Zayed Tower, Room 7125JB3, Baltimore, MD 21287, USA
* Corresponding author.
E-mail address: amlennon@jhmi.edu

surgpath.theclinics.com

| Abbreviations | |
| --- | --- |
| CEA | Carcinoembryonic antigen |
| CT | Computed tomography |
| EUS | Endoscopic ultrasound |
| FNA | Fine-needle aspiration |
| IPMN | Intraductal papillary mucinous neoplasm |
| LOH | Loss of heterozygosity |
| MCN | Mucinous cystic neoplasm |
| MRI | Magnetic resonance imaging |
| PCN | Pancreatic cystic neoplasm |
| SCA | Serous cystadenoma |
| SPN | Solid-pseudopapillary neoplasm |
| VHL | Von Hippel Lindau |

(SPNs) are low-grade malignant neoplasms, and surgical resection is recommended.[6] Invasive adenocarcinoma occurs in between 4% and 16% of surgically resected MCNs in modern studies.[7–9] Although some groups have recommended that asymptomatic MCNs may be followed,[10] many surgeons favor resection because these cysts have the potential for malignant transformation, surgery is curative, and if not undertaken patients require many years of surveillance.[11] The management of IPMNs depends on whether the main pancreatic duct is involved (main, or mixed-duct IPMN), which is associated with a higher risk of malignant transformation, with high-grade dysplasia or invasive adenocarcinoma identified in between 43% and 62% of patients who undergo surgical resection.[11] In contrast, branch-duct type IPMNs, in which there is no main duct involvement, have a much lower risk of malignant transformation, and in the absence of symptoms, or concerning features, usually undergo surveillance.[11]

Thus, the key question from a clinical perspective is whether a cyst is benign, has malignant potential, or harbors high-grade dysplasia or invasive carcinoma, as this dictates whether patients can be discharged, undergo surveillance, or require surgical intervention respectively (see Fig. 1).[10,11] The diagnosis of pancreatic cysts, and assessment of risk of malignant transformation, incorporates a number of factors, including clinical history, CT, MRI, and endoscopic ultrasonography (EUS). EUS allows detailed visualization of the cyst (Fig. 2A), and sampling of the cyst wall and fluid through EUS-guided fine-needle aspiration (EUS-FNA) (see Fig. 2). This is a relatively low-risk procedure with the most common adverse events being pancreatitis (1.1%) and abdominal pain (0.34%).[12] The addition of EUS and EUS-FNA to either CT or MRI has been shown to improve the overall accuracy for diagnosis of

pancreatic cysts.[13] Most of this additional benefit is from aspiration of cyst fluid, which can be sent for a range of tests, including cytology, biochemical, and molecular testing. This article focuses on the biochemical and molecular tests, whereas cyst fluid cytology is discussed in depth in the article (See Collins JA, Ali SZ, VandenBussche CJ: Pancreatic Cytopathology, in this issue).

## BIOCHEMICAL TESTS FOR CYST FLUID

## CARCINOEMBRYONIC ANTIGEN

### Identifying Intraductal Papillary Mucinous Neoplasms and Mucin Producing Cysts

Carcinoembryonic antigen (CEA) is currently considered the most accurate marker for differentiating mucin producing from non mucin producing cysts; that is, IPMNs and MCNs from other cyst types. The role of CEA was established in the multicenter, prospective cooperative study in 2004, which found that the accuracy of cyst fluid CEA was superior to EUS, cytology, or other tumor markers, including CA 72-4, CA 125, CA 19-9, and CA 15-3, for identifying mucin producing cysts.[14] However, since then, several issues with respect to CEA have arisen. The first is what is the optimal cutoff level to differentiate mucin producing from non-mucin producing cysts? The cooperative study identified the optimal level as 192 ng/mL, which was associated with 75% sensitivity, and 84% specificity for differentiating between mucin producing and non-mucin producing cysts, and this level is most commonly used in clinical practice and publications.[14] However, other groups have proposed alternative cutoffs. Using a higher cutoff level of greater than 800 ng/mL was shown in a meta-analysis to increase the specificity to 98%, although at the cost of lowering the sensitivity to 48%.[15] Similarly very low CEA levels of less than 5 ng/mL have a very high specificity of 95%, with 50% sensitivity, for non-mucin producing cysts, such as serous cystadenomas and pseudocysts.[15]

The second issue is that although the initial studies were very promising, more recent data have suggested that cyst fluid CEA is imperfect at differentiating mucin producing from non-mucin producing cysts. The cooperative study found CEA had a high sensitivity and specificity (75% and 84%, respectively), for identifying mucin producing cysts.[14] In contrast, more recent studies have suggested a lower accuracy, with a large prospective study reporting a lower sensitivity and specificity of only 63% and 62%, respectively.[16] These findings were confirmed in meta-analysis of 18 studies with 1438 patients, in which CEA had 63% sensitivity and 88% specificity for identifying mucin producing cysts.[17]

*Table 1*
**Classification of pancreatic cysts by pathologic type**

| | Epithelial Neoplasms | | | | | | | | Nonepithelial Neoplasms | Secondary Neoplasms (Metastases to the Pancreas)[c] | Non-neoplastic Tumors of the Exocrine Pancreas | Congenital Cyst |
|---|---|---|---|---|---|---|---|---|---|---|---|---|
| | **Exocrine Neoplasms** | | | | **Endocrine Neoplasms** | **Epithelial Neoplasms with Multiple Directions of Differentiation** | **Epithelial Neoplasms of Uncertain Direction of Differentiation** | **Miscellaneous** | **Extragastrointestinal Stromal Tumor[c]** | | | |
| *Serous neoplasms* | *Mucinous cystic neoplasms* | *Intraductal neoplasms* | *Invasive ductal adenocarcinoma* | *Acinar cell neoplasms* | Pancreatic neuroendocrine neoplasm[c] | Pancreatoblastoma[c] | Solid-pseudopapillary neoplasm | Teratoma[c] | Fibromatosis (desmoid)[c] | Choriocarcinoma[c] | Duodenal diverticulum | |
| Microcystic SCA | MCN[a] | IPMN[a] | Invasive ductal adenocarcinoma[c] | Acinar cell cystadenoma | | | | Lymphoepithelial cyst | Granular cell tumor[c] | | Endometriotic cyst[c] | |
| Macrocystic SCA | | Intraductal tubulopapillary neoplasm | | Acinar cell cystadenocarcinoma | | | | Epidermoid cyst in intrapancreatic heterotopic spleen | Leiomyoma[c] | | | Foregut cyst |
| Solid SCA | | | | | | | | | Lymphangioma | | Heterotopic pancreas[c] | |
| von-Hippel-Landau (VHL)-associated SCA | | | | | | | | | Lymphoma[c] | | Autoimmune pancreatitis[c] | |
| Serous cystadenocarcinoma[b] | | | | | | | | | Sarcoma[c] | | Parampullary duodenal wall cyst | |
| | | | | | | | | | Caverous hemangioma | | Hamartoma[c] | |

*Abbreviations:* IPMN, intraductal papillary mucinous neoplasms; MCN, mucinous cystic neoplasms; SCA, serous crystadenoma.

[a] These can be associated with low-grade, intermediate-grade, or high-grade dysplasia, or an associated invasive carcinoma.
[b] These are extremely rare.
[c] With cystic degeneration.

*Adapted from* Hruban RH, Pitman MB, Klimstra DS, editors. Tumors of the pancreas. American Registry of Pathology; 2007.

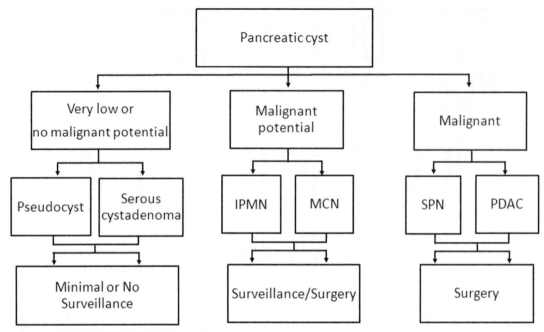

*Fig. 1.* Algorithm for the management of pancreatic cysts.

Finally, obtaining sufficient cyst fluid to assess CEA levels is often not possible, particularly in very small cysts, or if the fluid is very viscous. This issue was highlighted by a prospective European study in which CEA levels were obtained in only half of the cysts tested.[18]

### Carcinoembryonic Antigen Is Not Helpful in Identifying Cysts with High-Grade Dysplasia or Invasive Carcinoma

Some studies have suggested that a high cyst fluid CEA is associated with high-grade dysplasia or invasive cancer in IPMNs. However, these studies were small, retrospective, and there was significant overlap between the CEA level in IPMNs with low-, or intermediate-grade dysplasia and those with high-grade dysplasia or invasive carcinoma. In contrast, much larger studies, including a prospective study and a meta-analysis, have found no association between CEA level and the presence of high-grade dysplasia or invasive carcinoma.[14,19–21] Thus cyst fluid CEA level is not helpful in differentiating between benign and malignant pancreatic cysts.

### AMYLASE

### Excluding Pseudocysts

Cyst fluid amylase level can be useful in excluding a pseudocyst from other types of pancreatic cysts.

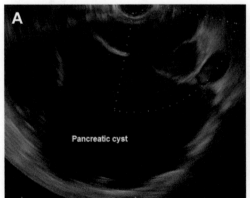
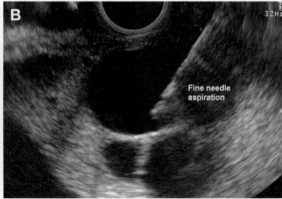

*Fig. 2.* Endoscopic ultrasound of a pancreatic cyst. (*A*) EUS image of a pancreatic cyst with thin septations. (*B*) EUS-guided FNA. The needle can be seen within the center of the cyst.

A large meta-analysis found a cyst fluid amylase level of less than 250 IU/L had a very high specificity of 98% for excluding pseudocysts.[15] In contrast, high cyst fluid amylase levels were found in numerous types of pancreatic cysts, including SCAs, IPMNs, and MCNs.

### High Amylase Levels Do Not Differentiate Intraductal Papillary Mucinous Neoplasms from Mucinous Cystic Neoplasms

One of the key questions is how to differentiate IPMNs from MCNs, as both have high cyst fluid CEA levels. On imaging, IPMNs communicate, or connect with the pancreatic duct, whereas MCNs have no communication. Theoretically, the communication between the main pancreatic duct and the cyst would cause IPMNs to have high cyst fluid amylase level, whereas MCNs should have a low amylase level. However, studies have shown that cyst fluid amylase level are similar in IPMNs and MCNs, and thus cannot be used to differentiate these 2 types of cysts.[22]

### OTHER MARKERS

Several other tumor markers, including CA 72-4, CA 125, CA 19-9, and CA 15-3 have been evaluated. However, the diagnostic accuracy of these tumor makers has been found to be inferior to cyst fluid CEA in distinguishing mucinous from nonmucinous cysts in a number of studies.[14,15] These markers are therefore not used in clinical practice.

### ACCURACY OF CYST FLUID MARKERS CURRENTLY USED IN CLINICAL PRACTICE

As can be seen, the currently available cyst fluid markers are imperfect at identifying cyst type, and cannot identify the presence of high-grade dysplasia or invasive carcinoma. This is highlighted by large surgical series, in which just over 20% of patients were found to have a benign cyst, such as an SCA or a pseudocyst,[23] whereas almost 80% of resected branch-duct IPMNs have either low, or intermediate-grade dysplasia,[24] and thus in retrospect, did not require surgical resection. Thus, better markers are required.

### MOLECULAR MARKERS

One of the problems with identifying mutations in pancreatic cysts is that the number of mutant alleles present is extremely low when compared with solid lesions, such as pancreatic ductal adenocarcinoma.[25] However, recent advances in molecular genetics, in particular the development

of techniques such as FastSeq sequencing, mean that mutant alleles present in very low levels can be identified.[26] In the following section we discuss the potential of molecular markers in pancreatic cyst fluid. There are many other promising markers, including mRNA and protein markers,[27–30] and a review of these markers is available elsewhere.[31]

In 2011, the group at Johns Hopkins lead by Bert Vogelstein analyzed the entire coding region of the genome of SCA, SPN, MCNs, and IPMNs using whole-exome sequencing.[25] There were two key findings: the first was that pancreatic cysts contained far fewer somatic mutations when compared with pancreatic ductal adenocarcinoma. The second was that each cyst type had a distinct mutational profile. SCAs contained a mutation in the von Hippel Lindau (VHL) gene. SPNs were found to have a single mutation in the CTNNB1 gene. Both IPMNs and MCNs had mutations in KRAS or RNF43, whereas IPMNs were found to harbor a mutation in GNAS, which was not identified in any other cyst type. This preliminary study was performed in pancreatic tissue, and in a subsequent study the group was able to show that the same mutations were identifiable in pancreatic cyst fluid.[32] In a recent, multicenter study involving 130 patients all of whom had undergone surgical resection, the molecular marker panel was expanded to include a larger number of genetic mutations, as well as assessing loss of heterozygosity (LOH) and aneuploidy. This study confirmed not only the ability of the molecular markers to accurately identify cyst type (Table 2), but also to identify the presence of high-grade dysplasia or invasive carcinoma in IPMNs, which was associated with the presence of mutations in SMAD4, TP53, LOH chromosome 17 (RNF43 or TP53 loci), or aneuploidy in chromosomes 5p, 8p, 13q, or 18q. In addition, the group developed a novel concept of combining molecular markers with clinical features to further improve the diagnostic accuracy of these markers, which increased the sensitivity and specificity further. One of the interesting results in this article was the ability of the molecular markers to correctly identify low-risk cysts. The markers correctly classified 56 of the 62 SCAs, and IPMNs with low-grade or intermediate-grade dysplasia. Thus, use of the molecular markers could potentially decrease the number of unnecessary surgical resections by 90%. The use of molecular markers in pancreatic cysts has been assessed by other groups, who have also found very promising results.[33–35] These, and the results from studies described previously are encouraging; however, larger studies, incorporating other cyst types, are required before

**Table 2**
Identification of cyst type using molecular marker

| Type of Cyst | Any of These *Present* | Any of These *Absent* | Sensitivity (95% CI) | Specificity (95% CI) |
|---|---|---|---|---|
| | | **Molecular Markers** | | |
| SCA | *VHL* chr3 LOH | *KRAS* *GNAS* *RNF43* chr5p aneu chr8p aneu | 100% (74%–100%) | 91% (84%–95%) |
| SPN | *CTNNB1* | *KRAS* *GNAS* *RNF43* chr18 LOH | 100% (69%–100%) | 100% (97%–100%) |
| MCN | None | *CTNNB1* *GNAS* chr3 LOH chr1q aneu chr22q aneu | 100% (74%–100%) | 75% (66%–82%) |
| IPMN | *GNAS* *RNF43* chr9 LOH chr1q aneu chr8p aneu | None | 76% (66%–84%) | 97% (85%–99.9%) |

*Abbreviations:* aneu, aneuploidy; chr, chromosome; CI, confidence intervals; IPMN, intraductal papillary mucinous neoplasms; MCN, mucinous cystic neoplasms; MPD, main pancreatic duct; SCA, serous crystadenoma; SPN, Solid-pseudopapillary neoplasm.

these molecular markers can be recommended in clinical practice. These studies are currently ongoing, and the results are expected to be available in 2016.

## PANCREATIC JUICE

One of the limitations of assessing pancreatic cyst fluid is that it requires EUS-FNA. Potential limitations are that a biopsy is invasive, only a portion of a cyst is sampled, and in cases of multiple pancreatic cysts, sampling of all cysts may not be feasible. An alternative approach is to analyze molecular markers in pancreatic juice collected from the duodenum. This avoids the potential adverse events of direct sampling of pancreatic fluid using FNA, and in addition, pancreatic juice may contain alterations present in multiple cysts throughout the pancreas, rather than a single cyst. The results from preliminary studies are promising. Kanda and colleagues[36] examined secretin-stimulated pancreatic juice collected from the duodenum during upper endoscopy, and identified *GNAS* mutations in 66% of IPMNs, which is similar to that observed in EUS-aspirated cyst fluid. In a further development of this technique, the same investigators examined the presence of *TP53* mutations, a known tumor suppressor gene that has been implicated in

progression of IPMNs, in duodenal samples of pancreatic juice.[37] They found that *TP53* mutations were detected in pancreatic juice in almost 70% of patients with pancreatic ductal adenocarcinoma, pancreatic intraepithelial neoplasias-3, or high-grade IPMN, but was not identified in individuals with benign cysts, or lower grades of dysplasia. These studies suggest the potential use of pancreatic juice for detecting mutations present in pancreatic cysts, and this technique may prove complementary to cyst fluid aspiration in the diagnostic workup of pancreatic cysts.

## CURRENT CLINICAL PRACTICE FOR THE ASSESSMENT OF PANCREATIC CYSTS

In our practice, we perform EUS-FNA of pancreatic cysts when it will alter management. Cyst fluid is currently sent for CEA and cytology. We also obtain cyst fluid amylase in cases in which there is clinical suspicion of a pseudocyst. We await further studies to validate the accuracy of the molecular markers, and to determine how to optimally combine them with the currently available tests. If these studies duplicate the results discussed previously, it is likely that molecular markers will become part, and may replace many of the currently used cyst fluid tests.

## SUMMARY

Pancreatic cyst fluid analysis provides important information that can be used to improve the diagnosis of pancreatic cysts. The results of cyst fluid analysis should be used in combination with clinical history and imaging to help guide management decisions. New molecular makers have shown promise, and are likely to become incorporated into clinical care in the near future.

## REFERENCES

1. Laffan TA, Horton KM, Klein AP, et al. Prevalence of unsuspected pancreatic cysts on MDCT. AJR Am J Roentgenol 2008;191:802–7.

2. Lee KS, Sekhar A, Rofsky NM, et al. Prevalence of incidental pancreatic cysts in the adult population on MR imaging. Am J Gastroenterol 2010;105: 2079–84.

3. Gaujoux S, Brennan MF, Gonen M, et al. Cystic lesions of the pancreas: changes in the presentation and management of 1,424 patients at a single institution over a 15-year time period. J Am Coll Surg 2011;212:590–600, [discussion: 600–3].

4. Lennon AM, Wolfgang C. Cystic neoplasms of the pancreas. J Gastrointest Surg 2013;17:645–53.

5. Jais B, Rebours V, Malleo G, et al. Serous cystic neoplasm of the pancreas: a multinational study of 2622 patients under the auspices of the International Association of Pancreatology and European Pancreatic Club (European Study Group on Cystic Tumors of the Pancreas). Gut 2016;65(2):305–12.

6. Law JK, Ahmed A, Singh VK, et al. A systematic review of solid-pseudopapillary neoplasms: are these rare lesions? Pancreas 2014;43:331–7.

7. Jang KT, Park SM, Basturk O, et al. Clinicopathologic characteristics of 29 invasive carcinomas arising in 178 pancreatic mucinous cystic neoplasms with ovarian-type stroma: implications for management and prognosis. Am J Surg Pathol 2015;39:179–87.

8. Yamao K, Yanagisawa A, Takahashi K, et al. Clinicopathological features and prognosis of mucinous cystic neoplasm with ovarian-type stroma: a multi-institutional study of the Japan Pancreas Society. Pancreas 2011;40:67–71.

9. Baker ML, Seeley ES, Pai R, et al. Invasive mucinous cystic neoplasms of the pancreas. Exp Mol Pathol 2012;93:345–9.

10. Del Chiaro M, Verbeke C, Salvia R, et al. European experts consensus statement on cystic tumours of the pancreas. Dig Liver Dis 2013;45:703–11.

11. Tanaka M, Fernandez-Del Castillo C, Adsay V, et al. International consensus guidelines 2012 for the management of IPMN and MCN of the pancreas. Pancreatology 2012;12:183–97.

12. Wang KX, Ben QW, Jin ZD, et al. Assessment of morbidity and mortality associated with EUS-guided FNA: a systematic review. Gastrointest Endosc 2011;73:283–90.

13. Khashab MA, Kim K, Lennon AM, et al. Should we do EUS/FNA on patients with pancreatic cysts? The incremental diagnostic yield of EUS over CT/MRI for prediction of cystic neoplasms. Pancreas 2013;42:717–21.

14. Brugge WR, Lewandrowski K, Lee-Lewandrowski E, et al. Diagnosis of pancreatic cystic neoplasms: a report of the cooperative pancreatic cyst study. Gastroenterology 2004;126:1330–6.

15. van der Waaij LA, van Dullemen HM, Porte RJ. Cyst fluid analysis in the differential diagnosis of pancreatic cystic lesions: a pooled analysis. Gastrointest Endosc 2005;62:383–9.

16. Al-Haddad M, Dewitt J, Sherman S, et al. Performance characteristics of molecular (DNA) analysis for the diagnosis of mucinous pancreatic cysts. Gastrointest Endosc 2014;79:79–87.

17. Anand N, Sampath K, Wu BU. Cyst features and risk of malignancy in intraductal papillary mucinous neoplasms of the pancreas: a meta-analysis. Clin Gastroenterol Hepatol 2013;11:913–21, [quiz: e59–60].

18. de Jong K, Poley JW, van Hooft JE, et al. Endoscopic ultrasound-guided fine-needle aspiration of pancreatic cystic lesions provides inadequate material for cytology and laboratory analysis: initial results from a prospective study. Endoscopy 2011;43:585–90.

19. Cizginer S, Turner BG, Bilge AR, et al. Cyst fluid carcinoembryonic antigen is an accurate diagnostic marker of pancreatic mucinous cysts. Pancreas 2011;40:1024–8.

20. Park WG, Mascarenhas R, Palaez-Luna M, et al. Diagnostic performance of cyst fluid carcinoembryonic antigen and amylase in histologically confirmed pancreatic cysts. Pancreas 2011;40: 42–5.

21. Ngamruengphong S, Bartel MJ, Raimondo M. Cyst carcinoembryonic antigen in differentiating pancreatic cysts: a meta-analysis. Dig Liver Dis 2013;45: 920–6.

22. Thornton GD, McPhail MJ, Nayagam S, et al. Endoscopic ultrasound guided fine needle aspiration for the diagnosis of pancreatic cystic neoplasms: a meta-analysis. Pancreatology 2013;13:48–57.

23. Valsangkar NP, Morales-Oyarvide V, Thayer SP, et al. 851 resected cystic tumors of the pancreas: a 33-year experience at the Massachusetts General Hospital. Surgery 2012;152:S4–12.

24. Sahora K, Mino-Kenudson M, Brugge W, et al. Branch duct intraductal papillary mucinous neoplasms: does cyst size change the tip of the scale? A critical analysis of the revised international consensus guidelines in a large single-institutional series. Ann Surg 2013;258:466–75.

25. Wu J, Jiao Y, Dal Molin M, et al. Whole-exome sequencing of neoplastic cysts of the pancreas reveals recurrent mutations in components of ubiquitin-dependent pathways. Proc Natl Acad Sci U S A 2011;108:21188–93.

26. Springer S, Wang Y, Dal Molin M, et al. A combination of molecular markers and clinical features improve the classification of pancreatic cysts. Gastroenterology 2015;149:1501–10.

27. Yip-Schneider MT, Wu H, Dumas RP, et al. Vascular endothelial growth factor, a novel and highly accurate pancreatic fluid biomarker for serous pancreatic cysts. J Am Coll Surg 2014;218:608–17.

28. Das KK, Xiao H, Geng X, et al. mAb Das-1 is specific for high-risk and malignant intraductal papillary mucinous neoplasm (IPMN). Gut 2014;63:1626–34.

29. Matthaei H, Wylie D, Lloyd MB, et al. miRNA biomarkers in cyst fluid augment the diagnosis and management of pancreatic cysts. Clin Cancer Res 2012;18:4713–24.

30. Zikos T, Pham K, Bowen R, et al. Cyst fluid glucose is rapidly feasible and accurate in diagnosing mucinous pancreatic cysts. Am J Gastroenterol 2015;110:909–14.

31. Maker AV, Carrara S, Jamieson NB, et al. Cyst fluid biomarkers for intraductal papillary mucinous neoplasms of the pancreas: a critical review from the international expert meeting on pancreatic branch-duct-intraductal papillary mucinous neoplasms. J Am Coll Surg 2015;220:243–53.

32. Wu J, Matthaei H, Maitra A, et al. Recurrent GNAS mutations define an unexpected pathway for pancreatic cyst development. Sci Transl Med 2011;3:92ra66.

33. Amato E, Molin MD, Mafficini A, et al. Targeted next-generation sequencing of cancer genes dissects the molecular profiles of intraductal papillary neoplasms of the pancreas. J Pathol 2014;233:217–27.

34. Singhi AD, Nikiforova MN, Fasanella KE, et al. Preoperative GNAS and KRAS testing in the diagnosis of pancreatic mucinous cysts. Clin Cancer Res 2014;20(16):4381–9.

35. Furukawa T, Kuboki Y, Tanji E, et al. Whole-exome sequencing uncovers frequent GNAS mutations in intraductal papillary mucinous neoplasms of the pancreas. Sci Rep 2011;1:161.

36. Kanda M, Knight S, Topazian MD, et al. Mutant GNAS detected in duodenal collections of secretin-stimulated pancreatic juice indicates the presence or emergence of pancreatic cysts. Gut 2012;62(7):1024–33.

37. Kanda M, Sadakari Y, Borges M, et al. Mutant TP53 in duodenal samples of pancreatic juice from patients with pancreatic cancer or high-grade dysplasia. Clin Gastroenterol Hepatol 2013;11(6):719–30.e5.

# Molecular Genetics of Pancreatic Neoplasms

Waki Hosoda, MD, PhD[a], Laura D. Wood, MD, PhD[b],*

## KEYWORDS

- Molecular genetics • Whole exome sequencing • Next-generation sequencing
- Pancreatic neoplasms • Mutation • Histologic type

---

### Key points

- Recent exome sequencing studies revealed that pancreatic neoplasms have characteristic genetic landscapes depending on the histologic types.

- Each histologic type of pancreatic neoplasms has its own distinct genetic changes of oncogenes and tumor suppressor genes, including mutations of KRAS, GNAS, RNF43, MEN1, DAXX, ATRX, CTNNB1, and VHL. These genes have the potential for adjunct diagnostic markers.

- Multiple exome sequencing studies have been performed against pancreatic ductal adenocarcinoma (PDAC), and they consistently showed that the genome of PDAC is highly diverse, harboring only 4 frequently mutated genes (KRAS, TP53, CDKN2A/P16, and SMAD4).

- The exome sequencing studies also revealed the presence of potentially targetable genetic mutations in a proportion of tumors, particularly in pancreatic ductal adenocarcinomas and acinar cell carcinomas.

---

## ABSTRACT

Pancreatic neoplasms have a wide range of histologic types with distinct clinical outcomes. Recent advances in high-throughput sequencing technologies have greatly deepened our understanding of pancreatic neoplasms. Now, the exomes of major histologic types of pancreatic neoplasms have been sequenced, and their genetic landscapes have been revealed. This article reviews the molecular changes underlying pancreatic neoplasms, with a special focus on the genetic changes that characterize the histologic types of pancreatic neoplasms. Emphasis is also made on the molecular features of key genes that have the potential for therapeutic targets.

Some of the histologic types occur in association with hereditary cancer-predisposing syndromes, which greatly contributed to the discovery of important molecular changes responsible for the development of pancreatic neoplasms. Recent advances in next-generation sequencing (NGS) have dramatically deepened our understanding of the molecular genetics of each pancreatic neoplasm, revealing that each has its own characteristic genetic changes. In addition, exome sequencing studies of pancreatic ductal adenocarcinoma (PDAC) have provided insights into evolution and genomic heterogeneity of cancer.[1] In this review, we summarize the recent results of the molecular genetics of pancreatic neoplasms, with a special emphasis on the correlation between histologic types and key genetic alterations, as well as on the potentially targetable genes discovered in some tumor types.

## OVERVIEW

Pancreatic neoplasms are one of the most intensively investigated human malignancies.

## DUCTAL ADENOCARCINOMA

The genetics of PDAC has been well studied, and we now know that PDAC is genetically a highly

---

[a] Department of Pathology, Johns Hopkins University, CRB-II 362, 1550 Orleans Street, Baltimore, MD 21231, USA; [b] Department of Pathology, Johns Hopkins University, CRB-II 345, 1550 Orleans Street, Baltimore, MD 21231, USA
* Corresponding author.
*E-mail address:* ldelong1@jhmi.edu

Surgical Pathology 9 (2016) 685–703
http://dx.doi.org/10.1016/j.path.2016.05.011

surgpath.theclinics.com

complicated tumor with a large number of point mutations, chromosomal structural variants, and epigenetic aberrations. Conventional and recent NGS studies consistently showed that PDAC has alterations of 4 genes: the oncogene KRAS, and the tumor suppressor genes TP53, CDKN2A/P16, and SMAD4.

KRAS is the most frequently altered oncogene in PDAC, with more than 90% of cases having activating mutations at codons 12, 13, or 61.[2–4] KRAS encodes a small GTPase protein, which is turned on and off by cycling between the GTP-bound active and GDP-bound inactive forms. KRAS protein serves as a transducer that couples with cell surface receptors (receptor tyrosine kinases), and, once activated, it stimulates a multitude of intracellular effector pathways including RAF-mitogen-activated kinase (MAPK), phosphoinositide-3-kinase (PI3K), and Ral guanine nucleotide dissociation stimulator (RalGDS) pathways. These effectors drive most of the hallmarks of cancer cells, such as proliferation, energy metabolism, antiapoptosis, remodeling of the tumor microenvironment, evasion of the immune system, cell migration, and metastasis.[5] Unfortunately, attempts to block the activity of mutated KRAS oncoprotein have been unsuccessful, and KRAS remains an undruggable cancer-related gene.[6]

The tumor suppressor gene TP53 is altered in 50% to 80% of PDACs.[7–13] The TP53 protein plays a central role in controlling growth, glucose metabolism, DNA repair, senescence, and apoptosis in response to many forms of cellular stress, including DNA damage, hypoxia, and nutrient deprivation.[14] The most common TP53 alterations are base substitutions or frameshift insertions/deletions in the DNA-binding domain, which is coupled with loss of the wild-type allele. Immunohistochemically, nuclear overexpression or complete loss of expression of the TP53 protein are closely associated with genetic alterations.[7]

The tumor suppressor gene CDKN2A/P16 is commonly altered in a variety of malignancies, and inactivation of CDKN2A/P16 is noted in 95% of PDACs. CDKN2A/P16 inactivation occurs by 3 mechanisms: homozygous deletion (40%), intragenic mutation coupled with loss of the second allele (40%), and promoter hypermethylation coupled with loss of the second allele (15%).[15–17] CDKN2A/P16 is located on chromosome 9p21, and its protein product P16 functions as a mediator of the RB signaling pathway. P16 inhibits CDK4/6-mediated phosphorylation of RB, thereby blocking the entry of cells into the S (DNA synthesis) phase of the cell cycle, and perturbation of the P16-CDK4/6-pRB pathway can lead to accelerated cell growth and proliferation.[18] Immunohistochemically, loss of nuclear expression of P16 is closely associated with inactivated CDKN2A/P16 via homozygous deletion; however, nuclear positivity was observed in a fraction of PDACs with promoter methylation or somatic mutation.[19,20] Although fluorescence in situ hybridization (FISH) is a common method for evaluating homozygous deletion of the CDKN2A locus, concordant loss of immunolabeling of both P16 and methylthioadenosine phosphorylase (MTAP) proteins, the latter located on the telomeric side of the same chromosome 9p21 locus, can be a surrogate marker for assessing homozygous deletion of CDKN2A.[21]

Alteration of the tumor suppressor gene SMAD4 (DPC4, MADH4) is observed in 30% to 60% of PDACs.[10–13,22–24] SMAD4 is inactivated by homozygous deletion or intragenic mutations coupled with loss of the other allele. This gene is mapped on chromosome 18q21, and its protein is a mediator of the TGF-beta signaling pathway. In non-neoplastic tissues, the TGF-beta pathway functions to maintain tissue homeostasis by controlling the proliferation of cells, including epithelial, endothelial, stromal, and immune cells, and its activation can lead to antiproliferative and apoptotic responses. Disruption of TGF-beta signaling in cancer cells causes not only a proliferative effect but also epithelial-mesenchymal transition as well as proangiogenic and immunosuppressive effects on the tumor microenvironment, all of which can promote cancer progression.[25] Loss of nuclear immunolabeling was shown to be highly correlated with genetic mutations and can be a useful marker for assessing SMAD4 alteration.[26] However, it should be noted that tumors with mutations occurring in a specific region of the SMAD4 gene (termed the mutation cluster region, located within the MH2 domain) exhibit strong nuclear staining for the SMAD4 protein.[24]

A correlation between loss of expression of SMAD4 and outcome of patients with PDAC has been examined by several studies. Initial studies reached opposite conclusions concerning the loss of SMAD4 immunolabeling and patient survival.[27–29] A recent genetic analysis showed that patients with PDAC with SMAD4 mutations had a poor prognosis.[30] Moreover, loss of SMAD4 expression has been correlated with an increased propensity of PDAC to metastasize widely rather than to develop a localized tumor.[31]

Exome sequencing studies have deepened our understanding of PDAC. The initial exome sequencing study by Jones and colleagues[10] analyzed 20,661 protein-coding genes in 24 PDACs and found an average of 48 nonsynonymous somatic mutations per tumor. Of these, 90% of the mutations were base substitutions. The genes with the highest mutation rates were the 4 well-known driver genes of PDAC (KRAS, TP53, CDKN2A/P16, and SMAD4), whereas the rest of the altered genes occurred far less frequently. Genes mutated in 2 or more patients constituted just 10% of the genes (148 genes). Many additional potential driver genes were identified; there was marked genetic heterogeneity between individual patients' tumors. However, when altered genes were classified in terms of cellular pathways and processes, most of the genes were categorized into 12 core signaling pathways.[10]

The study of Jones and colleagues[10] was followed by multiple whole exome/genome sequencing studies (Table 1).[11–13,32] These results reinforce the view that PDAC genome is highly diverse, characterized by frequent and consistent alterations of just 4 driver genes along with a long tail of less frequently mutated genes. Among the less commonly mutated genes, a limited number of genes were observed in multiple studies, such as ARID1A, TGFBR1, or MLL3. ARID1A was mutated in 2 or more patients throughout the exome sequencing studies of PDAC, with mutation rates ranging from 4% to 16%. ARID1A is a constituent of SWI/SNF complexes that functions as a regulator of chromatin remodeling. As part of the complexes, it remodels nucleosome structure and enables DNA-binding factors to gain access to DNA, thereby modulating transcription, synthesis, and repair.[33] Prognostically, one study showed that patients with PDAC with diminished ARID1A protein expression tended to have poor survival.[12]

Although tumors are often analyzed in bulk at a single time point, cancer is a heterogeneous, evolving disease, consisting of genetically distinct subclones that grow selectively by the acquisition of phenotypic advantage within a given tumor microenvironment.[34] Pathologists have been well aware of histologic and immunohistochemical heterogeneity among spatially different components of a tumor. Exome sequencing studies have impressively shown this intertumoral and intratumoral genomic diversity by detailing genetic mutations and chromosomal aberrations of multiple lesions in a patient.[35,36] Yachida and colleagues[35] investigated the genetic mutations of primary and metastatic lesions of PDAC within a patient and revealed that two-thirds of the mutations were present in all samples, and the remaining one-third of mutations were partially shared; the clone with omnipresent mutations are the parental clone, whereas the rest of clones with partially shared

mutations are subclones that evolved from the parental clone. Moreover, after examining multiple components in a primary tumor, they revealed that all mutations found in the metastatic deposits were also present in the primary tumor, suggesting that genetic alterations necessary for metastasis occur before the development of a metastatic lesion. Most importantly, using a mathematical model, the investigators estimated an average of 12 years from the birth of a parental clone to the initiating event of carcinogenesis and a further 7 years to the development of subclones that are capable of metastasis within the primary tumor.[35] Considering that most patients with PDAC are diagnosed with metastatic diseases, exploration of novel strategies for early detection within this time window is quite worthwhile to improve the outcome of this refractory cancer.

The PDAC genome is also characterized by highly complex chromosomal alterations. Traditional cytogenetic analysis, spectral karyotyping, comparative genomic hybridization (CGH), and more recent high-resolution microarray-based CGH consistently showed a number of chromosomal gains and losses in PDACs.[10,37–41] Recently, a deep whole genome sequencing study was performed by the International Cancer Genome Consortium.[13] The researchers investigated detailed structural variations, such as deletions, duplications, inversions, amplifications, and rearrangements, and found 11,868 somatic structural variants at an average of 119 variants per patient. Although 1200 structural variants were found that led to the joining of 2 gene loci, no recurrent gene fusions were detected. Remarkably, when they classified PDACs into 4 subtypes in terms of structural variation, they found that PDACs with the "unstable" subtype (characterized by marked genomic instability) had frequent BRCA1, BRCA2, and PALB2 mutations, as well as mutational signatures of carcinomas with BRCA1/2 mutations.[42] Breast carcinomas with BRCA1/2 mutations are sensitive to platinum-based and PARP-inhibitor therapy,[43] and, in fact, 2 patients with PDAC with this subtype showed an exceptional response to platinum-based therapy in their study, showing promise to treatment stratification of patients with PDAC.

Some genetic changes were highlighted via the analysis of variants of PDAC. Colloid carcinoma is characterized by frequent association with intraductal papillary mucinous neoplasm (IPMN), and molecular analysis supports the histologic observation; colloid carcinomas frequently harbor GNAS mutation, which is preferentially found in IPMNs among pancreatic neoplasms.[44–48] In addition, colloid carcinomas tend to have less frequent

Table 1
Whole exome/genome sequencing studies of pancreatic ductal adenocarcinoma

| Reference, year | Jones et al,[10] 2008 | Wang et al,[11] 2012 | ICGC (Biankin et al,[32] 2012) | Witkiewicz et al,[12] 2015 | ICGC (Waddell et al,[13] 2015) |
|---|---|---|---|---|---|
| Sequencing scope | Exome | Exome | Exome | Exome | Whole genome |
| Number of cases | 24 (Prevalence screen: 90) | 15 | 99 | 109 (including 11 adenosquamous carcinomas and 4 colloid carcinomas) | 100 |
| Stage (UICC) | IIB (n = 15) and IV (n = 9) | n.d. | I-II | I-II (n = 102), III (n = 6) and IV (n = 1) | I-II (n = 88), IV (n = 6) and uncertain (n = 6) |
| Average number of NSMs[a] per tumor | 48 | 73 (1 case was hypermutated [500 mutations]) | 20 | 67 (2 cases were hypermutated [400 mutations]) | 79 (2 cases were hypermutated [900 mutations]) |
| Alterations in PDAC-related genes | *KRAS* (100%: NSM)<br>*TP53* (83%: NSM, HD)<br>*CDKN2A* (75%: NSM, HD)<br>*SMAD4* (58%: NSM, HD) | *KRAS* (100%: NSM)<br>*TP53* (80%: NSM, LOH)<br>*CDKN2A* (67%: NSM, LOH, HD)<br>*SMAD4* (53%: NSM, LOH, HD) | *KRAS* (NSM in 95%)<br>*TP53* (NSM in 33%)<br>*CDKN2A* (NSM in 2%, deletion)<br>*SMAD4* (NSM in 16%, deletion) | *KRAS* (92%: NSM)<br>*TP53* (50%: NSM)<br>*CDKN2A* (41%: NSM, HD)<br>*SMAD4* (43%: NSM, HD) | *KRAS* (95%: NSM)<br>*TP53* (74%: NSM, structural variants)<br>*CDKN2A* (35%: NSM, structural variants)<br>*SMAD4* (31%: NSM, structural variants) |

| | | | | | |
|---|---|---|---|---|---|
| Other significantly mutated genes | • 148 mutated genes (in 2 or more patients) <br> • Other candidate cancer genes include, eg, MLL3, TGFBR2, PCDH15, CDH10, CTNNA2 | • 56 mutated genes (in 2 or more tumors) | • 79 mutated genes (in 2 or more patients) <br> • Other significantly mutated genes include, eg, MLL3, TGFBR2, ARID1A, ARID2, EPC1, ATM, SF3B1, ZIM2, MAP2K4, NALCN, SLC16A4, MAGEA6 | • 24 significantly mutated genes (occurring in >3.5% of cases) <br> • Other significantly mutated genes include, eg, FLG, ATXN1, ARID1A, COL14A1, RNF43, RP1L1, ITGAE, GLI3, GNAS, SPTA1 | • Integrated landscape of aberrations (including somatic mutations, copy number changes, and chromosomal variants) was illustrated <br> • An average of 119 structural variants per tumor <br> • No recurrent fusion genes <br> • 4 subtypes in terms of structural variation |
| Other major findings | Most altered genes were categorized into 12 core signaling pathways[a] | • One hypermutated case had MLH1 homozygous deletion and microsatellite instability <br> • A correlation between MLH1 allelic loss/homozygous deletion and genomic instability was suggested | In addition to the core signaling pathways shown by Jones et al,[10] genes of the axon guidance pathway were frequently altered (eg, genes: SLIT2, ROBO1, ROBO2, SEMA3A, SEMA3E) | • Hypermutated cases had alterations of DNA mismatch repair genes <br> • MYC amplification was associated with adenosquamous histology <br> • Potentially clinically actionable mutations/pathways were highlighted | PDACs with the "unstable" subtype were associated with deleterious mutations in the BRCA pathway genes (BRCA1, BRCA2, and PALB2) and the BRCA mutational signature[b] |

*Abbreviations:* HD, homozygous deletion; ICGC, International Cancer Genome Consortium; LOH, loss of heterozygosity; n.d., not described; NSM, nonsynonymous mutation.
[a] NSM mutations include missense, nonsense, splice site, translation start, translation stop, and indel mutations, all occurring in the amino acid coding sequence.
[b] BRCA mutational signature: a mathematical analysis of cancer genomes revealed that cancers have a characteristic pattern(s) of mutations, or "mutational signature" that is defined by the type of DNA damage and DNA repair processes. Among the possible 96 patterns of base substitutions, a pattern termed signature 3, defined by a more or less equal representation of all 96 mutations and associated with larger indels (4 bp–50 bp) with overlapping microhomology at breakpoint junctions, is associated with cancers harboring BRCA1/2 mutations. Signature 3 is commonly observed in cancers of the breast, ovary, and pancreas (see Ref.[42]).

*KRAS* mutations (50%) compared with conventional PDACs.[47,48] Adenosquamous carcinoma contains frequent alterations of *KRAS*, *TP53*, *CDKN2A/P16*, and *SMAD4* with similar prevalence to conventional PDAC.[49] Amplification of the *MYC* oncogene was reported to be associated with adenosquamous carcinoma.[12] Moreover, *UPF1*, encoding an RNA helicase important for nonsense-mediated RNA decay, was found to be frequently mutated in adenosquamous carcinomas in one study.[50]

Medullary carcinoma is a rare, histologically distinct subset of poorly differentiated adenocarcinomas. Medullary carcinoma is characterized by microsatellite instability (MSI) and less frequent *KRAS* mutations. Studies of 18 medullary carcinomas demonstrated that 67% had wild-type *KRAS* and 22% had MSI with loss of MLH1 expression.[51,52] PDACs with medullary morphology were also reported to have MSI and/or wild-type *KRAS*.[53–56] Several cases of pancreatic medullary carcinoma that occurred in patients with Lynch syndrome or carriers of germline mutations of mismatch repair genes were documented.[52,55,57] Although less well studied, the diagnosis of medullary carcinoma carries implications for the management of patients. In addition, *BRAF* mutations were reported in PDACs with medullary morphology and wild-type *KRAS*, suggesting the therapeutic potential of tyrosine kinase inhibitor therapy.[54]

## PANCREATIC INTRADUCTAL NEOPLASIA

A line of clinicopathological studies suggested that pancreatic intraductal neoplasia (PanIN) is the major precursor of PDAC. Molecular studies have supported this hypothesis by showing that (1) PanIN lesions have genetic abnormalities that are common to the adjacent PDACs, and (2) histologic progression of PanIN parallels the accumulation of molecular abnormalities.[58] However, studies of mutational analysis, particularly those of tumor suppressor genes, are limited, and the genetic features, particularly those of PanIN-3, remain to be elucidated.

Telomere shortening and *KRAS* mutation are the earliest genetic events in PanIN. Telomere shortening was observed in 90% of PanIN-1A lesions and in 96% of all PanIN lesions.[59] A recent study also showed that telomere shortening occurs in PanIN-1, and the degree of shortening increases as the grade of PanIN rises.[60] *KRAS* is frequently mutated in PanIN-1 lesions. An early study showed that the rate of *KRAS* mutations increases as the degree of dysplasia rises (36%, 44%, and 87% of PanIN-1A, 1B, and 2–3 lesions,

respectively).[61] Recent studies using highly sensitive detection assays demonstrated that *KRAS* mutations were detected in 80% to 90% of PanIN-1 lesions.[47,62] These results suggest that *KRAS* mutation is crucial for the initiation of PanIN.

Abnormalities in the tumor suppressor genes *CDKN2A/P16*, *TP53*, and *SMAD4*, which are frequently targeted in PDAC, are also noted in PanIN. Loss of expression of P16 was observed in 5% to 30% of PanIN-1, 16% to 55% of PanIN-2, and 40% to 83% of PanIN-3.[63–65] Homozygous deletion of *CDKN2A*, assessed by concordant loss of expression of the P16 and MTAP proteins, was shown to be present in 8% of PanIN lesions (mostly PanIN-3).[66] Promoter hypermethylation of *CDKN2A/P16* was detected in 15% of PanIN-1, 5% of PanIN-2, and 21% of PanIN-3 lesions.[67] Taken together, inactivation of *CDKN2A/P16* is considered to play a role in PanIN development.

*SMAD4* and *TP53* alterations appear to be involved in late events in PanIN development. Immunohistochemically, abnormal expressions of the TP53 and SMAD4 proteins were observed in 40% and 30% to 54% of PanIN-3 lesions, respectively, but the expressions of both proteins were almost retained in PanIN-1/-2 lesions.[65,68,69] A recent exome sequencing study of PanIN-2/-3 lesions showed that *TP53* was mutated in 4/15 lesions.[70] *SMAD4* mutations were not detected. A study of loss of heterozygosity (LOH) using microsatellite markers was performed to examine allelic losses of gene loci of *CDKN2A* (9p), *TP53* (17p) and *SMAD4* (18q) in PanIN and associated PDAC; no allelic losses of 3 chromosomal arms were found in PanIN-1, whereas allelic losses were frequent in PanIN-3, seen in 87% (13/15) of lesions at 9p, 60% (6/10) of lesions at 17p, and 88% (14/16) of lesions at 18q.[69]

Exome sequencing of 10 PDAC and 15 adjacent PanIN-2 and PanIN-3 lesions was performed in an attempt to examine the genetic correlation between the invasive carcinoma and the preinvasive component.[70] The investigators found 1053 somatic mutations in 937 genes in PDACs and adjacent PanIN lesions. There was a trend toward fewer mutations in PanIN-2 (an average of 30 mutations) compared with invasive carcinoma (an average of 49 mutations). Surprisingly, PanIN-3 showed 63 mutations on average per lesion, and the commonality of mutations between PanIN-3 and adjacent invasive carcinoma ranged from 34% to 96%, with 10 of 15 PanIN lesions showing commonality of greater than 50%.

It should be noted that there is one critical issue in the molecular study of PanIN: the genetics of high-grade PanIN (PanIN-3 or carcinoma in situ) has been analyzed mostly using pancreatectomy specimens for PDAC. Although it is reasonable to examine the genetic changes by comparing a noninvasive carcinoma with an invasive one to highlight the factors of malignant transition, the histologic distinction between genuine high-grade PanIN and cancerization of pancreatic ducts is sometimes difficult, and the interpretation of the genetic analysis of the noninvasive component may not be reliable in some lesions. Because of the rarity of high-grade PanIN (≤5%) in the resected specimens without PDAC,[61,71–73] very few studies reported molecular characteristics of high-grade PanIN without associated PDAC, hampering a definitive conclusion.

## INTRADUCTAL PAPILLARY MUCINOUS NEOPLASMS

IPMN is another important precursor of PDAC. Molecular studies supported the notion that IPMN develops an invasive carcinoma through the progression from low-grade IPMN to high-grade IPMN by showing that genetic abnormalities important for the development of PDAC are also found in high-grade IPMN and that genetic changes accumulate with increasing cytoarchitectural atypia.

PDAC-related genes were altered in IPMN and are thus considered to play a role in the development of IPMN. KRAS mutations are present in 50% to 80% of IPMNs.[45,47,48,74–77] KRAS mutations are frequently noted in 60% to 90% of low-grade IPMNs, indicating that mutated KRAS is important in the initiation of IPMN development.

Aberration of TP53 is most commonly noted in high-grade IPMN and is thus considered important for the malignant progression of IPMN. Overexpression or complete loss of expression of TP53 protein was reported in 50% to 80% of high-grade IPMNs and invasive IPMNs, but not in low-grade IPMNs.[65,76,78] Recent NGS studies showed that somatic mutations of TP53 were observed in 0% to 20% of high-grade IPMNs/invasive IPMNs but were rare in low-grade and intermediate-grade IPMNs.[46,48,79] LOH studies using polymerase chain reaction (PCR)-based microsatellite markers showed allelic loss of 17p in 15% to 40% of IPMNs (mostly high-grade IPMNs).[80,81] However, a study using high-density array CGH did not show frequent allelic loss of 17p in IPMNs.[82]

Inactivation of CDKN2A/P16 is involved in the development of IPMN. Loss of P16 expression was noted in 28% to 62% of IPMNs and in 53% to 63% of invasive IPMNs. Of these, loss of expression was observed in 10% to 50% of low-grade and intermediate-grade IPMNs.[46,65,83,84] Genetic analysis of CDKN2A/P16 revealed that aberrations appear to be confined to high-grade IPMNs; 3 sequencing studies using NGS revealed that somatic mutations of CDKN2A/P16 were rare (0%, 2%),[46,79] or infrequent (seen in only 20% of high-grade IPMNs).[48] LOH studies using PCR-based microsatellite markers identified allelic loss of 9p in 18% to 62% of IPMNs.[80,81] However, studies using high-throughput methods (array CGH and digital karyotyping) did not find recurrent loss at the 9p21 locus.[79,82] Promoter hypermethylation is another important mechanism of gene silencing of CDKN2A/P16, and one study showed that hypermethylation was detected in 22% of high-grade IPMNs but not in low-grade IPMNs.[85] Taken together, inactivation of CDKN2A/P16 in IPMN is mediated by the same 3 mechanisms as PDAC and is important in the later events of IPMN progression.

In contrast to the previously mentioned 3 PDAC-related genes, SMAD4 inactivation appears to be involved in the transition to invasive IPMN. Immunohistochemical studies consistently reported that expression of the SMAD4 protein is mostly retained in preinvasive IPMNs, whereas loss of expression is noted in one-third of invasive IPMNs.[46,65,83,86] Studies using NGS revealed that somatic mutations of SMAD4 were rare in IPMN.[46,48,79] On the other hand, chromosomal loss of the SMAD4 locus (18q21) appears to be present before the development of invasive IPMN. LOH studies using PCR-based microsatellite markers detected allelic loss of 18q in 20% to 38% of IPMNs,[80,81] and a recent study using array CGH showed recurrent loss of 18q in intermediate-grade IPMNs (2/5) and in high-grade or invasive IPMNs (5/8).[82]

The discovery of frequent involvement of GNAS in IPMN deepened our understanding of pancreatic neoplasms. Wu and colleagues[45] performed an elaborate experiment to capture frequently mutated genes from cyst fluids of IPMN. After sequencing 169 genes commonly altered in human cancers, they successfully identified hotspot mutations of GNAS codon 201 in 66% of IPMNs. Furukawa and colleagues[87] also found frequent GNAS mutations in 41% of IPMNs. Other studies followed, confirming that GNAS mutations are specific to IPMN and are rare in other pancreatic neoplasms.[45,47,79,87] GNAS encodes the stimulatory G-protein α-subunit (Gsα) of the heterotrimeric G-protein, and codon 201 missense mutations constitutively activate the GNAS protein and increase the level of cyclic AMP.[88,89] Both GNAS and KRAS are most commonly targeted in

IPMN, with more than 90% of cases having one or both mutations.[45–47] Of the 4 IPMN subtypes, GNAS mutations are most prevalent in the intestinal subtype and are observed in 70% to 100% of cases.[45,47,48,90]

Whole exome sequencing has identified other frequently mutated genes in IPMN. Eight high-grade IPMNs were sequenced, and a total of 211 nonsynonymous mutations with an average of 27 mutations per tumor were found.[79] Of 6 genes that were mutated in 2 or more cases, 4 genes (KRAS [63%, 5/8], GNAS [63%, 5/8], RNF43 [75%, 6/8], and APC [25%, 2/8]) were identified as potential driver genes. The RNF43 gene is located on chromosome 17q22, and it encodes a protein with intrinsic E3 ubiquitin ligase activity. Frequent inactivating mutations (ie, nonsense and frameshift mutations) and accompanied LOH of the gene locus indicate that RNF43 functions as a tumor suppressor gene in IPMN and mucinous cystic neoplasm (MCN). Studies by other groups also confirmed recurrent RNF43 mutations in 14% to 18% of IPMNs.[46,48] Intriguingly, recent exome sequencing studies of PDAC found that RNF43 mutations are also seen in approximately 10% of PDACs.[12,13,91] Other cancer-related genes reported in IPMN include BRAF, molecules of the PI3K pathway (PIK3CA, PTEN, and AKT1) and STK11/LKB1, although the prevalence of these mutations is low (<10%).[46,92–97]

Intraductal tubulopapillary neoplasm (ITPN) is a rare subtype of intraductal neoplasm with distinctive histologic and immunohistochemical features.[98] Although examined cases are limited, ITPN seems to have different molecular traits from those of IPMN, including rare KRAS mutations (1/14, 0/4), occasional PIK3CA mutations (3/14, 0/4), and rare GNAS mutations (0/14, 1/4).[46,95] It is surprising that most ITPNs rarely exhibited mutations of common cancer-related genes, even though ITPN often shows high-grade histology.[46] Further studies would clarify the molecular features of this rare subtype of intraductal tumor.

## MUCINOUS CYSTIC NEOPLASM

MCN, the third precursor of PDAC, is a mucin-producing neoplasm with distinctive clinicopathological features. Like IPMNs, MCNs contain alterations in genes commonly mutated in PDAC, and an NGS study revealed frequent alterations of RNF43 in MCN.

KRAS mutations are reported in 6% to 50% of MCNs, with mutations observed from low-grade lesions.[45,47,99–101] The mutation frequency tends to rise as the grade increases; one study showed KRAS mutations in 20% (2/10) of low-grade, 33% (3/9) of intermediate-grade, and 89% (8/9) of high-grade MCNs or invasive MCNs.[99] Abrogation of TP53 function occurs late in the progression of MCN; overexpression of the TP53 protein was noted in high-grade MCNs and invasive MCNs but not in low-grade and intermediate-grade MCNs.[99,102] In parallel, TP53 mutations were found in high-grade MCNs (2/5) and invasive MCNs (5/7), but not in low-grade MCNs (0/3).[79,103] CDKN2A/P16 inactivation has been suggested by past data, but the number of cases is limited and its relevance is not clear. Genetic mutations of CDKN2A/P16 were rarely observed in MCNs.[79,103] Promotor hypermethylation was reported in low-grade/intermediate-grade MCNs (14%, 2/14) and invasive MCNs (43%, 3/7).[100,103] SMAD4 seems to play a role in the progression of MCN, particularly in the transition to invasive carcinoma. Loss of expression of SMAD4 was examined in 36 MCNs in one study, which revealed that all MCNs including high-grade MCNs retained SMAD4 expression whereas most invasive MCNs (6/7) showed loss of SMAD4 expression.[104] Recent NGS studies did not find somatic mutations of SMAD4.[79] Other minor alterations of cancer-related genes reported in MCN include LOH of 3p25 (VHL locus) (2/12) and PIK3CA mutation (1/15).[100,105]

A whole exome sequencing study of 8 MCNs (3 low-grade and 5 high-grade MCNs) revealed 128 somatic mutations in 115 genes, with an average of 16 nonsynonymous mutations per tumor.[79] KRAS was the most frequently targeted (6/8), followed by RNF43 (4/8) and TP53 (2/8). GNAS, which is frequently targeted in IPMNs, did not show mutations in MCNs, and this result was supported by other studies.[45,47]

## NEUROENDOCRINE TUMOR

Although familial cancer-predisposing syndromes account for a small proportion of all human cancers, they have provided important insights into the identification of responsible genes in both familial and sporadic cancers. Multiple endocrine neoplasia-type 1 (MEN1) is a good example, and Pittman and colleagues provide an excellent review of familial syndromes affecting the pancreas elsewhere in this issue (see Pittman ME, Brosens LA, Wood LD: Genetic Syndromes with Pancreatic Manifestations, in this issue). In addition to its involvement in familial tumors, the tumor suppressor gene MEN1 is commonly inactivated in patients with sporadic pancreatic neuroendocrine tumors (PanNETs) via somatic mutations coupled with loss of the wild-type allele. Somatic mutations of MEN1 has been reported in 25% to 44% of sporadic PanNETs.[106–110] In addition, allelic loss of the MEN1 locus (11q13) was reported in 30% to 70% of PanNETs.[107,108,111–114]

Dysregulation of the PI3K/AKT/mTOR pathway is another important characteristic of PanNETs. This pathway controls most hallmarks of cancer, including cell cycle, survival, metabolism, motility, and genetic instability, and constituent molecules are frequently altered in a broad range of human cancers.[115] Among these, genetic alterations of PTEN, TSC2, and PIK3CA were noted in PanNETs. PanNETs contain a number of recurrent chromosomal gains and losses, among which loss of 10q (where PTEN is located) and loss of 16p (where TSC2 is located) were noted in 25% and 36% of cases, respectively.[116,117] Perren and colleagues[118] investigated both PTEN mutations and allelic loss of 10p23, and found that 36% (8/22) of PanNETs have allelic loss of 10q23, although 3% (1/33) had somatic mutations. An exome sequencing study, however, revealed that PTEN, TSC2, and PIK3CA mutations were found in 7.3%, 8.8%, and 1.0% of PanNETs, respectively.[110] Expression microarray revealed that the TSC2 and PTEN transcripts were downregulated in most PanNETs, and low expression levels of these transcripts were associated with shorter disease-free and overall survival.[119] In total, 15% of PanNETs have mutations of mammalian target of rapamycin (mTOR) pathway genes, providing a rationale for the application of mTOR inhibitors for PanNETs. Inhibitors of the mTOR pathway, such as everolimus have shown great promise in the treatment of PanNETs in clinical trials, but treatment response has not yet been linked to mutation status.[120]

An exome sequencing study revealed novel recurrent somatic mutations of the DAXX or ATRX genes in 25% and 18% of PanNETs, respectively.[110] Mutations of both genes were considered inactivating because most mutations were nonsense mutations or insertion/deletions. In addition, immunolabeling of DAXX or ATRX (positive for nuclei in normal cells) was lost in Pan-NETs harboring somatic mutations.[110,121] Both DAXX and ATRX proteins play a role in chromatin remodeling. They interact with each other and together function as a histone chaperone for the deposition of the histone variant H3.3 into telomeric and pericentromeric heterochromatin.[122,123] In this exome sequencing study DAXX and ATRX were mutated in a mutually exclusive manner, supporting the hypothesis that both proteins function within the same pathway.

Furthermore, a striking link between DAXX or ATRX mutations and unique telomere phenotype was discovered. Cancers commonly express telomerase to maintain the length of telomeres so that they can divide indefinitely. However, in a small proportion of cancers, telomere loss is compensated by a telomerase independent mechanism, termed ALT (alternative lengthening of telomeres).[124] Heaphy and colleagues[121] found, using telomere-specific FISH, that there is a strong correlation between PanNETs with DAXX or ATRX mutations and ALT phenotype. Although the mechanism and relevance of the ALT phenotype in PanNETs are not yet understood fully, a correlation between the ALT phenotype and chromosomal instability in PanNETs was suggested by one study.[125] The ALT phenotype is present in only 3% of all human tumors.[126] DAXX or ATRX mutations are suggested to be late events in PanNET development, at least in patients with MEN1 syndrome: no PanNET nodules less than 0.5 cm in diameter (microadenomas) showed either the ALT phenotype or loss of immunostaining of DAXX or ATRX proteins in syndromic patients.[127]

Most studies of PanNETs have not stratified the tumors by hormone secretion status; however, insulinomas in particular have been studied in depth by Cao and colleagues,[128] who investigated the exomes of 10 insulinomas. After examining additional tumors for validation, they found a recurrent hot-spot mutation of T372R in the YY1 gene in 30% (34/113) of sporadic insulinomas, and this result was confirmed by other groups (13% to 33%).[129,130] The YY1 protein is a transcription factor, responsible for the regulation of mitochondrial function and insulin/insulinlike growth factor signaling that is crucial for pancreatic beta-cell survival and insulin secretion. Cromer and colleagues[129] have shown a unique effect of T372R mutation on YY1 gene function: the T372R missense mutation changes the DNA-binding specificity of this transcription factor, conferring a new binding activity not present in the wild-type gene product. Increased expression of genes not normally regulated by the YY1 protein includes ADCY1 and CACNA2D2, which are involved in cAMP and $Ca^{2+}$ signaling, respectively, and play a role in insulin secretion, suggesting a contribution to insulinoma pathogenesis.

In addition to small point mutations, novel gene alterations are suggested as a potential tumor suppressor of PanNETs. Based on the past LOH studies, Ohki and colleagues[131] identified frequent allelic loss at chromosome 1q31 (72%), on which the PHLDA3 gene is located. Although no PHLDA3 mutation was detected, the promoter of the PHLDA3 gene was hypermethylated in PanNETs with LOH of the PHLDA3 locus in 7 of 7 cases, suggesting that *PHLDA3* plays a role as a tumor suppressor gene in PanNETs.

The genetic landscape of PanNETs depicted by exome sequencing is that PanNETs have 8 to 23 somatic mutations per tumor with a mean of 16.[110] Two studies of exome sequencing of insulinomas also showed small numbers of somatic mutations (an average of 8.0 and 3.7 mutations per tumor).[128,129] Four PDAC-related genes (*KRAS*, *TP53*, *CDKN2A/P16* and *SMAD4*) were only very rarely mutated in PanNETs. In addition, multiple LOH studies revealed that a number of chromosomal gains and losses are present in sporadic PanNETs.[132]

## SEROUS CYSTADENOMA

Studies of von Hippel-Lindau (VHL) disease contributed greatly to the molecular understanding of serous cystadenoma (SCA), a benign, slow-growing cystic neoplasm. Early genetic studies and a recent study using NGS consistently showed that the tumor suppressor gene *VHL* is commonly mutated in SCA via somatic mutations and LOH of the wild-type allele. Sporadic SCAs frequently harbor allelic loss of 3p25 (the *VHL* locus), which is observed in 40% to 70% of cases.[100,133,134] A high-resolution LOH assay (digital karyotyping) also showed that allelic loss of 3p was detected in 88% (7/8) of cases.[79] In addition, somatic mutations of *VHL* were detected in 10% to 22% of SCAs examined by conventional methods[133,134] and in 50% (4/8) of SCAs examined by NGS.[79] Moreover, a study reported that epigenetic silencing of the *VHL* gene was detected in a minority of cases (7%, 1/14).[100]

Whole exome sequencing of 8 SCAs showed an average of 10 nonsynonymous mutations per tumor, and *VHL* was the most frequently mutated gene.[79] In addition, PDAC-related genes (*KRAS*, *TP53*, *CDKN2A/P16*, and *SMAD4*), IPMN-related genes (*GNAS*, *RNF43*), PanNET-related genes (*MEN1*, *DAXX* and *ATRX*), and *CTNNB1*, which is frequently mutated in solid-pseudopapillary neoplasm (SPN) and pancreatoblastoma, are all wild-type in SCA, supporting the notion that SCA is a distinct type of tumor in the pancreas.[47,79,100,134–136]

## ACINAR CELL CARCINOMA

Accumulating evidence of the molecular genetics of acinar cell carcinomas (ACCs) supports the notion that ACC is different from PDAC and PanNET. Moreover, ACC has been thought to be characterized by alterations of the APC/beta-catenin pathway. However, recent sequencing studies revealed other recurrently mutated genes and fusion genes, leading us to renew our understanding of this rare neoplasm.

Studies by several groups consistently showed that ACCs rarely have mutations of *KRAS*, which is almost invariably mutated in PDACs.[47,137–143] Although mutations of *TP53* and *SMAD4* were rarely detected in the early studies,[137,139,140,144] recent studies using NGS revealed that ACCs contain mutations of *TP53* and *SMAD4* at low frequencies (*TP53* in 14% to 23% of cases and *SMAD4* in 14% to 19% of cases).[142,145] *CDKN2A/P16* mutations (14%) and homozygous deletions (19%) were also detected in the NGS studies of ACC.[142,145]

LOH studies consistently showed that ACC is characterized by high degrees of chromosomal instability, with a large number of chromosomal gains and losses.[141,143,146,147]

Alterations in the APC/β-catenin pathway have been reported in 24% of ACCs, and include activating mutations of *CTTNB1* or inactivating mutations of *APC*.[148] Recent studies by Furlan and colleagues[141] confirmed this, showing that mutations of *CTTNB1* and *APC* were found in 13% (3/23) and 7% (2/29) of cases, respectively. Furthermore, they showed more frequent involvement of allelic loss of 5q (the *APC* locus) (48%, 12/25) and promoter hypermethylation of the *APC* gene (56%, 24/43). As they found decreased levels of APC mRNA in cases with LOH, they suggested that allelic loss and promoter methylation play a major role in the inactivation of *APC*.

Exome sequencing studies have revealed that ACC is characterized by a large number of somatic mutations (an average of 98 and 131 mutations per tumor in 2 studies), with no apparent "mountains" in its genetic landscape.[142,149] Whole exome sequencing of 21 pancreatic carcinomas with acinar cell differentiation revealed that no genes were mutated in more than 20% of the tumors. Frequently mutated cancer-related genes included *SMAD4* (19%, 4/21), *JAK1* (19%, 4/21), *BRAF* (14%, 3/21), *RB1* (14%, 3/21), *TP53* (14%, 3/21), *APC* (10%, 2/21), *ARID1A* (10%, 2/21), *GNAS* (10%, 2/21), *MLL3* (10%, 2/21), and *PTEN* (10%, 2/21), as well as homozygous deletion of *CDKN2A/P16* (19%, 4/21). Their results were confirmed by another targeted sequencing study, in which PDAC-related genes (*TP53*, *SMAD4*, and *CDKN2A*), as well as *CTNNB1, APC*, and *RB1* were mutated recurrently but with low frequency (10% to 20%).[145]

A targeted sequencing study of 44 ACCs also revealed frequent alterations of the *BRCA2* gene (20%, 9/44).[145] Notably, genes related to DNA repair (eg, *BRCA1/2, PALB2, ATM, MSH1/2*) were mutated in 45% of the cases. The recurrent involvement of BRCA2 mutations was confirmed by another whole exome sequencing study.[149] Another outstanding discovery of ACC genetics is the presence of recurrent gene rearrangements. RNA sequencing found rearrangements involving BRAF or RAF1 in 23% (10/44) of ACCs.[145] The most prevalent fusion protein was SND1-BRAF, and in vitro experiments showed that SND1-BRAF-transformed cells resulted in constitutive activation of the MAPK pathway and exhibited sensitivity to treatment with MEK inhibitor.

Overall, ACC is genetically complex and highly heterogeneous. Although no frequently mutated genes ("mountains") were detected, almost half of the patients with ACC contained somatic mutations that are potentially targetable, including mutations in BRCA1/2, PALB2, BRAF, and JAK1. Indeed, a patient with ACC with a BRCA2 mutation who responded dramatically to platinum-based chemotherapy was documented.[149]

## PANCREATOBLASTOMA

Pancreatoblastoma is a rare pancreatic neoplasm with acinar cell differentiation, occurring most commonly in children. Abraham and colleagues[150] first revealed recurrent genetic alterations of pancreatoblastoma based on an insightful observation. By focusing on the clinicopathological findings that pancreatoblastoma can occur in patients with familial adenomatous polyposis and Beckwith-Wiedemann syndrome, they hypothesized that the molecular pathogenesis of pancreatoblastoma may involve the genetic loci targeted in these syndromes.[151,152] They identified recurrent activating mutations of CTNNB1 and inactivating mutations of APC in 67% (6/9) of cases. Frequent loss of 11p was also noted (6/7).[150,153] Jiao and colleagues performed a whole exome sequencing study of 2 cases of pancreatoblastoma.[142] The cases contained 17 and 18 somatic mutations per tumor, and both pancreatoblastomas had CTNNB1 mutations and SMAD4 mutations.

## SOLID-PSEUDOPAPILLARY NEOPLASM

SPN has distinctive histologic and molecular characteristics. Early studies revealed that 83% to 90% of SPNs have CTNNB1 exon 3 mutations in addition to aberrant nuclear expression of beta-catenin.[154,155] Cyclin D1, a cell cycle regulator of the G1/S transition and that lies in the downstream of Wnt/beta-catenin pathway, is overexpressed in SPN.[154,155]

For PDAC-related genes, no KRAS mutations were noted.[47,79,139,155] Strong nuclear expression of TP53 protein and/or somatic mutations of TP53 were rare in SPN.[79,139,155] However, pleomorphic variant of SPN showed strong TP53 immunostaining in more than half of cases (65%, 11/17), and was shown to harbor TP53 mutations in some cases (3/9).[156] CDKN2A and SMAD4 are retained in SPN.[79,139,155]

Chromosomal alterations in SPN have been investigated by multiple groups. A recent array CGH study of 12 SPNs showed that SPN generally had no chromosomal changes or a low number of chromosomal changes; one-third of the cases (4/12) had no changes, and the remaining two-thirds of the cases had 4 common chromosomal gains at 13q, 17q, 1q, and 8q.[157]

The SPN genome is stable, with few mutations and chromosomal copy number changes except one "mountain" (CTNNB1). Whole exome sequencing of 8 SPNs revealed that the genome of SPN contained an average of just 2.9 mutations per tumor.[79] CTNNB1 mutations were targeted in all cases (8/8). In addition, chromosomal structural changes were not observed in 7/8 of SPNs.[79]

## DIAGNOSTIC AND THERAPEUTIC IMPLICATIONS

Currently, the exomes of the major histologic types of pancreatic neoplasms have been sequenced and their genetic characteristics are known (Table 2). KRAS mutation is prevalent in ductal neoplasms including PDAC, IPMN, and MCN. GNAS is highly specific to IPMN, and 90% of IPMNs have KRAS and/or GNAS mutations. RNF43 is frequently mutated in IPMN and MCN as well as in a small fraction of PDACs. MEN1, DAXX, and ATRX are specifically mutated in PanNET; CTNNB1 is specifically mutated in SPN, pancreatoblastoma and a small proportion of ACCs; and VHL is specifically mutated in SCA. ACC can have a variety of cancer-related genes in addition to APC/CTTNB1. The recent discoveries of the YY1 T372R mutation and the BRAF/RAF1 translocation may also have potential diagnostic utility once evidence has been accumulated.

Based on these pieces of information, some of the genetic alterations can be applied to the practice of surgical pathology. KRAS mutation analysis is considered a useful adjunct to the histologic diagnosis of PDAC, particularly when diagnosing small tissues obtained by endoscopic ultrasound-guided fine needle aspiration (EUS-FNA).[158] Genetic analysis of a panel of genes including KRAS, GNAS, RNF43, VHL, and CTNNB1 and an LOH/aneuploidy analysis of chromosomes 3, 9, 17, and 18 revealed that these were promising

**Table 2**
**Frequently mutated genes in pancreatic neoplasms**

| Histology | Gene Symbol | Prevalence | Major Alterations | Reference |
|---|---|---|---|---|
| PDAC | KRAS | >90% | Missense mutation (hot spots: codons 12, 13 and 61) | [2–4] and others |
| | TP53 | 50%–80% | NSM, LOH | [7–13] |
| | CDKN2A/P16 | 95% | NSM, LOH, homozygous deletion, methylation | [15–17] |
| | SMAD4 | 30%–60% | NSM, LOH, homozygous deletion | [10–13,22–24] |
| IPMN | KRAS | 50%–80% | Missense mutation (hot spots: codons 12, 13, and 61) | [45,47,48,74–77] |
| | TP53 | HGD/invasive carcinoma | NSM, LOH | [46,48,79] |
| | GNAS | 41%–66% | Missense mutation (hot spot: codon 201) | [45,47,79,87] |
| | RNF43 | 14%–75% | NSM, LOH | [45,46,48] |
| MCN | KRAS | 6%–50% | Missense mutation (hot spots: codons 12, 13, and 61) | [45,47,99–101] |
| | TP53 | HGD/invasive carcinoma | NSM | [79,103] |
| | RNF43 | 50% | NSM, LOH | [79] |
| SCA | VHL | 10%–50% | NSM, LOH, methylation | [79,100,133,134] |
| SPN | CTNNB1 | 83%–100% | NSM (hot spot: exon 3) | [79,154,155] |
| PanNET | MEN1 | 25%–44% | NSM, LOH | [106–110] |
| | DAXX/ATRX | 43% | NSM | [110] |
| | Genes in mTOR pathway | 15% | | [110,118] |
| | PTEN | 3%–7% | NSM, LOH | [110,118] |
| | TSC2 | 9% | NSM, LOH | [110] |
| | PIK3CA | 1% | NSM | [110] |
| Insulinoma | YY1 | 13%–33% | Missense mutation (hot spot: codon 372) | [128–130] |
| ACC | APC/CTNNB1 | 10%–24% | | [141,142,145,148] |
| | APC | 2%–18% | NSM, LOH, methylation (56%) | [141,142,145,148] |
| | CTNNB1 | 0%–13% | NSM (hot spot: exon 3) | [141,142,145,148] |
| | Common cancer-related genes[a] | 10%–20% (per gene) | NSM | [142,145] |
| | DNA repair genes | 45% | NSM | [145] |
| | BRCA2 | 20% | NSM | [145,149] |
| | BRAF/RAF1 fusion | 23% | Translocation | [145] |
| Pancreatoblastoma | APC/CTNNB1 | 67% | NSM, LOH (APC) | [142,150,153] |

*Abbreviations:* ACC, acinar cell carcinoma; HGD, high-grade dysplasia; IGD, intermediate-grade dysplasia; IPMN, intraductal papillary mucinous neoplasm; LGD, low-grade dysplasia; LOH, loss of heterozygosity; MCN, mucinous cystic neoplasm; mTOR, mammalian target of rapamycin; NSM, nonsynonymous mutation; PanNET, pancreatic neuroendocrine tumor; PDAC, pancreatic ductal adenocarcinoma; SCA, serous cystadenoma; SPN, solid-pseudopapillary neoplasm.
[a] Common cancer-related genes include, eg, SMAD4, TP53, CDKN2A, JAK1, BRAF, RB1, ARID1A, GNAS, MLL3, PTEN.

markers for distinguishing pancreatic cystic neoplasms using cyst fluids (for details, see the review article by Ngamruengphong S, Lennon AM: Analysis of Pancreatic Cyst Fluid, in this issue).[159]

Histologic diagnosis currently provides the most solid basis for clinical decision-making in chemotherapy for patients with pancreatic malignancies, and no genetic biomarkers are available to stratify patients for treatment purposes. However, some genetic alterations show the potential for markers of good response to treatment. For example, patients with PDAC or ACC harboring mutations of DNA double-strand break repair (BRCA1, BRCA2, and PALB2) were documented to respond dramatically to chemotherapy, including mitomycin C, platinum-based drugs, and PARP inhibitors.[13,149,160,161] Defining biomarkers of responsiveness to these drugs is expected to alter the current treatments of PDAC and ACC, and a phase III clinical trial is under way to investigate the efficacy of the PARP-inhibitor Olaparib on PDAC with *BRCA* mutations. In addition, a series of sequencing studies revealed that potentially actionable genetic changes, such as *BRAF*, molecules of the Wnt/beta-catenin pathway (eg, *RNF43, AXIN1/2, APC*), *PIK3CA, HER2* amplification, and *JAK1*, are present in a fraction of PDACs and ACCs.[12,142,145,162,163] As genomic approaches become more widely available and sequencing studies continue to identify clinically relevant subsets of tumors (eg, with differing prognosis, response to therapy), genomic analysis of patient samples will become a key component of personalized medicine. Surgical pathologists will play a critical role in the implementation of these analyses into standard clinical practice. As such, knowledge of these alterations will be critical for the effective practice of pathology in the era of personalized medicine so as to provide the best possible care for patients with pancreatic neoplasms.

## REFERENCES

1. Vogelstein B, Papadopoulos N, Velculescu VE, et al. Cancer genome landscapes. Science 2013; 339:1546–58.
2. Almoguera C, Shibata D, Forrester K, et al. Most human carcinomas of the exocrine pancreas contain mutant c-K-ras genes. Cell 1988;53: 549–54.
3. Smit VT, Boot AJ, Smits AM, et al. KRAS codon 12 mutations occur very frequently in pancreatic adenocarcinomas. Nucleic Acids Res 1988;16: 7773–82.
4. Hruban RH, van Mansfeld AD, Offerhaus GJ, et al. K-ras oncogene activation in adenocarcinoma of the human pancreas. A study of 82 carcinomas using a combination of mutant-enriched polymerase chain reaction analysis and allele-specific oligonucleotide hybridization. Am J Pathol 1993;143: 545–54.
5. Pylayeva-Gupta Y, Grabocka E, Bar-Sagi D. RAS oncogenes: weaving a tumorigenic web. Nat Rev Cancer 2011;11:761–74.
6. Berndt N, Hamilton AD, Sebti SM. Targeting protein prenylation for cancer therapy. Nat Rev Cancer 2011;11:775–91.
7. Scarpa A, Capelli P, Mukai K, et al. Pancreatic adenocarcinomas frequently show p53 gene mutations. Am J Pathol 1993;142:1534–43.
8. Pellegata NS, Sessa F, Renault B, et al. K-ras and p53 gene mutations in pancreatic cancer: ductal and nonductal tumors progress through different genetic lesions. Cancer Res 1994;54:1556–60.
9. Redston MS, Caldas C, Seymour AB, et al. p53 mutations in pancreatic carcinoma and evidence of common involvement of homocopolymer tracts in DNA microdeletions. Cancer Res 1994;54: 3025–33.
10. Jones S, Zhang X, Parsons DW, et al. Core signaling pathways in human pancreatic cancers revealed by global genomic analyses. Science 2008;321:1801–6.
11. Wang L, Tsutsumi S, Kawaguchi T, et al. Whole-exome sequencing of human pancreatic cancers and characterization of genomic instability caused by MLH1 haploinsufficiency and complete deficiency. Genome Res 2012;22:208–19.
12. Witkiewicz AK, McMillan EA, Balaji U, et al. Whole-exome sequencing of pancreatic cancer defines genetic diversity and therapeutic targets. Nat Commun 2015;6:6744.
13. Waddell N, Pajic M, Patch AM, et al. Whole genomes redefine the mutational landscape of pancreatic cancer. Nature 2015;518:495–501.
14. Bieging KT, Mello SS, Attardi LD. Unravelling mechanisms of p53-mediated tumour suppression. Nat Rev Cancer 2014;14:359–70.
15. Caldas C, Hahn SA, da Costa LT, et al. Frequent somatic mutations and homozygous deletions of the p16 (MTS1) gene in pancreatic adenocarcinoma. Nat Genet 1994;8:27–32.
16. Schutte M, Hruban RH, Geradts J, et al. Abrogation of the Rb/p16 tumor-suppressive pathway in virtually all pancreatic carcinomas. Cancer Res 1997; 57:3126–30.
17. Ueki T, Toyota M, Sohn T, et al. Hypermethylation of multiple genes in pancreatic adenocarcinoma. Cancer Res 2000;60:1835–9.
18. Kim WY, Sharpless NE. The regulation of INK4/ARF in cancer and aging. Cell 2006;127:265–75.
19. Geradts J, Hruban RH, Schutte M, et al. Immunohistochemical p16INK4a analysis of archival tumors with deletion, hypermethylation, or mutation of the CDKN2/MTS1 gene. A comparison of four commercial antibodies. Appl Immunohistochem Mol Morphol 2000;8:71–9.
20. Ohtsubo K, Watanabe H, Yamaguchi Y, et al. Abnormalities of tumor suppressor gene p16 in pancreatic carcinoma: immunohistochemical and genetic findings compared with clinicopathological parameters. J Gastroenterol 2003;38:663–71.
21. Hustinx SR, Hruban RH, Leoni LM, et al. Homozygous deletion of the MTAP gene in invasive adenocarcinoma of the pancreas and in periampullary cancer: a potential new target for therapy. Cancer Biol Ther 2005;4:83–6.

22. Hahn SA, Schutte M, Hoque AT, et al. DPC4, a candidate tumor suppressor gene at human chromosome 18q21.1. Science 1996;271:350–3.

23. Hahn SA, Hoque AT, Moskaluk CA, et al. Homozygous deletion map at 18q21.1 in pancreatic cancer. Cancer Res 1996;56:490–4.

24. Iacobuzio-Donahue CA, Song J, Parmiagiani G, et al. Missense mutations of MADH4: characterization of the mutational hot spot and functional consequences in human tumors. Clin Cancer Res 2004;10:1597–604.

25. Siegel PM, Massague J. Cytostatic and apoptotic actions of TGF-beta in homeostasis and cancer. Nat Rev Cancer 2003;3:807–21.

26. Wilentz RE, Su GH, Dai JL, et al. Immunohistochemical labeling for dpc4 mirrors genetic status in pancreatic adenocarcinomas: a new marker of DPC4 inactivation. Am J Pathol 2000;156:37–43.

27. Tascilar M, Skinner HG, Rosty C, et al. The SMAD4 protein and prognosis of pancreatic ductal adenocarcinoma. Clin Cancer Res 2001;7:4115–21.

28. Biankin AV, Morey AL, Lee CS, et al. DPC4/Smad4 expression and outcome in pancreatic ductal adenocarcinoma. J Clin Oncol 2002;20:4531–42.

29. Toga T, Nio Y, Hashimoto K, et al. The dissociated expression of protein and messenger RNA of DPC4 in human invasive ductal carcinoma of the pancreas and their implication for patient outcome. Anticancer Res 2004;24:1173–8.

30. Blackford A, Serrano OK, Wolfgang CL, et al. SMAD4 gene mutations are associated with poor prognosis in pancreatic cancer. Clin Cancer Res 2009;15:4674–9.

31. Iacobuzio-Donahue CA, Fu B, Yachida S, et al. DPC4 gene status of the primary carcinoma correlates with patterns of failure in patients with pancreatic cancer. J Clin Oncol 2009;27:1806–13.

32. Biankin AV, Waddell N, Kassahn KS, et al. Pancreatic cancer genomes reveal aberrations in axon guidance pathway genes. Nature 2012;491:399–405.

33. Wilson BG, Roberts CW. SWI/SNF nucleosome remodellers and cancer. Nat Rev Cancer 2011;11:481–92.

34. Burrell RA, McGranahan N, Bartek J, et al. The causes and consequences of genetic heterogeneity in cancer evolution. Nature 2013;501:338–45.

35. Yachida S, Jones S, Bozic I, et al. Distant metastasis occurs late during the genetic evolution of pancreatic cancer. Nature 2010;467:1114–7.

36. Campbell PJ, Yachida S, Mudie LJ, et al. The patterns and dynamics of genomic instability in metastatic pancreatic cancer. Nature 2010;467:1109–13.

37. Mahlamaki EH, Hoglund M, Gorunova L, et al. Comparative genomic hybridization reveals frequent gains of 20q, 8q, 11q, 12p, and 17q, and losses of 18q, 9p, and 15q in pancreatic cancer. Genes Chromosomes Cancer 1997;20:383–91.

38. Aguirre AJ, Brennan C, Bailey G, et al. High-resolution characterization of the pancreatic adenocarcinoma genome. Proc Natl Acad Sci U S A 2004;101:9067–72.

39. Holzmann K, Kohlhammer H, Schwaenen C, et al. Genomic DNA-chip hybridization reveals a higher incidence of genomic amplifications in pancreatic cancer than conventional comparative genomic hybridization and leads to the identification of novel candidate genes. Cancer Res 2004;64:4428–33.

40. Griffin CA, Morsberger L, Hawkins AL, et al. Molecular cytogenetic characterization of pancreas cancer cell lines reveals high complexity chromosomal alterations. Cytogenet Genome Res 2007;118:148–56.

41. Harada T, Chelala C, Bhakta V, et al. Genome-wide DNA copy number analysis in pancreatic cancer using high-density single nucleotide polymorphism arrays. Oncogene 2008;27:1951–60.

42. Alexandrov LB, Nik-Zainal S, Wedge DC, et al. Signatures of mutational processes in human cancer. Nature 2013;500:415–21.

43. Farmer H, McCabe N, Lord CJ, et al. Targeting the DNA repair defect in BRCA mutant cells as a therapeutic strategy. Nature 2005;434:917–21.

44. Seidel G, Zahurak M, Iacobuzio-Donahue C, et al. Almost all infiltrating colloid carcinomas of the pancreas and periampullary region arise from in situ papillary neoplasms: a study of 39 cases. Am J Surg Pathol 2002;26:56–63.

45. Wu J, Matthaei H, Maitra A, et al. Recurrent GNAS mutations define an unexpected pathway for pancreatic cyst development. Sci Transl Med 2011;3:92ra66.

46. Amato E, Molin MD, Mafficini A, et al. Targeted next-generation sequencing of cancer genes dissects the molecular profiles of intraductal papillary neoplasms of the pancreas. J Pathol 2014;233:217–27.

47. Hosoda W, Sasaki E, Murakami Y, et al. GNAS mutation is a frequent event in pancreatic intraductal papillary mucinous neoplasms and associated adenocarcinomas. Virchows Arch 2015;466:665–74.

48. Tan MC, Basturk O, Brannon AR, et al. GNAS and KRAS mutations define separate progression pathways in intraductal papillary mucinous neoplasm-associated carcinoma. J Am Coll Surg 2015;220:845–54.e1.

49. Brody JR, Costantino CL, Potoczek M, et al. Adenosquamous carcinoma of the pancreas harbors KRAS2, DPC4 and TP53 molecular alterations similar to pancreatic ductal adenocarcinoma. Mod Pathol 2009;22:651–9.

50. Liu C, Karam R, Zhou Y, et al. The UPF1 RNA surveillance gene is commonly mutated in pancreatic

adenosquamous carcinoma. Nat Med 2014;20: 596–8.

51. Goggins M, Offerhaus GJ, Hilgers W, et al. Pancreatic adenocarcinomas with DNA replication errors (RER+) are associated with wild-type K-ras and characteristic histopathology. Poor differentiation, a syncytial growth pattern, and pushing borders suggest RER+. Am J Pathol 1998;152:1501–7.

52. Wilentz RE, Goggins M, Redston M, et al. Genetic, immunohistochemical, and clinical features of medullary carcinoma of the pancreas: a newly described and characterized entity. Am J Pathol 2000;156:1641–51.

53. Yamamoto H, Itoh F, Nakamura H, et al. Genetic and clinical features of human pancreatic ductal adenocarcinomas with widespread microsatellite instability. Cancer Res 2001;61:3139–44.

54. Calhoun ES, Jones JB, Ashfaq R, et al. BRAF and FBXW7 (CDC4, FBW7, AGO, SEL10) mutations in distinct subsets of pancreatic cancer: potential therapeutic targets. Am J Pathol 2003;163: 1255–60.

55. Maple JT, Smyrk TC, Boardman LA, et al. Defective DNA mismatch repair in long-term (> or =3 years) survivors with pancreatic cancer. Pancreatology 2005;5:220–7, [discussion: 7–8].

56. Laghi L, Beghelli S, Spinelli A, et al. Irrelevance of microsatellite instability in the epidemiology of sporadic pancreatic ductal adenocarcinoma. PLoS One 2012;7:e46002.

57. Banville N, Geraghty R, Fox E, et al. Medullary carcinoma of the pancreas in a man with hereditary nonpolyposis colorectal cancer due to a mutation of the MSH2 mismatch repair gene. Hum Pathol 2006;37:1498–502.

58. Feldmann G, Beaty R, Hruban RH, et al. Molecular genetics of pancreatic intraepithelial neoplasia. J Hepatobiliary Pancreat Surg 2007;14:224–32.

59. van Heek NT, Meeker AK, Kern SE, et al. Telomere shortening is nearly universal in pancreatic intraepithelial neoplasia. Am J Pathol 2002;161:1541–7.

60. Matsuda Y, Ishiwata T, Izumiyama-Shimomura N, et al. Gradual telomere shortening and increasing chromosomal instability among PanIN grades and normal ductal epithelia with and without cancer in the pancreas. PLoS One 2015;10:e0117575.

61. Lohr M, Kloppel G, Maisonneuve P, et al. Frequency of K-ras mutations in pancreatic intraductal neoplasias associated with pancreatic ductal adenocarcinoma and chronic pancreatitis: a meta-analysis. Neoplasia 2005;7:17–23.

62. Kanda M, Matthaei H, Wu J, et al. Presence of somatic mutations in most early-stage pancreatic intraepithelial neoplasia. Gastroenterology 2012; 142:730–3.e9.

63. Wilentz RE, Geradts J, Maynard R, et al. Inactivation of the p16 (INK4A) tumor-suppressor gene in pancreatic duct lesions: loss of intranuclear expression. Cancer Res 1998;58:4740–4.

64. Rosty C, Geradts J, Sato N, et al. p16 inactivation in pancreatic intraepithelial neoplasias (PanINs) arising in patients with chronic pancreatitis. Am J Surg Pathol 2003;27:1495–501.

65. Furukawa T, Fujisaki R, Yoshida Y, et al. Distinct progression pathways involving the dysfunction of DUSP6/MKP-3 in pancreatic intraepithelial neoplasia and intraductal papillary-mucinous neoplasms of the pancreas. Mod Pathol 2005;18:1034–42.

66. Hustinx SR, Leoni LM, Yeo CJ, et al. Concordant loss of MTAP and p16/CDKN2A expression in pancreatic intraepithelial neoplasia: evidence of homozygous deletion in a noninvasive precursor lesion. Mod Pathol 2005;18:959–63.

67. Fukushima N, Sato N, Ueki T, et al. Aberrant methylation of preproenkephalin and p16 genes in pancreatic intraepithelial neoplasia and pancreatic ductal adenocarcinoma. Am J Pathol 2002;160: 1573–81.

68. Wilentz RE, Iacobuzio-Donahue CA, Argani P, et al. Loss of expression of Dpc4 in pancreatic intraepithelial neoplasia: evidence that DPC4 inactivation occurs late in neoplastic progression. Cancer Res 2000;60:2002–6.

69. Luttges J, Galehdari H, Brocker V, et al. Allelic loss is often the first hit in the biallelic inactivation of the p53 and DPC4 genes during pancreatic carcinogenesis. Am J Pathol 2001;158:1677–83.

70. Murphy SJ, Hart SN, Lima JF, et al. Genetic alterations associated with progression from pancreatic intraepithelial neoplasia to invasive pancreatic tumor. Gastroenterology 2013;145:1098–109.e1.

71. Abraham SC, Wilentz RE, Yeo CJ, et al. Pancreaticoduodenectomy (Whipple resections) in patients without malignancy: are they all 'chronic pancreatitis'? Am J Surg Pathol 2003;27:110–20.

72. Andea A, Sarkar F, Adsay VN. Clinicopathological correlates of pancreatic intraepithelial neoplasia: a comparative analysis of 82 cases with and 152 cases without pancreatic ductal adenocarcinoma. Mod Pathol 2003;16:996–1006.

73. Konstantinidis IT, Vinuela EF, Tang LH, et al. Incidentally discovered pancreatic intraepithelial neoplasia: what is its clinical significance? Ann Surg Oncol 2013;20:3643–7.

74. Z'Graggen K, Rivera JA, Compton CC, et al. Prevalence of activating K-ras mutations in the evolutionary stages of neoplasia in intraductal papillary mucinous tumors of the pancreas. Ann Surg 1997;226:491–8, [discussion: 498–500].

75. Schonleben F, Qiu W, Remotti HE, et al. PIK3CA, KRAS, and BRAF mutations in intraductal papillary mucinous neoplasm/carcinoma (IPMN/C) of the pancreas. Langenbecks Arch Surg 2008;393: 289–96.

76. Chadwick B, Willmore-Payne C, Tripp S, et al. His-tologic, immunohistochemical, and molecular clas-sification of 52 IPMNs of the pancreas. Appl Immunohistochem Mol Morphol 2009;17:31–9.

77. Kuboki Y, Shimizu K, Hatori T, et al. Molecular bio-markers for progression of intraductal papillary mucinous neoplasm of the pancreas. Pancreas 2015;44:227–35.

78. Satoh K, Shimosegawa T, Moriizumi S, et al. K-ras mutation and p53 protein accumulation in intraduc-tal mucin-hypersecreting neoplasms of the pancreas. Pancreas 1996;12:362–8.

79. Wu J, Jiao Y, Dal Molin M, et al. Whole-exome sequencing of neoplastic cysts of the pancreas re-veals recurrent mutations in components of ubiquitin-dependent pathways. Proc Natl Acad Sci U S A 2011;108:21188–93.

80. Fujii H, Inagaki M, Kasai S, et al. Genetic progres-sion and heterogeneity in intraductal papillary-mucinous neoplasms of the pancreas. Am J Pathol 1997;151:1447–54.

81. Abe T, Fukushima N, Brune K, et al. Genome-wide al-lelotypes of familial pancreatic adenocarcinomas and familial and sporadic intraductal papillary mucinous neoplasms. Clin Cancer Res 2007;13:6019–25.

82. Fritz S, Fernandez-del Castillo C, Mino-Kenudson M, et al. Global genomic analysis of intraductal papil-lary mucinous neoplasms of the pancreas reveals significant molecular differences compared to ductal adenocarcinoma. Ann Surg 2009;249:440–7.

83. Biankin AV, Biankin SA, Kench JG, et al. Aberrant p16(INK4A) and DPC4/Smad4 expression in intra-ductal papillary mucinous tumours of the pancreas is associated with invasive ductal adenocarci-noma. Gut 2002;50:861–8.

84. Mohri D, Asaoka Y, Ijichi H, et al. Different subtypes of intraductal papillary mucinous neoplasm in the pancreas have distinct pathways to pancreatic cancer progression. J Gastroenterol 2012;47:203–13.

85. Sato N, Ueki T, Fukushima N, et al. Aberrant methyl-ation of CpG islands in intraductal papillary mucinous neoplasms of the pancreas. Gastroenter-ology 2002;123:365–72.

86. Iacobuzio-Donahue CA, Klimstra DS, Adsay NV, et al. Dpc-4 protein is expressed in virtually all human intraductal papillary mucinous neoplasms of the pancreas: comparison with conventional ductal adenocarcinomas. Am J Pathol 2000;157:755–61.

87. Furukawa T, Kuboki Y, Tanji E, et al. Whole-exome sequencing uncovers frequent GNAS mutations in intraductal papillary mucinous neoplasms of the pancreas. Sci Rep 2011;1:161.

88. Weinstein LS, Liu J, Sakamoto A, et al. Minireview: GNAS: normal and abnormal functions. Endocri-nology 2004;145:5459–64.

89. Komatsu H, Tanji E, Sakata N, et al. A GNAS muta-tion found in pancreatic intraductal papillary mucinous neoplasms induces drastic alterations of gene expression profiles with upregulation of mucin genes. PLoS One 2014;9:e87875.

90. Dal Molin M, Matthaei H, Wu J, et al. Clinicopatho-logical correlates of activating GNAS mutations in intraductal papillary mucinous neoplasm (IPMN) of the pancreas. Ann Surg Oncol 2013;20(12):3802–8.

91. Dal Molin M, Zhang M, de Wilde RF, et al. Very long-term survival following resection for pancre-atic cancer is not explained by commonly mutated genes: results of whole-exome sequencing anal-ysis. Clin Cancer Res 2015;21:1944–50.

92. Schonleben F, Qiu W, Bruckman KC, et al. BRAF and KRAS gene mutations in intraductal papillary mucinous neoplasm/carcinoma (IPMN/IPMC) of the pancreas. Cancer Lett 2007;249:242–8.

93. Schonleben F, Qiu W, Ciau NT, et al. PIK3CA muta-tions in intraductal papillary mucinous neoplasm/carcinoma of the pancreas. Clin Cancer Res 2006;12:3851–5.

94. Lubezky N, Ben-Haim M, Marmor S, et al. High-throughput mutation profiling in intraductal papil-lary mucinous neoplasm (IPMN). J Gastrointest Surg 2011;15:503–11.

95. Yamaguchi H, Kuboki Y, Hatori T, et al. The discrete nature and distinguishing molecular features of pancreatic intraductal tubulopapillary neoplasms and intraductal papillary mucinous neoplasms of the gastric type, pyloric gland variant. J Pathol 2013;231:335–41.

96. Garcia-Carracedo D, Turk AT, Fine SA, et al. Loss of PTEN expression is associated with poor prognosis in patients with intraductal papillary mucinous neo-plasms of the pancreas. Clin Cancer Res 2013;19:6830–41.

97. Sato N, Rosty C, Jansen M, et al. STK11/LKB1 Peutz-Jeghers gene inactivation in intraductal papillary-mucinous neoplasms of the pancreas. Am J Pathol 2001;159:2017–22.

98. Yamaguchi H, Shimizu M, Ban S, et al. Intraductal tubulopapillary neoplasms of the pancreas distinct from pancreatic intraepithelial neoplasia and intra-ductal papillary mucinous neoplasms. Am J Surg Pathol 2009;33:1164–72.

99. Jimenez RE, Warshaw AL, Z'Graggen K, et al. Sequential accumulation of K-ras mutations and p53 overexpression in the progression of pancreatic mucinous cystic neoplasms to malignancy. Ann Surg 1999;230:501–9, [discussion: 9–11].

100. Kim SG, Wu TT, Lee JH, et al. Comparison of epige-netic and genetic alterations in mucinous cystic neoplasm and serous microcystic adenoma of pancreas. Mod Pathol 2003;16:1086–94.

101. Kuboki Y, Shiratori K, Hatori T, et al. Association of epidermal growth factor receptor and mitogen-activated protein kinase with cystic neoplasms of the pancreas. Mod Pathol 2010;23:1127–35.

102. Zamboni G, Scarpa A, Bogina G, et al. Mucinous cystic tumors of the pancreas: clinicopathological features, prognosis, and relationship to other mucinous cystic tumors. Am J Surg Pathol 1999; 23:410–22.

103. Gerdes B, Wild A, Wittenberg J, et al. Tumor-suppressing pathways in cystic pancreatic tumors. Pancreas 2003;26:42–8.

104. Iacobuzio-Donahue CA, Wilentz RE, Argani P, et al. Dpc4 protein in mucinous cystic neoplasms of the pancreas: frequent loss of expression in invasive carcinomas suggests a role in genetic progression. Am J Surg Pathol 2000;24:1544–8.

105. Garcia-Carracedo D, Chen ZM, Qiu W, et al. PIK3CA mutations in mucinous cystic neoplasms of the pancreas. Pancreas 2014;43:245–9.

106. Zhuang Z, Vortmeyer AO, Pack S, et al. Somatic mutations of the MEN1 tumor suppressor gene in sporadic gastrinomas and insulinomas. Cancer Res 1997;57:4682–6.

107. Wang EH, Ebrahimi SA, Wu AY, et al. Mutation of the MENIN gene in sporadic pancreatic endocrine tumors. Cancer Res 1998;58:4417–20.

108. Hessman O, Lindberg D, Skogseid B, et al. Mutation of the multiple endocrine neoplasia type 1 gene in nonfamilial, malignant tumors of the endocrine pancreas. Cancer Res 1998;58:377–9.

109. Corbo V, Dalai I, Scardoni M, et al. MEN1 in pancreatic endocrine tumors: analysis of gene and protein status in 169 sporadic neoplasms reveals alterations in the vast majority of cases. Endocr Relat Cancer 2010;17:771–83.

110. Jiao Y, Shi C, Edil BH, et al. DAXX/ATRX, MEN1, and mTOR pathway genes are frequently altered in pancreatic neuroendocrine tumors. Science 2011;331:1199–203.

111. Beghelli S, Pelosi G, Zamboni G, et al. Pancreatic endocrine tumours: evidence for a tumour suppressor pathogenesis and for a tumour suppressor gene on chromosome 17p. J Pathol 1998;186: 41–50.

112. Chung DC, Brown SB, Graeme-Cook F, et al. Localization of putative tumor suppressor loci by genome-wide allelotyping in human pancreatic endocrine tumors. Cancer Res 1998;58:3706–11.

113. Gortz B, Roth J, Krahenmann A, et al. Mutations and allelic deletions of the MEN1 gene are associated with a subset of sporadic endocrine pancreatic and neuroendocrine tumors and not restricted to foregut neoplasms. Am J Pathol 1999;154:429–36.

114. Moore PS, Missiaglia E, Antonello D, et al. Role of disease-causing genes in sporadic pancreatic endocrine tumors: MEN1 and VHL. Genes Chromosomes Cancer 2001;32:177–81.

115. Liu P, Cheng H, Roberts TM, et al. Targeting the phosphoinositide 3-kinase pathway in cancer. Nat Rev Drug Discov 2009;8:627–44.

116. Speel EJ, Richter J, Moch H, et al. Genetic differences in endocrine pancreatic tumor subtypes detected by comparative genomic hybridization. Am J Pathol 1999;155:1787–94.

117. Rigaud G, Missiaglia E, Moore PS, et al. High resolution allelotype of nonfunctional pancreatic endocrine tumors: identification of two molecular subgroups with clinical implications. Cancer Res 2001;61:285–92.

118. Perren A, Komminoth P, Saremaslani P, et al. Mutation and expression analyses reveal differential subcellular compartmentalization of PTEN in endocrine pancreatic tumors compared to normal islet cells. Am J Pathol 2000;157:1097–103.

119. Missiaglia E, Dalai I, Barbi S, et al. Pancreatic endocrine tumors: expression profiling evidences a role for AKT-mTOR pathway. J Clin Oncol 2010; 28:245–55.

120. Yao JC, Shah MH, Ito T, et al. Everolimus for advanced pancreatic neuroendocrine tumors. N Engl J Med 2011;364:514–23.

121. Heaphy CM, de Wilde RF, Jiao Y, et al. Altered telomeres in tumors with ATRX and DAXX mutations. Science 2011;333:425.

122. Lewis PW, Elsaesser SJ, Noh KM, et al. Daxx is an H3.3-specific histone chaperone and cooperates with ATRX in replication-independent chromatin assembly at telomeres. Proc Natl Acad Sci U S A 2010;107:14075–80.

123. Clynes D, Higgs DR, Gibbons RJ. The chromatin remodeller ATRX: a repeat offender in human disease. Trends Biochem Sci 2013;38:461–6.

124. Bryan TM, Englezou A, Dalla-Pozza L, et al. Evidence for an alternative mechanism for maintaining telomere length in human tumors and tumor-derived cell lines. Nat Med 1997;3:1271–4.

125. Marinoni I, Kurrer AS, Vassella E, et al. Loss of DAXX and ATRX are associated with chromosome instability and reduced survival of patients with pancreatic neuroendocrine tumors. Gastroenterology 2014;146:453–60.e5.

126. Heaphy CM, Subhawong AP, Hong SM, et al. Prevalence of the alternative lengthening of telomeres telomere maintenance mechanism in human cancer subtypes. Am J Pathol 2011;179: 1608–15.

127. de Wilde RF, Heaphy CM, Maitra A, et al. Loss of ATRX or DAXX expression and concomitant acquisition of the alternative lengthening of telomeres phenotype are late events in a small subset of MEN-1 syndrome pancreatic neuroendocrine tumors. Mod Pathol 2012;25:1033–9.

128. Cao Y, Gao Z, Li L, et al. Whole exome sequencing of insulinoma reveals recurrent T372R mutations in YY1. Nat Commun 2013;4:2810.

129. Cromer MK, Choi M, Nelson-Williams C, et al. Neomorphic effects of recurrent somatic mutations in Yin Yang 1 in insulin-producing adenomas. Proc Natl Acad Sci U S A 2015;112:4062–7.

130. Lichtenauer UD, Di Dalmazi G, Slater EP, et al. Frequency and clinical correlates of somatic Ying Yang 1 mutations in sporadic insulinomas. J Clin Endocrinol Metab 2015;100:E776–82.

131. Ohki R, Saito K, Chen Y, et al. PHLDA3 is a novel tumor suppressor of pancreatic neuroendocrine tumors. Proc Natl Acad Sci U S A 2014;111:E2404–13.

132. Jonkers YM, Ramaekers FC, Speel EJ. Molecular alterations during insulinoma tumorigenesis. Biochim Biophys Acta 2007;1775:313–32.

133. Vortmeyer AO, Lubensky IA, Fogt F, et al. Allelic deletion and mutation of the von Hippel-Lindau (VHL) tumor suppressor gene in pancreatic microcystic adenomas. Am J Pathol 1997;151:951–6.

134. Moore PS, Zamboni G, Brighenti A, et al. Molecular characterization of pancreatic serous microcystic adenomas: evidence for a tumor suppressor gene on chromosome 10q. Am J Pathol 2001;158:317–21.

135. Ishikawa T, Nakao A, Nomoto S, et al. Immunohistochemical and molecular biological studies of serous cystadenoma of the pancreas. Pancreas 1998;16:40–4.

136. Yamaguchi K, Chijiiwa K, Noshiro H, et al. Ki-ras codon 12 point mutation and p53 mutation in pancreatic diseases. Hepatogastroenterology 1999;46:2575–81.

137. Hoorens A, Lemoine NR, McLellan E, et al. Pancreatic acinar cell carcinoma. An analysis of cell lineage markers, p53 expression, and Ki-ras mutation. Am J Pathol 1993;143:685–98.

138. Terhune PG, Heffess CS, Longnecker DS. Only wild-type c-Ki-ras codons 12, 13, and 61 in human pancreatic acinar cell carcinomas. Mol Carcinog 1994;10:110–4.

139. Moore PS, Orlandini S, Zamboni G, et al. Pancreatic tumours: molecular pathways implicated in ductal cancer are involved in ampullary but not in exocrine nonductal or endocrine tumorigenesis. Br J Cancer 2001;84:253–62.

140. de Wilde RF, Ottenhof NA, Jansen M, et al. Analysis of LKB1 mutations and other molecular alterations in pancreatic acinar cell carcinoma. Mod Pathol 2011;24:1229–36.

141. Furlan D, Sahnane N, Bernasconi B, et al. APC alterations are frequently involved in the pathogenesis of acinar cell carcinoma of the pancreas, mainly through gene loss and promoter hypermethylation. Virchows Arch 2014;464:553–64.

142. Jiao Y, Yonescu R, Offerhaus GJ, et al. Whole-exome sequencing of pancreatic neoplasms with acinar differentiation. J Pathol 2014;232:428–35.

143. Bergmann F, Aulmann S, Sipos B, et al. Acinar cell carcinomas of the pancreas: a molecular analysis in a series of 57 cases. Virchows Arch 2014;465:661–72.

144. Terhune PG, Memoli VA, Longnecker DS. Evaluation of p53 mutation in pancreatic acinar cell carcinomas of humans and transgenic mice. Pancreas 1998;16:6–12.

145. Chmielecki J, Hutchinson KE, Frampton GM, et al. Comprehensive genomic profiling of pancreatic acinar cell carcinomas identifies recurrent RAF fusions and frequent inactivation of DNA repair genes. Cancer Discov 2014;4:1398–405.

146. Rigaud G, Moore PS, Zamboni G, et al. Allelotype of pancreatic acinar cell carcinoma. Int J Cancer 2000;88:772–7.

147. Taruscio D, Paradisi S, Zamboni G, et al. Pancreatic acinar carcinoma shows a distinct pattern of chromosomal imbalances by comparative genomic hybridization. Genes Chromosomes Cancer 2000;28:294–9.

148. Abraham SC, Wu TT, Hruban RH, et al. Genetic and immunohistochemical analysis of pancreatic acinar cell carcinoma: frequent allelic loss on chromosome 11p and alterations in the APC/beta-catenin pathway. Am J Pathol 2002;160:953–62.

149. Furukawa T, Sakamoto H, Takeuchi S, et al. Whole exome sequencing reveals recurrent mutations in BRCA2 and FAT genes in acinar cell carcinomas of the pancreas. Sci Rep 2015;5:8829.

150. Abraham SC, Wu TT, Klimstra DS, et al. Distinctive molecular genetic alterations in sporadic and familial adenomatous polyposis-associated pancreatoblastomas: frequent alterations in the APC/beta-catenin pathway and chromosome 11p. Am J Pathol 2001;159:1619–27.

151. Giardiello FM, Petersen GM, Brensinger JD, et al. Hepatoblastoma and APC gene mutation in familial adenomatous polyposis. Gut 1996;39:867–9.

152. Blaker H, Hofmann WJ, Rieker RJ, et al. Beta-catenin accumulation and mutation of the CTNNB1 gene in hepatoblastoma. Genes Chromosomes Cancer 1999;25:399–402.

153. Kerr NJ, Fukuzawa R, Reeve AE, et al. Beckwith-Wiedemann syndrome, pancreatoblastoma, and the wnt signaling pathway. Am J Pathol 2002;160:1541–2, [author reply: 1542].

154. Tanaka Y, Kato K, Notohara K, et al. Frequent beta-catenin mutation and cytoplasmic/nuclear accumulation in pancreatic solid-pseudopapillary neoplasm. Cancer Res 2001;61:8401–4.

155. Abraham SC, Klimstra DS, Wilentz RE, et al. Solid-pseudopapillary tumors of the pancreas are genetically distinct from pancreatic ductal adenocarcinomas and almost always harbor beta-catenin mutations. Am J Pathol 2002;160:1361–9.

156. Kim SA, Kim MS, Kim MS, et al. Pleomorphic solid pseudopapillary neoplasm of the pancreas: degenerative change rather than high-grade malignant potential. Hum Pathol 2014;45:166–74.

157. Rund CR, Moser AJ, Lee KK, et al. Array comparative genomic hybridization analysis of solid pseudopapillary neoplasms of the pancreas. Mod Pathol 2008;21:559–64.

158. Fuccio L, Hassan C, Laterza L, et al. The role of K-ras gene mutation analysis in EUS-guided FNA cytology specimens for the differential diagnosis of pancreatic solid masses: a meta-analysis of prospective studies. Gastrointest Endosc 2013;78:596–608.

159. Springer S, Wang Y, Dal Molin M, et al. A combination of molecular markers and clinical features improve the classification of pancreatic cysts. Gastroenterology 2015;149:1501–10.

160. Villarroel MC, Rajeshkumar NV, Garrido-Laguna I, et al. Personalizing cancer treatment in the age of global genomic analyses: PALB2 gene mutations and the response to DNA damaging agents in pancreatic cancer. Mol Cancer Ther 2011;10:3–8.

161. Kaufman B, Shapira-Frommer R, Schmutzler RK, et al. Olaparib monotherapy in patients with advanced cancer and a germline BRCA1/2 mutation. J Clin Oncol 2015;33:244–50.

162. Jiang X, Hao HX, Growney JD, et al. Inactivating mutations of RNF43 confer Wnt dependency in pancreatic ductal adenocarcinoma. Proc Natl Acad Sci U S A 2013;110:12649–54.

163. Chantrill LA, Nagrial AM, Watson C, et al. Precision medicine for advanced pancreas cancer: the Individualized Molecular Pancreatic Cancer Therapy (IMPaCT) trial. Clin Cancer Res 2015;21:2029–37.

# Genetic Syndromes with Pancreatic Manifestations

 CrossMark

Meredith E. Pittman, MD[a], Lodewijk A.A. Brosens, MD, PhD[b],
Laura D. Wood, MD, PhD[c],*

## KEYWORDS

- Pancreatic cancer • Genetics • Familial syndromes

## Key points

- Familial pancreatic cancer accounts for approximately 10% of pancreatic ductal adenocarcinomas (PDACs). Although PDAC is a feature of several well-described genetic syndromes and rare germline mutations underlying familial PDAC have recently been identified, the genetic basis for most familial PDAC remains unknown.

- In addition to repeated bouts of pancreatitis, patients with familial pancreatitis (caused by germline mutations in *CFTR*, *PRSS1*, or *SPINK1*) have a markedly increased risk of PDAC, presumably due to repeated rounds of injury and repair in the pancreas.

- Nonductal pancreatic neoplasms also occur in several well-described genetic syndromes and are a key cause of morbidity and mortality in some patients.

## ABSTRACT

Although the pancreas is affected by only a small fraction of known inherited disorders, several of these syndromes predispose patients to pancreatic adenocarcinoma, a cancer that has a consistently dismal prognosis. Still other syndromes are associated with neuroendocrine tumors, benign cysts, or recurrent pancreatitis. Because of the variability of pancreatic manifestations and outcomes, it is important for clinicians to be familiar with several well-described genetic disorders to ensure that patients are followed appropriately. The purpose of this review was to briefly describe the hereditary syndromes that are associated with pancreatic disorders and neoplasia.

## OVERVIEW

Pancreatic adenocarcinoma (PDAC) remains the fourth leading cause of cancer deaths for both men and women in the United States.[1] It is estimated that at least 10% of all pancreatic adenocarcinoma is familial, and a subset of familial PDAC occurs in the setting of well-defined hereditary cancer predisposition syndromes,[2] some of which are widely recognized for other cancer types, such as breast cancer with *BRCA2* mutations, and colon cancer in Lynch syndrome. Because the risk of PDAC rises rapidly (sixfold) when 2 first-degree relatives are affected, it is important to recognize these families for counseling and/or surveillance.[3] Adenocarcinoma is not the only pancreatic manifestation of systemic genetic syndromes (**Table 1**).

The authors have no financial disclosures.

[a] Department of Pathology and Laboratory Medicine, Weill Cornell Medical College, Starr 1031A, 525 East 68th Street, New York, NY 10065, USA; [b] Department of Pathology, University Medical Center Utrecht, Heidelberglaan 100, 3584 CX, Utrecht, The Netherlands; [c] Department of Pathology, The Sol Goldman Pancreatic Cancer Research Center, Johns Hopkins University School of Medicine, CRB2 Room 345, 1550 Orleans Street, Baltimore, MD 21231, USA
* Corresponding author.
*E-mail address:* ldwood@jhmi.edu

Surgical Pathology 9 (2016) 705–715
http://dx.doi.org/10.1016/j.path.2016.05.012

**Table 1**
Genetic syndromes with pancreatic manifestations

| Syndrome | Gene (Chromosome) | Pancreatic Disease |
|---|---|---|
| Familial atypical multiple mole melanoma syndrome (FAMMM) | *CDKN2A* (9p21) | PDAC |
| Hereditary breast and ovarian cancer syndromes | *BRCA1* (17q21) *BRCA2* (13q12) *PALB2* (16p12) | PDAC |
| Lynch syndrome (hereditary nonpolyposis colon cancer) | *MLH1* (3p21) *MSH2* (2p21) *MSH6* (2p16) *PMS2* (7p22) | PDAC |
| Familial adenomatous polyposis (FAP) | *APC* (5q21-22) | PDAC Acinar cell carcinoma Pancreatoblastoma |
| Peutz-Jeghers (PJS) | *STK11/LKB1* (19p13) | PDAC Acinar cell carcinoma IPMN |
| | *ATM* (11q22-23) | PDAC |
| Cystic fibrosis | *CFTR* (7q31) | Pancreatic insufficiency Pancreatitis |
| Hereditary pancreatitis | *PRSS1* (7q34) *SPINK1* (5q32) | Pancreatitis Pseudotumors PDAC |
| Multiple endocrine neoplasia, type 1 (MEN1) | *MEN1* (11q13) | PanNET |
| Von-Hippel Lindau | *VHL* (3p25) | Serous cystadenoma PanNET |
| Neurofibromatosis, type 1 (NF1) | *NF1* (17q11) | PanNET (somatostatinoma) |
| Tuberous sclerosis complex | *TSC1* (9q34) *TSC2* (16p13) | PanNET |
| Beckwith-Wiedemann | Chromosome 11 | Pancreatoblastoma |
| McCune-Albright syndrome | *GNAS* (20q13) | IPMN |

*Abbreviations:* IPMN, intraductal papillary mucinous neoplasm; PanNET, pancreatic neuroendocrine tumor; PDAC, pancreatic ductal adenocarcinoma.

Other neoplasms can involve the pancreas, such as neuroendocrine tumors or pancreatoblastomas. Still other patients inherit a disposition to exocrine pancreatic failure or repeated bouts of pancreatitis. The purpose of this review was to give an overview of the pancreatic manifestations within these syndromic settings.

## HEREDITARY CANCER SYNDROMES ASSOCIATED WITH PANCREATIC DUCTAL ADENOCARCINOMA

### FAMILIAL ATYPICAL MULTIPLE MOLE MELANOMA SYNDROME

The Familial Atypical Multiple Mole Melanoma Syndrome (FAMMM) is generally characterized by patients who have a high count of total body nevi, nevi with atypical features, and melanoma in themselves or relatives, although there is variability in phenotypic expression. FAMMM is inherited as an autosomal dominant condition due to a mutation in the *CDKN2A* gene on chromosome 9p21. *CDKN2A* encodes the p16 protein, an inhibitor of the cyclin D1-cyclin-dependent kinase complex. By inhibiting this complex, p16 prevents phosphorylation of the retinoblastoma protein, effectively acting as a tumor suppressor through regulation of the cell cycle.[4,5]

Although melanoma is the most common cancer in patients with FAMMM, these patients are at increased risk for other cancers as well, with pancreatic adenocarcinoma being the second most common malignancy. Although the risk for PDAC in these families does not vary by gender, it does vary considerably by geographic location. Families with FAMMM in Europe and North America have an association with PDAC; however, pancreatic cancer is not associated with FAMMM in Australian families.[6] This variability in FAMMM phenotype and penetrance can be traced to the founder mutation in each location. For example, the p16 Leiden mutation, a 19 base pair germline deletion that causes a truncated protein, is common in Dutch families.[7] Patients with p16 Leiden have a relative risk of 46 for pancreatic cancer. Similar PDAC risk is also seen in patients with the common Swedish founder mutation (113insArg), and patients with the Italian "Liguria" founder mutation (Gly101Trp) have approximately 10 times the risk of PDAC compared with controls.[8]

FAMMM patients usually have conventional PDAC on histologic examination. Other variations in pancreatic carcinoma that have been reported include adenosquamous carcinoma and undifferentiated carcinoma with osteoclastlike giant cells (Fig. 1). In the latter, the reported patient was a known carrier of the p16 Leiden mutation. DNA analysis showed p16 deletion in the malignant cells while the giant cells retained p16 expression, consistent with the hypothesis that the intratumoral giant cells are reactive and non-neoplastic.[9]

## HEREDITARY BREAST AND OVARIAN CANCER SYNDROMES (BRCA1 AND BRCA2)

Families with mutations in the Fanconi anemia gene pathway are at increased risk for malignancy, as the proteins encoded by these genes, including BRCA1, BRCA2, and PALB2, are responsible for repairing breaks in DNA.[2] Mutations in BRCA2 are highly associated with both breast and ovarian carcinoma, especially in patients of Ashkenazi Jewish (AJ) decent.[10] BRCA2 mutations are also linked to an increased risk of pancreatic carcinoma, with one US study of "sporadic" PDAC showing that these cancers may actually occur in up to 7% of patients who carry germline BRCA2 mutations.[11] A European study of 26 patients with familial PDAC (defined as 2 first-degree relatives with PDAC) found that 19% of these families carried a frameshift or unclassified mutation in BRCA2. Despite this finding, most of the families in this PDAC cohort did not meet criteria for familial breast or ovarian cancer.[12] Risk for pancreatic cancer is also increased for patients who have germline mutations in the "partner and localizer of BRCA2" gene, or PALB2.[13] These families have truncating mutations that may predispose to breast cancer as well.[14]

In contrast to BRCA2 and PALB2, the tumor suppressor BRCA1 has a less direct association with pancreatic adenocarcinoma. Still, there is growing evidence that patients with BRCA1 mutations are at increased risk for PDAC. As previously mentioned, the prevalence of BRCA mutations in patients of AJ decent is known to be increased, and AJ patients with PDAC carry recognized BRCA1 and BRCA2 mutations.[10] A recent study of 159 patients with PDAC who underwent genetic testing found germline mutations of BRCA1 in 4 individuals. Two were of AJ descent, and 2 were not. Surprisingly, it was the non-AJ patients who had early-onset PDAC at age 50 or younger,[15] a finding that provides additional evidence for the risk association with BRCA1.

Determining the BRCA1, BRCA2, or PALB2 status of a patient with PDAC is important not just for

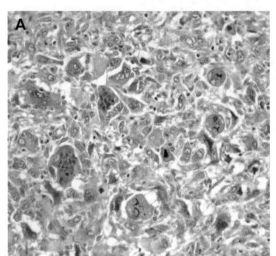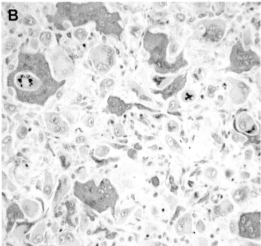

Fig. 1. Undifferentiated carcinoma with osteoclastlike giant cells (×40). (A) A slide stained with hematoxylin-eosin (H&E) slide of an undifferentiated carcinoma. Note the bizarre atypia of the singly nucleated malignant cells and the multinucleated giant cells that react to the malignancy. (B) A CD68 immunostain highlights the multinucleated cells, confirming that they are reactive rather than malignant.

prognosis, but also for screening and treatment. Currently, guidelines recommend pancreatic screening of patients who have both known germline *BRCA2* mutations and a family member with PDAC.[3] Additionally, nonpancreatic *BRCA*-associated cancers have shown some sensitivity to platinum agents and poly (ADP-ribose) polymerase (PARP) inhibitors. These inhibitors cause fatal DNA breaks in cells that lack functional BRCA1 or BRCA2 proteins.[16] Clinical trials are ongoing to determine the combination of therapy that will be best for patients with PDAC with these mutations.

## LYNCH SYNDROME

Patients with Lynch syndrome, also known as Hereditary Non-Polyposis Colorectal Cancer Syndrome, primarily come to clinical attention due to a family history of colorectal and/or endometrial carcinoma, although they are at increased risk for a variety of carcinomas at other sites. The underlying abnormality in Lynch syndrome is a germline mutation in 1 of the 4 genes involved in DNA mismatch repair pathways: *MLH1, MSH2, MSH6,* and *PMS2*. Deficiency in one of these pathways increases the likelihood of errors in DNA repair, and these errors can be detected in areas of repetitive DNA sequences. The resulting "microsatellite instability" can be detected by polymerase chain reaction amplification of the tumor cells. Alternatively, immunohistochemistry for the DNA mismatch repair proteins will show loss of protein expression in neoplastic cells.

Although not originally recognized as part of Lynch syndrome,[17] risk for PDAC appears to be increased in some families with mismatch repair deficiency.[15] In some patients, PDAC may be the initial manifestation of a mismatch repair deficiency within a family.[13] Most PDAC in patients with Lynch syndrome will be of the conventional type, but on occasion the histologic growth pattern of these microsatellite unstable PDACs take on the same "medullary" phenotype; that is, typical of Lynch syndrome colorectal carcinomas: a poorly differentiated carcinoma with a syncytial growth pattern, extensive necrosis, and brisk intratumoral lymphocytic infiltrate (**Fig. 2**).[18] The importance of recognizing patients with Lynch syndrome–associated carcinomas may be greater now than ever because of the promising new treatment regimens, including immunotherapy drugs such as PD-1 inhibitors, currently under study for microsatellite unstable malignancies.[19]

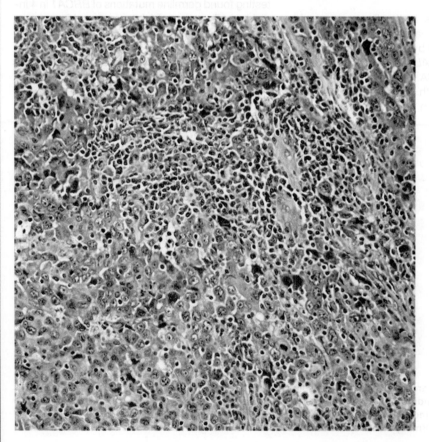

*Fig. 2.* Poorly differentiated pancreatic adenocarcinoma with medullary features (×20). Note the syncytial, sheetlike growth of the malignant cells and prominent lymphocytic infiltrate. This patient was known to have Lynch syndrome.

## FAMILIAL ADENOMATOUS POLYPOSIS

Familial adenomatous polyposis (FAP) occurs as a result of a germline mutation in the *APC* gene on chromosome 5q. Mutations are autosomal dominant, and most cause truncation of the APC protein, a tumor suppressor that functions in the Wnt/β-catenin pathway to degrade β-catenin. Patients with FAP have innumerable adenomas in the large intestine and undergo prophylactic colectomy shortly after adolescence. As patients age, they also develop multiple adenomas within the stomach and small intestine, often in the ampullary area. Most rare "pancreatic cancers" that arise in patients with FAP, then, are more likely of duodenal or ampullary origin than true PDAC.[20] Moreover, the primary pancreatic tumors that have been reported in patients with FAP are rare tumors including endocrine carcinomas, acinar cell carcinoma, and pancreatoblastoma, instead of PDAC. Screening for PDAC is not recommended for patients with FAP.[21]

## PEUTZ-JEGHERS SYNDROME

Peutz-Jeghers syndrome (PJS) is another autosomal dominant tumor predisposition syndrome characterized by intestinal polyps and melanocytic macules on oral mucosa. The underlying abnormality is a germline mutation in *STK11/LKB1* on chromosome 19p. Most mutations result in a truncated protein with a resulting loss of tumor suppressive activity.[22] In up to 90% of individuals with a family history or clinical evidence of PJS, identifiable *STK11/LKB1* mutations, either deletions or point mutations, can be found.[23]

Gastrointestinal polyps are the most common feature of PJS. These polyps are usually benign hamartomatous polyps with characteristic branching architecture on histology. Although in rare cases these polyps do undergo the adenomatous dysplasia-carcinoma sequence, it remains a matter of debate whether these polyps are the obligate precursor lesions of colorectal cancer in these patients.[24] Patients with PJS are at risk for not only gastrointestinal malignancies, but also neoplasms of the breast, lung, ovary, uterus, and pancreas.[20] Overall, patients with PJS have an approximately 10% chance of developing pancreatic carcinoma by age 70,[22] and current recommendations are to screen all patients with PJS, regardless of family history of PDAC.[3] As with FAP, these patients are also at risk for duodenal and ampullary malignancies, which must be separated from PDAC. Although most pancreatic tumors in PJS are conventional PDAC, acinar cell carcinoma has also been described.[25] Additionally, intraductal papillary mucinous neoplasms (IPMN), a precursor of PDAC, with loss of heterozygosity of the wild-type *STK11/LKB1* allele, have been reported in PJS (**Fig. 3**).[26]

## ATM GENE MUTATIONS

The ataxia-telangiectasia syndrome, caused by biallelic germline mutations in the *ATM* gene on chromosome 11, is a rare disorder with primarily neurologic and immunologic manifestations. The ATM protein is similar to BRCA1 and BRCA2 in that it functions to correct DNA double-stranded breakage, and patients with the syndrome have increased risk of malignancy.

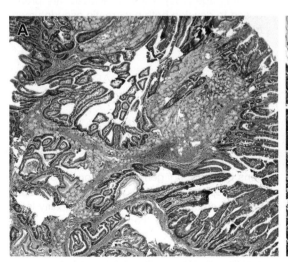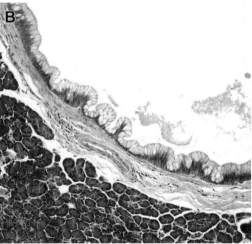

*Fig. 3.* PJS. (*A*) Sections of a characteristic duodenal hamartomatous polyp in a patient with PJS. Note the benign overgrowth of both epithelial elements and the smooth muscle, so that epithelial islands are formed encircled by the branching muscle fibers (×4). (*B*) From the same patient, a portion of an IPMN, gastric subtype, with low-grade dysplasia (×20).

Intriguingly, heterozygous germline mutations in *ATM* also play a role in familial cancer predisposition. Such mutations segregated with disease in 2 familial pancreatic cancer kindreds, and the PDACs demonstrated loss of heterozygosity of the wild-type allele. In an analysis of an additional 166 familial pancreatic cancer probands, 4 (2.6%) were found to have deleterious germline heterozygous *ATM* mutations, and these mutations occurred in the most severely affected families. Taken together, these results suggest that *ATM* acts as an inherited tumor suppressor gene in a small fraction of familial pancreatic cancers.[27]

## MCCUNE-ALBRIGHT SYNDROME

McCune-Albright syndrome (MAS) is a rare disorder and the only one in this review that is not heritable. Instead, activating mutations in *GNAS1* occur early in development, so that patients with MAS have mosaicism for the mutant and wild-type gene. Characteristic findings in MAS include café-au-lait spots, polycystic fibrous dysplasia, and precocious puberty.[28]

Approximately two-thirds of IPMNs of the pancreas have also been shown to have activating mutations of *GNAS*.[29] Perhaps unsurprisingly, then, a recent study of 19 adult patients with MAS who underwent MRI found that 3 (15%) of these individuals had an IPMN, a prevalence far above the estimated 25 per 100,000 persons.[28] Because IPMN is known to be a precursor to PDAC, screening of adult patients for pancreatobiliary disease is prudent in this patient population.[28]

## HEREDITARY SYNDROMES ASSOCIATED WITH PANCREATIC EXOCRINE DYSFUNCTION

### CYSTIC FIBROSIS

Cystic fibrosis (CF) is the most common recessive genetic disease in the Caucasian population and is caused by a variety of mutations in the *CFTR* gene.[30] *CFTR* encodes a chloride ion channel that allows for transport across cell membranes. Loss or dysfunction of the channel results in production of viscous mucous that clogs passageways and damages epithelium rather than providing a fluid protective barrier. CF is best known for its pulmonary manifestations secondary to abnormal mucous production, but chronic dysfunction of the digestive tract is also common.

Although it is estimated that less than 10% of acinar (exocrine) pancreatic tissue is necessary to maintain pancreatic sufficiency, pancreatic insufficiency occurs in most patients with CF. The CFTR channel is normally expressed in pancreatic ductal epithelium. Without the appropriate ion exchange, pancreatic secretions become more acidic and less watery, causing both obstruction of ducts and damage to the ductal and acinar epithelium. Patients with pancreatic insufficiency are able to adequately digest most carbohydrates and proteins, but lipid digestion is markedly impaired, causing steatorrhea and deficiency of fat-soluble vitamins.[31]

A subset of patients with CF has less deleterious mutations in the *CFTR* gene. These individuals are able to maintain pancreatic sufficiency; however, precisely because they maintain exocrine function, they are at increased risk for developing acute pancreatitis in the setting of an obstructed duct. In a study of more than 10,000 patients with CF, slightly more than 1% developed acute pancreatitis, predominantly in patients with pancreatic sufficiency. Unfortunately, most patients with CF patients with 1 episode of pancreatitis go on to relapse and ultimately develop chronic pancreatitis.[32] It is thought that the chronic inflammation in these patients accounts for the increased risk of PDAC in some patients with CF.[30]

## HEREDITARY PANCREATITIS

An excellent review of hereditary pancreatitis is provided elsewhere in this issue (see Stram M, Liu S, Singhi AD: Chronic Pancreatitis, in this issue). Briefly, hereditary pancreatitis is a syndrome caused by mutations in *PRSS1* or *SPINK1*, genes involved in the production and inactivation of the pancreatic enzyme trypsinogen. Patients have recurrent bouts of pancreatitis beginning at a young age (<30). These individuals are predisposed to develop both pancreatic pseudotumors, from the chronic fibrosis, and pancreatic adenocarcinoma, secondary to chronic injury.[2,33]

## HEREDITARY SYNDROMES ASSOCIATED WITH NONDUCTAL PANCREATIC NEOPLASIA

### MULTIPLE ENDOCRINE NEOPLASIA, TYPE 1

Multiple endocrine neoplasia, type 1 (MEN1) is an autosomal dominant syndrome caused by mutations in the *MEN1* gene located on chromosome 11q. Despite extensive work with the menin protein, the complete range of its functionality is still unknown, and more than 1300 causative mutations have been identified. Patients with this syndrome characteristically develop tumors of the parathyroid glands, the anterior pituitary gland, and the endocrine pancreas (**Fig. 4**).[34,35]

MEN1 is the most frequent genetic syndrome associated with pancreatic neuroendocrine

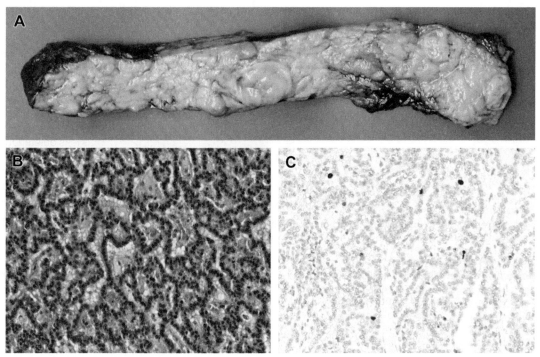

*Fig. 4.* PanNET in MEN1. (*A*) Surgical resection of a pancreatic tail from a patient with MEN1 that shows yellow-tan lobulated pancreatic parenchyma with multiple, fleshy pale pink neuroendocrine tumors. (*B*) An H&E-stained slide of one of the tumors showing a beautiful reticulated pattern of growth. (*C*) An immunostain for Ki-67 shows that the tumor has a low proliferative rate and would be considered a well-differentiated PanNET grade 1.

tumors (PanNETs), and up to 70% of patients with MEN1 will develop a macroscopic (radiologically visible) PanNET in their lifetime. It is thought that 100% of patients with MEN1 have microscopic neuroendocrine tumors within the pancreas. The age of diagnosis for a macroscopic PanNET in MEN1 is usually less than 50 years. Although most PanNETs in MEN1 are nonfunctional, symptomatic (hormone-secreting) gastrinomas and insulinomas are also seen in a substantial percentage of these patients.[35] Of note, as in FAP where many "pancreatic" tumors actually arise from the duodenum or ampulla, the functional gastrinoma in a patient with MEN1 may be located not within the pancreas, but in the duodenum. Care must be taken during surgery and the gross dissection of the resected specimen to investigate the duodenal tissue and all lymph nodes because duodenal gastrinomas are known to metastasize to paraduodenal lymph nodes even when small.[36] Almost all patients with MEN1 eventually die from complications of their disease, often related to PanNET metastases or comorbidities.[35]

## VON-HIPPEL LINDAU

Von-Hippel Lindau (VHL) is an autosomal dominant syndrome that predisposes patients to PanNET,

pancreatic serous cystadenomas, brain and spinal cord hemangioblastomas, adrenal pheochromocytomas, and renal cysts and clear cell carcinomas. The causative mutations occur in the *VHL* gene on chromosome 3p25 that encodes the VHL tumor suppressor protein. The VHL protein normally functions to degrade hypoxia-inducible factor, which, in the active state, promotes angiogenesis.[37]

In the pancreas, serous cystadenomas are the most common manifestation of VHL (**Fig. 5**). Although these are benign cysts without risk of risk of malignant transformation, they are often multiple and can be associated with diffuse replacement of the gland or ductal obstruction secondary to simple mass effect. Additionally, the presence of serous cystadenomas can be the initial presentation of de novo VHL disease in patients who do not have familial disease.[38]

PanNETs occur in approximately 10% of patients with VHL, and in contrast to MEN1, the tumors are solitary and nonfunctional. For this reason, PanNETs are often detected in VHL on routine surveillance abdominal imaging, which is recommended primarily because of the risk of renal cell carcinoma in VHL. PanNETs with clear cell features as well as combined serous endocrine neoplasms can occur in patients with VHL but are very rare in the nonsyndromic setting. Although PanNETs in VHL can be

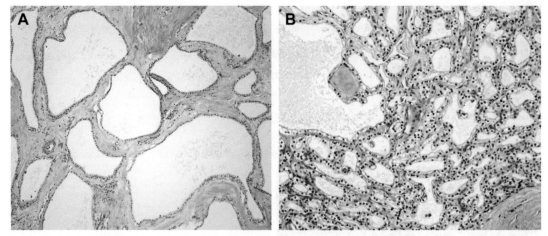

*Fig. 5.* Serous cystadenoma in VHL. (*A*) Irregular, medium-sized cystic spaces filled with clear, serous fluid and lined by small cells with clear cytoplasm and regular round nuclei (×10). (*B*) Microcystic variant (×40).

indolent, some grow rapidly and cause symptoms secondary to their size. Additionally, risk for metastasis increases when the PanNET is larger than 3 cm. Still, death from PanNET in this patient population is extremely rare.[35,38]

## NEUROFIBROMATOSIS TYPE 1

Neurofibromatosis type 1 (NF1), also known as von Recklinghausen disease, is a common autosomal dominant condition (1:2500 in the United Kingdom) caused by a mutation in the *NF1* gene on chromosome 17q. Under normal conditions, the neurofibromin 1 protein is a tumor suppressor that inhibits the Ras protein and therefore hinders cell growth. The primary manifestations of NF1 are pigmented skin lesions (café-au-lait spots) and nerve sheath tumors called neurofibromas, although the phenotypic expression of the disease can vary even between members of the same family.[39]

A rare feature of NF1 is the presence of a particular type of functional neuroendocrine tumor known as a somatostatinoma (Fig. 6). Although these can be found in the pancreas, they are more commonly located in the duodenum or periampullary region where they may cause pancreatic obstruction and mimic a pancreatic neoplasm. The histologic findings of a somatostatinoma can be quite characteristic: glandular formation and psammomatous calcifications.[40] Although these tumors are associated with increased morbidity in patients with NF1, they are not a significant cause of mortality in this population.[35]

## TUBEROUS SCLEROSUS COMPLEX

A final syndrome associated with PanNETs is tuberous sclerosis (TS). TS is an autosomal dominant condition caused by mutations in either *TSC1*, which encodes hamartin, or *TSC2*,

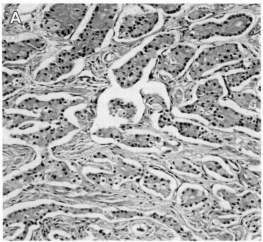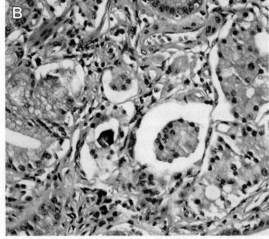

*Fig. 6.* Somatostatin-producing pancreatic neuroendocrine tumor (somatostatinoma). (*A*) Note the amphophilic cytoplasm of the neoplastic cells and the small nuclei (×20). (*B*) A characteristic calcification, a psammoma body, within the somatostatinoma (×40).

which encodes tuberin. These proteins are necessary for regulation of cell growth via the phosphoinositide 3-kinase pathway. Although most tumors associated with TS are benign, they cause significant morbidity due to their predominant locations in the skin and brain. Patients with TS often experience seizures and developmental delay. A rare manifestation of TS is the presence of PanNETs, which may be functional or nonfunctional.[35]

## BECKWITH-WIEDEMANN

Unlike the previously discussed syndromes, Beckwith-Wiedemann syndrome (BWS) is associated with a different type of pancreatic malignancy, the pancreatoblastoma. The genetic mechanism underlying BWS is complex but most often involves chromosome 11. BWS can be caused by abnormal genetic imprinting, a defect in gene regulation by methylation of a region of chromosome 11. Another common cause of BWS is paternal uniparental disomy, where the region of interest on both copies of chromosome 11 is inherited from the father, and no copies are from the mother. In many cases of BWS, however, the mechanism of disease is unknown.[41]

BWS is considered an overgrowth syndrome. Patients characteristically have hemihypertrophy, macroglossia, and intra-abdominal tumors. Pancreatoblastoma is the most common pediatric pancreatic malignancy, and in BWS, these tumors are often congenital.[42] Because of their size in the neonate, pancreatoblastomas often come to clinical attention as a palpable abdominal mass; up to half have metastasized to the liver at the time of diagnosis. On histologic review, pancreatoblastomas are very cellular neoplasms with uniform polygonal cells and interspersed squamoid nests (Fig. 7).

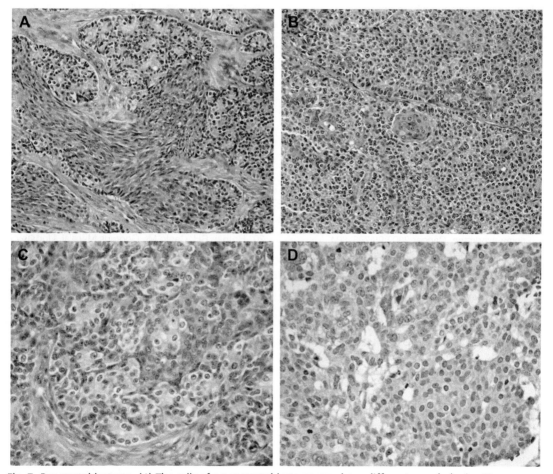

*Fig. 7.* Pancreatoblastoma. (*A*) The cells of a pancreatoblastoma may have different morphologies. Here, we see both a spindled "streaming" growth pattern in the center surrounded by round, regular cells that appear to have acinar morphology. The nests of tumor are surrounded by a fibrotic stroma (×20). (*B*) Solid growth of neuroendocrine-appearing cells with a characteristic squamoid nest in the center of the field (×20). (*C, D*) High magnification of neoplastic cells with pale cytoplasm and nucleoli (×40).

"Normal" constituents of the pancreas, including acinar and endocrine cells, may be present in pancreatoblastoma. At a genetic level, pancreatoblastomas show loss of 11p, and also may have alterations of the *APC* pathway.[21]

## SUMMARY

The pancreas is affected by a variety of hereditary syndromes. In some, such as CF, pancreatic dysfunction is a common and severe manifestation of the disease process. In other syndromes, such as TS, pancreatic neoplasia is rare and does not significantly contribute to disease burden. Perhaps the most important syndromes, however, are those in which pancreatic adenocarcinoma may develop because of the morbidity and mortality involved. Knowing the spectrum of pancreatic disease is important to understand the risk that individual patients have for disease, and to offer genetic counseling and surveillance where appropriate.

## REFERENCES

1. Siegel RL, Miller KD, Jemal A. Cancer statistics, 2015. CA Cancer J Clin 2015;65:5–29.
2. Rustgi AK. Familial pancreatic cancer: genetic advances. Genes Dev 2014;28:1–7.
3. Canto MI, Harinck F, Hruban RH, et al. International cancer of the pancreas screening (CAPS) consortium summit on the management of patients with increased risk for familial pancreatic cancer. Gut 2013;62:339–47.
4. Rulyak SJ, Brentnall TA, Lynch HT, et al. Characterization of the neoplastic phenotype in the familial atypical multiple-mole melanoma-pancreatic carcinoma syndrome. Cancer 2003;98:798–804.
5. Okamoto A, Demetrick DJ, Spillare EA, et al. Mutations and altered expression of p16INK4 in human cancer. Proc Natl Acad Sci U S A 1994;91:11045–9.
6. Goldstein AM, Chan M, Harland M, et al. Features associated with germline CDKN2A mutations: a GenoMEL study of melanoma-prone families from three continents. J Med Genet 2007;44:99–106.
7. Gruis NA, van der Velden PA, Sandkuijl LA, et al. Homozygotes for CDKN2 (p16) germline mutation in Dutch familial melanoma kindreds. Nat Genet 1995;10:351–3.
8. de Snoo FA, Bishop DT, Bergman W, et al. Increased risk of cancer other than melanoma in CDKN2A founder mutation (p16-Leiden)-positive melanoma families. Clin Cancer Res 2008;14:7151–7.
9. Koorstra JB, Maitra A, Morsink FH, et al. Undifferentiated carcinoma with osteoclastic giant cells (UCOCGC) of the pancreas associated with the familial atypical multiple mole melanoma syndrome (FAMMM). Am J Surg Pathol 2008;32:1905–9.
10. Stadler ZK, Salo-Mullen E, Patil SM, et al. Prevalence of BRCA1 and BRCA2 mutations in Ashkenazi Jewish families with breast and pancreatic cancer. Cancer 2012;118:493–9.
11. Goggins M, Schutte M, Lu J, et al. Germline BRCA2 gene mutations in patients with apparently sporadic pancreatic carcinomas. Cancer Res 1996;56:5360–4.
12. Hahn SA, Greenhalf B, Ellis I, et al. BRCA2 germline mutations in familial pancreatic carcinoma. J Natl Cancer Inst 2003;95:214–21.
13. Salo-Mullen EE, O'Reilly EM, Kelsen DP, et al. Identification of germline genetic mutations in patients with pancreatic cancer. Cancer 2015;121(24): 4382–8.
14. Jones S, Hruban RH, Kamiyama M, et al. Exomic sequencing identifies PALB2 as a pancreatic cancer susceptibility gene. Science 2009;324:217.
15. Kastrinos F, Mukherjee B, Tayob N, et al. Risk of pancreatic cancer in families with Lynch syndrome. JAMA 2009;302:1790–5.
16. Lowery MA, Kelsen DP, Stadler ZK, et al. An emerging entity: pancreatic adenocarcinoma associated with a known BRCA mutation: clinical descriptors, treatment implications, and future directions. Oncologist 2011;16:1397–402.
17. Watson P, Lynch HT. Extracolonic cancer in hereditary nonpolyposis colorectal cancer. Cancer 1993; 71:677–85.
18. Wilentz RE, Goggins M, Redston M, et al. Genetic, immunohistochemical, and clinical features of medullary carcinoma of the pancreas: a newly described and characterized entity. Am J Pathol 2000;156: 1641–51.
19. Le DT, Uram JN, Wang H, et al. PD-1 blockade in tumors with mismatch-repair deficiency. N Engl J Med 2015;372:2509–20.
20. Hruban RH, Canto MI, Goggins M, et al. Update on familial pancreatic cancer. Adv Surg 2010;44: 293–311.
21. Abraham SC, Wu TT, Klimstra DS, et al. Distinctive molecular genetic alterations in sporadic and familial adenomatous polyposis-associated pancreatoblastomas: frequent alterations in the APC/beta-catenin pathway and chromosome 11p. Am J Pathol 2001;159:1619–27.
22. Hearle N, Schumacher V, Menko FH, et al. Frequency and spectrum of cancers in the Peutz-Jeghers syndrome. Clin Cancer Res 2006;12: 3209–15.
23. de Leng WW, Jansen M, Carvalho R, et al. Genetic defects underlying Peutz-Jeghers syndrome (PJS) and exclusion of the polarity-associated MARK/Par1 gene family as potential PJS candidates. Clin Genet 2007;72:568–73.
24. Jansen M, de Leng WW, Baas AF, et al. Mucosal prolapse in the pathogenesis of Peutz-Jeghers polyposis. Gut 2006;55:1–5.

25. de Wilde RF, Ottenhof NA, Jansen M, et al. Analysis of LKB1 mutations and other molecular alterations in pancreatic acinar cell carcinoma. Mod Pathol 2011; 24:1229–36.

26. Sato N, Rosty C, Jansen M, et al. STK11/LKB1 Peutz-Jeghers gene inactivation in intraductal papillary-mucinous neoplasms of the pancreas. Am J Pathol 2001;159:2017–22.

27. Roberts NJ, Jiao Y, Yu J, et al. ATM mutations in patients with hereditary pancreatic cancer. Cancer Discov 2012;2:41–6.

28. Gaujoux S, Salenave S, Ronot M, et al. Hepatobiliary and pancreatic neoplasms in patients with McCune-Albright syndrome. J Clin Endocrinol Metab 2014; 99:E97–101.

29. Dal Molin M, Matthaei H, Wu J, et al. Clinicopathological correlates of activating GNAS mutations in intraductal papillary mucinous neoplasm (IPMN) of the pancreas. Ann Surg Oncol 2013;20:3802–8.

30. Neglia JP, FitzSimmons SC, Maisonneuve P, et al. The risk of cancer among patients with cystic fibrosis. Cystic Fibrosis and Cancer Study Group. N Engl J Med 1995;332:494–9.

31. Li L, Somerset S. Digestive system dysfunction in cystic fibrosis: challenges for nutrition therapy. Dig Liver Dis 2014;46:865–74.

32. De Boeck K, Weren M, Proesmans M, et al. Pancreatitis among patients with cystic fibrosis: correlation with pancreatic status and genotype. Pediatrics 2005;115:e463–9.

33. Klöppel G. Chronic pancreatitis, pseudotumors and other tumor-like lesions. Mod Pathol 2007;20(Suppl 1):S113–31.

34. Byström C, Larsson C, Blomberg C, et al. Localization of the MEN1 gene to a small region within chromosome 11q13 by deletion mapping in tumors. Proc Natl Acad Sci U S A 1990;87: 1968–72.

35. Jensen RT, Berna MJ, Bingham DB, et al. Inherited pancreatic endocrine tumor syndromes: advances in molecular pathogenesis, diagnosis, management, and controversies. Cancer 2008;113:1807–43.

36. Pipeleers-Marichal M, Somers G, Willems G, et al. Gastrinomas in the duodenums of patients with multiple endocrine neoplasia type 1 and the Zollinger-Ellison syndrome. N Engl J Med 1990; 322:723–7.

37. Lonser RR, Glenn GM, Walther M, et al. von Hippel-Lindau disease. Lancet 2003;361:2059–67.

38. Hammel PR, Vilgrain V, Terris B, et al. Pancreatic involvement in von Hippel–Lindau disease. Gastroenterology 2000;119:1087–95.

39. Reynolds RM, Browning GG, Nawroz I, et al. Von Recklinghausen's neurofibromatosis: neurofibromatosis type 1. Lancet 2003;361:1552–4.

40. Burke AP, Sobin LH, Shekitka KM, et al. Somatostatin-producing duodenal carcinoids in patients with von Recklinghausen's neurofibromatosis. A predilection for black patients. Cancer 1990;65:1591–5.

41. Weksberg R, Smith AC, Squire J, et al. Beckwith–Wiedemann syndrome demonstrates a role for epigenetic control of normal development. Hum Mol Genet 2003;12:R61–8.

42. Drut R, Jones MC. Congenital pancreatoblastoma in Beckwith-Wiedemann syndrome: an emerging association. Pediatr Pathol 1988;8:331–9.

# *Moving?*

## Make sure your subscription moves with you!

To notify us of your new address, find your **Clinics Account Number** (located on your mailing label above your name), and contact customer service at:

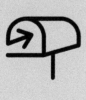

**Email: journalscustomerservice-usa@elsevier.com**

**800-654-2452** (subscribers in the U.S. & Canada)
**314-447-8871** (subscribers outside of the U.S. & Canada)

**Fax number: 314-447-8029**

**Elsevier Health Sciences Division**
**Subscription Customer Service**
**3251 Riverport Lane**
**Maryland Heights, MO 63043**

# Moving?

## Make sure your subscription moves with you!

To notify us of your new address, find your Clinics Account Number (located on your mailing label above your name), and contact customer service at:

**Email: journalscustomerservice-usa@elsevier.com**

**800-654-2452** (subscribers in the U.S. & Canada)
**314-447-8871** (subscribers outside of the U.S. & Canada)

**Fax number: 314-447-8029**

**Elsevier Health Sciences Division**
**Subscription Customer Service**
**3251 Riverport Lane**
**Maryland Heights, MO 63043**

*To ensure uninterrupted delivery of your subscription,
please notify us at least 4 weeks in advance of move.

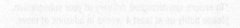

Printed and bound by CPI Group (UK) Ltd, Croydon, CR0 4YY

03/10/2024

01040304-0014